Lung Cancer

Guest Editor

MARK J. KRASNA, MD

SURGICAL ONCOLOGY CLINICS OF NORTH AMERICA

www.surgonc.theclinics.com

Consulting Editor

NICHOLAS J. PETRELLI, MD

October 2011 • Volume 20 • Number 4

SAUNDERS an imprint of ELSEVIER, Inc.

W.B. SAUNDERS COMPANY
A Division of Elsevier Inc.

1600 John F. Kennedy Boulevard ● Suite 1800 ● Philadelphia, PA 19103-2899

http://www.theclinics.com

SURGICAL ONCOLOGY CLINICS OF NORTH AMERICA Volume 20, Number 4
October 2011 ISSN 1055-3207, ISBN-13: 978-1-4557-0804-8

Editor: Jessica McCool
Developmental Editor: Donald Mumford

Surgical Oncology Clinics of North America (ISSN 1055-3207) is published quarterly by Elsevier Inc., 360 Park Avenue South, New York, NY 10010-1710. Months of publication are January, April, July, and October. Business and Editorial Offices: 1600 John F. Kennedy Blvd., Ste. 1800, Philadelphia, PA 19103-2899. Customer Service Office: 3251 Riverport Lane, Maryland Heights, MO 63043. Periodicals postage paid at New York, NY and additional mailing offices. Subscription prices are $241.00 per year (US individuals), $357.00 (US institutions) $119.00 (US student/resident), $277.00 (Canadian individuals), $444.00 (Canadian institutions), $171.00 (Canadian student/resident), $346.00 (foreign individuals), $444.00 (foreign institutions), and $171.00 (foreign student/resident). Foreign air speed delivery is included in all *Clinics* subscription prices. All prices are subject to change without notice. **POSTMASTER**: Send address changes to *Surgical Oncology Clinics of North America*, Elsevier Health Science Division, Subscription Customer Service, 3251 Riverport Lane, Maryland Heights, MO 63043. **Customer Service: 1-800-654-2452 (US and Canada). 314-447-8871 (outside U.S. and Canada). Fax: 314-447-8029. E-mail: journalscustomerservice-usa@elsevier.com** (for print support); **journalsonline support-usa@elsevier.com** (for online support).

Reprints. For copies of 100 or more, of articles in this publication, please contact the Commercial Reprints Department, Elsevier Inc., 360 Park Avenue South, New York, New York 10010-1710. Tel. 212-633-3813; Fax: 212-462-1935; E-mail: reprints@elsevier.com.

Surgical Oncology Clinics of North America is covered in *MEDLINE/PubMed (Index Medicus)* and *EMBASE/ Excerpta Medica, Current Contents/Clinical Medicine, and ISI/BIOMED.*

Printed and bound by CPI Group (UK) Ltd, Croydon, CR0 4YY

Transferred to Digital Print 2011

Contributors

CONSULTING EDITOR

NICHOLAS J. PETRELLI, MD
Bank of America Endowed Medical Director, Helen F. Graham Cancer Center
at Christiana Care Health System, Newark, Delaware; Professor of Surgery,
Thomas Jefferson University, Philadelphia, Pennsylvania

GUEST EDITOR

MARK J. KRASNA, MD
Corporate Medical Director, Meridian Helath System, Neptune, New Jersey

AUTHORS

NASSER K. ALTORKI, MD
Professor and Chief, Division of Thoracic Surgery, Department of Cardinthoracic Surgery,
Weill Cornell Medical College, New York, New York

THOMAS BAUER, MD
Chief, Thoracic Surgery, Helen F. Graham Cancer Center, Christiana Care; Adjunct
Assistant Professor of Biological Sciences, University of Delaware, Newark, Delaware;
Associate Professor of Surgery, Jefferson Medical College, Philadelphia, Pennsylvania

RAPHAEL BUENO, MD
Division of Thoracic Surgery, Brigham and Women's Hospital, Boston, Massachusetts

ROBERT J. CERFOLIO, MD
Professor of Surgery, Chief Section of Thoracic Surgery, JH Estes Endowed Chair of Lung
Cancer Research, University of Alabama, Birmingham, Alabama

AARON M. CHENG, MD
Division of Cardiothoracic Surgery, University of Washington School of Medicine, Seattle,
Washington

MELISSA H. COLEMAN, MD
Division of Thoracic Surgery, Brigham and Women's Hospital, Boston, Massachusetts

BENEDICT D.T. DALY, MD
Professor and Chairman of Cardiothoracic Surgery, Boston University School of Medicine;
Chief of Cardiothoracic Surgery, Boston Medical Center, Boston, Massachusetts

ANTONIO D'ANDRILLI, MD
Assistant Professor of Thoracic Surgery, Department of Thoracic Surgery, Sant'Andrea
Hospital, University LaSapienza, Rome, Italy

MARCELO C. DASILVA, MD
Division of Thoracic Surgery, Brigham and Women's Hospital, Boston, Massachusetts

CAROLYN M. DRESLER, MD, MPA
Director, Tobacco Prevention and Cessation Program, State of Arkansas Department of Health, Little Rock, Arkansas

ZHEN FAN, MD
Pathologist, Department of Pathology, St Joseph Pathology Associates, St Joseph Medical Center, Towson, Maryland

ZIV GAMLIEL, MD, FACS
Chief, Thoracic Surgery, St Joseph Medical Center, Towson, Maryland

SETH D. GOLDSTEIN, MD
Resident, General Surgery, Johns Hopkins University School of Medicine, Baltimore, Maryland

PETER GOLDSTRAW, MB, FRCS
Honorary Consultant in Thoracic Surgery, Academic Department of Thoracic Surgery, Royal Brompton Hospital; Emeritus Professor of Thoracic Surgery, National Heart and Lung Institute, Imperial College, London, United Kingdom; President, International Association for the Study of Lung Cancer, Aurora, Colorado

LYALL A. GORENSTEIN, MD
Assistant Clinical Professor of Surgery, Columbia University; Director of Minimally Invasive Thoracic Surgery, New York Presbyterian Hospital, New York, New York

MARK J. KRASNA, MD
Corporate Medical Director, Meridian Helath System, Neptune, New Jersey

DAARON MCFIELD, MD
Department of Surgery, Christiana Care, Newark, Delaware

CECILIA MENNA, MD
Resident of Thoracic Surgery, Department of Thoracic Surgery, Sant'Andrea Hospital, University LaSapienza, Rome, Italy

ERINO A. RENDINA, MD
Professor and Chief, Department of Thoracic Surgery, Sant'Andrea Hospital, University LaSapienza, Rome, Italy

RICHARD SCHRAEDER, MD
Medical Oncologist, Department of Medicine, St. Joseph Cancer Institute, St. Joseph Medical Center, Towson, Maryland

JOSHUA R. SONETT, MD
Edward C & Anne K Weiskopf Professor of Clinical Surgical Oncology, Director of Thoracic Surgery, New York Presbyterian Hospital, New York, New York

MATTHEW A. STELIGA, MD
Assistant Professor of Surgery, Division of Cardiothoracic Surgery, University of Arkansas for Medical Sciences, Little Rock, Arkansas

BRENDON M. STILES, MD
Assistant Professor, Division of Thoracic Surgery, Department of Cardiothoracic Surgery, Weill Cornell Medical College, New York, New York

DAVID J. SUGARBAKER, MD
Chief, Division of Thoracic Surgery, Brigham and Women's Hospital, Boston, Massachusetts

FEDERICO VENUTA, MD
Professor of Thoracic Surgery, Department of Thoracic Surgery, Policlinico Umberto I, Sant'Andrea Hospital, University LaSapienza, Rome, Italy

DOUGLAS E. WOOD, MD
Division of Cardiothoracic Surgery, University of Washington School of Medicine, Seattle, Washington

STEPHEN C. YANG, MD
The Arthur B. and Patricia B. Modell Professor of Surgery, Professor and Chief, Division of Thoracic Surgery, Johns Hopkins University School of Medicine, Baltimore, Maryland

Contents

The link between smoking and development of lung cancer has been demonstrated, not only for smokers but also for those exposed to secondhand smoke. Despite the obvious carcinogenic effects of tobacco smoking, not all smokers develop lung cancer, and conversely some nonsmokers can develop lung cancer in the absence of other environmental risk factors. A multitude of genetic factors are beginning to be explored that interact with environmental exposure to alter the risk of developing this deadly disease. By more fully appreciating the complex interrelationship between genetics and other risks the development of lung cancer can be more completely understood.

Lung cancer is a global health burden and is among the most common and deadly of all malignancies worldwide. Early detection of resectable and potentially curable disease may reduce the overall death rate from lung cancer. However, at the present time, screening for lung cancer is not recommended by most clinical societies and health care agencies in the United States. This article discusses the history of, and rationale for, lung cancer screening, addresses optimization of screening protocols, and describes our current approach for the evaluation of small pulmonary nodules referred for surgical management.

Lung cancer classification is of paramount importance in determining the treatment for oncologic patients. Most lung cancers are non–small cell lung carcinomas (NSCLC), which are further subclassified into squamous cell carcinoma, adenocarcinoma, and large cell carcinoma. Lung neuroendocrine tumors are subclassified into typical carcinoid, atypical carcinoid, small cell carcinoma, and large cell neuroendocrine carcinoma. In NSCLC in particular, the histologic classification and tumor mutation analysis are central to today's targeted therapy and personalized treatment. This article discusses the current diagnostic criteria for classification of NSCLC and lung neuroendocrine tumors and implications for oncologic treatment.

treatment of patients with stages I and II NSCLC. Anatomic lobectomy combined with hilar and mediastinal lymphadenectomy constitutes the oncologic basis of surgical resection. The surgical data favor video-assisted thoracic surgery (VATS) lobectomy over open lobectomy and have established VATS lobectomy as a gold standard in the surgical resection of early-stage NSCLC. However, the role of sublobar pulmonary resection, either anatomic segmentectomy or nonanatomic wedge resection, in patients with subcentimeter nodules may become important.

Over the last 30 years neoadjuvant treatment of stage IIIA non–small cell lung cancer (NSCLC) followed by surgical resection for stage IIIB disease has significantly improved the overall results of treatment for patients with stage III NSCLC as well as for those with locally invasive tumors. Different chemotherapy regimens have been used, although in most studies some combination of drugs that include cisplatin is the standard. Radiation when given as part of the induction protocol appears to offer a higher rate of resection and complete resection, and higher doses of radiation are associated with better nodal downstaging. Resection in patients with persistent N2 disease and pneumonectomy following induction therapy remain controversial. Resection in patients with persistent N2 disease and pneumonectomy following induction therapy remain controversial.

Infiltration by lung tumor of adjacent anatomic structures including major vessels, main bronchi, and chest wall not only influences the oncologic severity of the disease but also increases the technical complexity of surgery, requiring extended resections and demanding reconstructive procedures. Completeness of resection represents in every case one of the main factors influencing the long-term outcome of patients. Technical and oncologic aspects of extended operations, including resection of Pancoast tumors and chest wall, bronchovascular sleeve resections, and en bloc resections of major thoracic vessels, are reported in this article.

Complete surgical resection is the main therapy for early-stage non-small cell lung cancer. Survival rates remain, at best, 80% for stage IA, necessitating the development of effective systemic therapy. Several large randomized control trials and meta-analyses provide evidence for the use of adjuvant chemotherapy for stage I to III, and are the basis for the standards of care. Cisplatin-based adjuvant chemotherapy regimens have shown 4% to 15% survival advantage at 5 years. Given this modest survival benefit, research is focused on the identification of prognostic and

predictive markers to aid in the selection of appropriate adjuvant chemotherapy regimens.

Conventional treatment for small cell lung cancer (SCLC) is currently thoracic radiation and combination chemotherapy, and surgery has been traditionally stated to have little to no role in disease management. However,
a growing body of literature suggests that early-stage SCLC may be more
amenable to local control following resection, with surgery being an important component of multimodality therapy. This article attempts to summarize what is currently known about early-stage SCLC, and outlines the
methods by which this controversy is actively being investigated.

Pulmonary symptoms from advanced-stage lung cancer often require palliative treatments for compassionate patient care. Although many of these
symptoms can result from complications of advanced lung cancer treatment regimens (ie, radiation/chemotherapy-induced lung toxicity) or the
patient's underlying comorbid conditions and poor constitution, a significant number of patients have symptoms that originate from the primary
tumor itself or from locoregional metastases within the thoracic cavity.
These complications from advanced-stage lung cancer can be a serious
threat to life and require appropriate intervention.

RELATED INTEREST

PET Clinics, July 2011 (Vol. 6, Issue 3)
PET Imaging of Thoracic Disease
Drew A. Toriglan, MD, and Abass Alavi, MD, *Guest Editors*
Available at: http://www.pet.theclinics.com/

VISIT THE CLINICS ONLINE!

Access your subscription at:
www.theclinics.com

Foreword

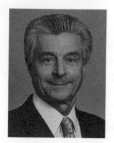

Nicholas J. Petrelli, MD
Consulting Editor

This issue of the *Surgical Oncology Clinics of North America* is devoted to lung cancer. The guest editor is Mark J. Krasna, MD. Dr Krasna has been the Medical Director of The Cancer Institute at St Joseph's Towson and Physician Advisor, Cancer Care for the Catholic Health Initiatives. Previously, he had been Director of the General Thoracic Surgery Department at the University of Maryland School of Medicine and Chief of Thoracic and Cardiovascular Surgery at the Baltimore Veteran's Administration Medical Center. Dr Krasna's career has spanned the gamut of the treatment and prevention of lung cancer. His career has centered around clinical trials and the multidisciplinary care team approach of the cancer patient. As principal investigator of the National Cancer Institute Community Cancer Centers program at St Joseph's Towson Cancer Institute, he led the project, evaluating outcomes from the multidisciplinary team approach to patients with lung and colorectal cancer. This will be the first prospective outcomes evaluation of multidisciplinary cancer care to be reported in the literature.

Dr Krasna has assembled a group of talented individuals for this edition of the *Surgical Oncology Clinics of North America*. This edition discusses pathology, the updated staging system, epidemiology, molecular markers, and surgical palliation among other topics for lung cancer. The gamut of such discussion is illustrated by the article by Cheng and Wood entitled, "Surgical and Endoscopic Palliation of Advanced Lung Cancer." This article gives detailed descriptions of the treatment for airway obstruction, malignant pleural effusions, and hemoptysis.

Although lung cancer is a preventable cancer, it still is responsible for the majority of cancer deaths in the United States. Prevention is the key, but once the lung cancer has been established, patients need talented individuals like those in this issue of the *Surgical Oncology Clinics of North America* to make sure they get high-quality multidisciplinary care.

Surg Oncol Clin N Am 20 (2011) xiii–xiv
doi:10.1016/j.soc.2011.08.002
1055-3207/11/$ – see front matter © 2011 Elsevier Inc. All rights reserved.

surgonc.theclinics.com

I thank Dr Mark Krasna and his colleagues for this outstanding issue of the *Clinics* and encourage the readers to share this information with all of their trainees and colleagues.

Respectfully,

Nicholas J. Petrelli, MD
Helen F. Graham Cancer Center
4701 Ogletown-Stanton Road, Suite 1213
Newark, DE 19713, USA

E-mail address:
npetrelli@christianacare.org

Preface
Lung Cancer

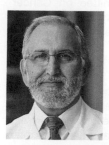

Mark J. Krasna, MD
Guest Editor

This issue of the *Surgical Oncology Clinics of North America* is dedicated to a thorough review of lung cancer. This disease, often referred to as "the forgotten cancer" (hence the "clear" survivor ribbon), is actually one of the most important of malignancies, causing major illness affecting over 1.5 million patients worldwide, and most importantly, killing more men and women than the next three cancers combined. With such a high impact on the health and financial burden to North American and worldwide patients, one could reasonably have expected improvements over the years, such as we have seen in breast and prostate cancer. Unfortunately, the advances made in screening for those diseases, as well as use of hormone treatment and molecular targeted therapies, have led to successes unrivaled as yet in lung cancer.

This *Surgical Oncology Clinics of North America* issue, however, is timely, coming after the newest revision in the staging of lung cancer, new diagnostic and screening modalities and pathologic definitions, and, of course, progress in surgical management strategies. Given the "shrinking global distances," we have assembled a panel of experts from around the world, who bring local, regional, and global perspective on their subject matter.

Drs Fan and Schraeder provide a thorough, yet concise overview of the newest pathologic definitions using the WHO criteria for non-small cell lung cancer (NSCLC), with an emphasis on the importance of immunostaining on clinical decision-making.

Dr Dresler and coworkers introduce the epidemiology of the incidence and prevalence of NSCLC and relate it to the smoking burden and its impact on society in North America and across the globe.

Dr Altorki and colleagues update the recent series of screening trials, which have finally shown unequivocally the value of screening computed tomography in high-risk patients for lung cancer. Drs Sugarbaker and colleagues provide a thoughtful

Surg Oncol Clin N Am 20 (2011) xv–xvi
doi:10.1016/j.soc.2011.08.004
1055-3207/11/$ – see front matter © 2011 Elsevier Inc. All rights reserved.

surgonc.theclinics.com

and complete algorithm to the workup of the patient with lung cancer, from both the diagnostic and the physiologic perspective. I would also encourage readers to review the recently released "Ontario Guidelines on NSCLC."

Dr Goldstraw, who led the revision of the Union Internationale Contra Canceur (International union against cancer) and American Joint Committee on Cancer systems under the auspices of the International Society for the Study of Lung Cancer, gives a superb overview of the new staging system, highlighting the changes and the clinical implications.

Dr Bauer and coworkers discuss the recent progress made in the "noninvasive" and "minimally invasive" approaches to staging and diagnosis of lung cancer. This is followed by Dr Gamliel's thorough description of the use of surgical staging and re-staging of NSCLC, following in the tradition of Pearson and Ginsberg.

Dr Sonett and coworkers describe the approaches to early stage lung cancer with an emphasis on the use of video-assisted thoracoscopic surgery and newer robotic techniques. Drs Rendina and colleagues dive into their vast experience with major extensive en bloc and sleeve resections for locally advanced NSCLC. Dr Daly and colleagues have pooled their experiences that have defined the successful use of multimodality in the treatment of stage 3 NSCLC, changing the face of this disease and making the word "cure" a real option for these patients.

Dr Wood discusses the important issue of palliation for patients who are not curative candidates, but in whom some improvement in quality of life is possible. Dr Bueno rounds out the discussion on NSCLC with an emphasis on the newest data for the value of adjuvant therapy using chemo and/or molecular targeted therapy for all but the very earliest stages (Ia) of this dreaded disease.

Finally, Dr Yang and coworkers describe the intriguing new approach to utilizing surgery as one of the modalities for treating patients with small-cell lung cancer.

I hope you enjoy this volume and benefit from the expert opinions and experiences included. I wish to thank Dr Nick Petrelli, my good friend and mentor, for giving me this opportunity to edit this issue of the *Surgical Oncology Clinics*.

Mark J. Krasna, MD
Meridian Health System
Neptune, NJ, USA

E-mail address:
mkrasna@meridianhealth.com

Epidemiology of Lung Cancer: Smoking, Secondhand Smoke, and Genetics

Matthew A. Steliga, MD[a],*, Carolyn M. Dresler, MD, MPA[b]

KEYWORDS

- Lung cancer • Tobacco • Smoking • Secondhand smoke
- Epidemiology • Genetics

The cause of lung cancer is multifactorial with genetic risk and lifestyle and environmental exposure risks. The rates of lung cancer globally have been changing, and continue to change, remarkably over the past 100 years. Lung cancer is currently the leading cause of cancer death in men and women (**Fig. 1**), accounting for more than 157,300 deaths in the United States during 2010, and more than 1.3 million deaths worldwide (**Fig. 2**). The rise of the lung cancer epidemic over the past 100 years correlates with the increased acceptance of smoking tobacco and the commercialization and mass production of tobacco during the same time period. Despite the known and proved carcinogenic risk of tobacco exposure, most lifelong smokers do not develop lung cancer, and conversely there are infrequent lifelong never-smokers who develop lung cancer in the absence of identifiable carcinogenic exposure. The complex interrelationships between smoking, other environmental carcinogens, and genetic risk are becoming better defined and have been shown to have synergistic, not simply additive impact on the development of lung cancer. By evaluating and understanding these relationships, future efforts at identifying high-risk individuals may lead to earlier detection, and by appreciating the risk of secondhand smoke and other environmental carcinogens, future efforts to reduce exposure may gain support in the battle against this deadly disease.

HISTORICAL PERSPECTIVE OF SMOKING

The tobacco plant is native to the Americas, and before the European discovery of the Americas, tobacco was unknown in the rest of the world. After Europeans were

The authors have no conflicts or potential conflicts to disclose.
[a] Division of Cardiothoracic Surgery, University of Arkansas for Medical Sciences, 4301 West Markham Street #713, Little Rock, AR 72205, USA
[b] Tobacco Prevention and Cessation Program, State of Arkansas Department of Health, 4815 West Markham Street #3, Little Rock, AR 72205-3867, USA
* Corresponding author.
E-mail address: MASteliga@uams.edu

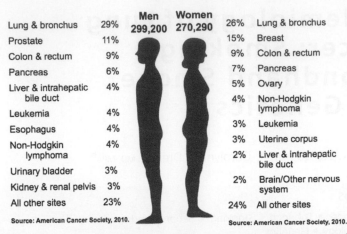

Men 299,200		Women 270,290	
Lung & bronchus	29%	26%	Lung & bronchus
Prostate	11%	15%	Breast
Colon & rectum	9%	9%	Colon & rectum
Pancreas	6%	7%	Pancreas
Liver & intrahepatic bile duct	4%	5%	Ovary
		4%	Non-Hodgkin lymphoma
Leukemia	4%		
Esophagus	4%	3%	Leukemia
Non-Hodgkin lymphoma	4%	3%	Uterine corpus
		2%	Liver & intrahepatic bile duct
Urinary bladder	3%		
Kidney & renal pelvis	3%	2%	Brain/Other nervous system
All other sites	23%	24%	All other sites

Source: American Cancer Society, 2010.

Source: American Cancer Society, 2010.

Fig. 1. Lung cancer remains the primary cause of cancer death in men and women in the United States. (*From* American Cancer Society Facts and Figures. Available at: http://www. cancer.org/Research/CancerFactsFigures/CancerFactsFigures/cancer–facts–and–figures–2010. Accessed March 12, 2011; with permission.)

introduced to tobacco and nicotine addiction, tobacco use grew in popularity, but much of tobacco use was in the form of chew tobacco, pipe tobacco, cigars, or snuff. Cigars and pipe tobacco produce smoke that is highly alkaline, of relatively large particle size, and irritating to the airways, and thus usually lead to buccal and pharyngeal absorption rather than pulmonary alveolar exposure. In the 1800s cigarettes were handmade and not common. The Bonsack machine (**Fig. 3**), patented in 1881, which could roll 12,000 cigarettes per hour, revolutionized the efficiency of the tobacco industry and led to a rise in the cheap accessibility of the cigarette after 1900. Cigarettes are often smoked with deeper inhalation and greater exposure of the lung to nicotine and carcinogens. Modern engineering of the cigarette has included the addition of anti-irritants, such as menthol and other chemicals, to allow deeper inhalation of nicotine and carcinogens to the lung parenchyma. The deep inhalation of nicotine from a cigarette provides a rapid rise and peak in nicotine levels to the brain within seconds. This is a much more rapid rise and peak than that from chew tobacco or pipe tobacco, in which the nicotine is slowly absorbed via buccal and pharyngeal mucosal surfaces. The cigarette not only is an extremely efficient nicotine delivery device, but the rapidity of the delivery leads to a much more addictive form of tobacco use. Today, with globalization of farming, manufacturing, marketing, and shipping, tobacco use is prevalent in nearly every society across the globe with most industrialized societies reporting at least a 20% smoking rate, and some countries (eg, Russia, Ukraine, and Belarus) reporting a 60% to 70% smoking rate among men, and an 82% rate of men in Afghanistan (**Fig. 4**). It is unsurprising that the rates of lung cancer reflect this, and are significantly higher in geographic areas with a higher rate of smoking. In addition, over the past 100 years changes in public health, such as air and water quality improvements, sanitation, immunization, and antibiotics, have led to a longer lifespan in industrialized nations. Lung cancer most often arises after decades of carcinogen exposure, with the average lung cancer patient more than 65 years old at time of diagnosis. The complex combination of rapidly rising widespread cigarette use and improvements in other areas of public health has led to a large population of individuals exposed to decades of carcinogen exposure who live long enough, in turn, to develop lung cancer.

A   United States of America: Both sexes
Estimated number of cancer deaths, all ages (total: 565,644)

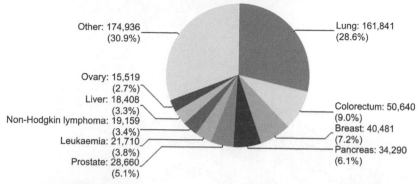

Other: 174,936
(30.9%)

Ovary: 15,519
(2.7%)
Liver: 18,408
(3.3%)
Non-Hodgkin lymphoma: 19,159
(3.4%)
Leukaemia: 21,710
(3.8%)
Prostate: 28,660
(5.1%)

Lung: 161,841
(28.6%)

Colorectum: 50,640
(9.0%)
Breast: 40,481
(7.2%)
Pancreas: 34,290
(6.1%)

B   World: Both sexes
Estimated number of cancer deaths, all ages (total: 7,564,802)

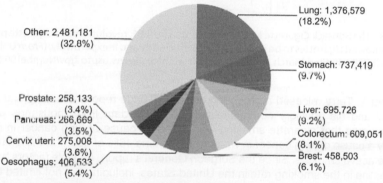

Other: 2,481,181
(32.8%)

Prostate: 258,133
(3.4%)
Pancreas: 266,669
(3.5%)
Cervix uteri: 275,008
(3.6%)
Oesophagus: 406,533
(5.4%)

Lung: 1,376,579
(18.2%)

Stomach: 737,419
(9.7%)

Liver: 695,726
(9.2%)
Colorectum: 609,051
(8.1%)
Brest: 458,503
(6.1%)

Fig. 2. (*A*) United States: estimated cancer deaths 2008 graph generated on http://globocan.
iarc.fr. (*B*) Worldwide: estimated cancer deaths 2008 graph generated on http://globocan.
iarc.fr. (*From* World Health Organization, International Agency for Research on Cancer. Accessed March 12, 2011; with permission.)

HISTORICAL PERSPECTIVE: CHANGES IN THE SMOKING EPIDEMIC

As a junior medical student, Alton Ochsner and his class were summoned to witness an autopsy of a patient who had died of a rare disease: primary lung carcinoma. The year was 1919, and indeed it was rare at the time; he did not witness another case for the next several years, even as a thoracic surgeon. Seventeen years later, he witnessed eight cases in a 6-month time span. He noted many of these patients were male veterans of World War I who had a history of smoking. It is now well accepted that tobacco smoke leads to multiple diseases including lung cancer,[1] but this was not common knowledge nor accepted at the time. His report with DeBakey in 1939[2] was one of the first to suggest a link between cigarette smoking and lung cancer, yet his views were not widely accepted nor respected. At one point when Ochsner, as a faculty member, entered a classroom of medical students to deliver a lecture, the entire class intentionally lit up cigarettes.[3] Cigarette smoking continued to rise in the United States during the 1950s and 1960s, despite significant epidemiologic observational studies linking tobacco and lung cancer. In 1964, Surgeon General

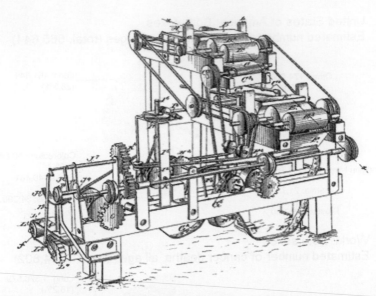

Fig. 3. The Bonsack Cigarette Machine, patented in 1881, revolutionized cigarette production and allowed cigarettes to be mass-produced efficiently and inexpensively. (*From* United States Patent 238,640 filed March 8 1881. Available at: http://www.uspto.gov/Number00238640.)

Luther L. Terry released a groundbreaking 387-page report "Smoking and Health."[4] Terry and his advisory committee had compiled data from thousands of articles concluding that cigarette smoking was indeed a cause of lung cancer in men, and likely a cause of lung cancer in women. At the time 46% of adults in the United States were active smokers. Since the Surgeon General's report, multiple factors have led to a decline in the smoking rate in the United States, including but not limited to restriction on sales to minors, advertising restrictions, increased taxation, warning labels, and increasing bans on smoking in public areas. Further research has led to reinforced evidence of the link between smoking and lung cancer and development of nonneoplastic diseases, such as chronic bronchitis, emphysema, cardiovascular disease, and cerebrovascular disease. Despite oceans of evidence of the negative impact of smoking, and increasing limitations and taxation, approximately 20% of the current adult United States population continues to smoke.

CHANGES IN LUNG CANCER RATES OVER TIME

In 1919, when Ochsner was a medical student, the death rate from lung cancer was less than 5 per 100,000, and rose throughout the next 65 to 70 years. It was not until the early 1990s that the lung cancer death rate reached a plateau at more than 90 per 100,000 and subsequently began to decline for men (**Fig. 5**A). The lung cancer death rate for women, however, continued to rise through the 1990s, and seems to be currently reaching its plateau at approximately 40 per 100,000 (see **Fig. 5**B). The United States has the highest rate of lung cancer for women of any country in the world with approximately 43.2 deaths per 100,000.[5] The number of deaths in the lung cancer epidemic is appalling, especially when one considers the perspective that lung cancer takes more lives than breast, prostate, and colorectal cancers combined, and that most lung cancer deaths are preventable. Unfortunately, lung cancer is often

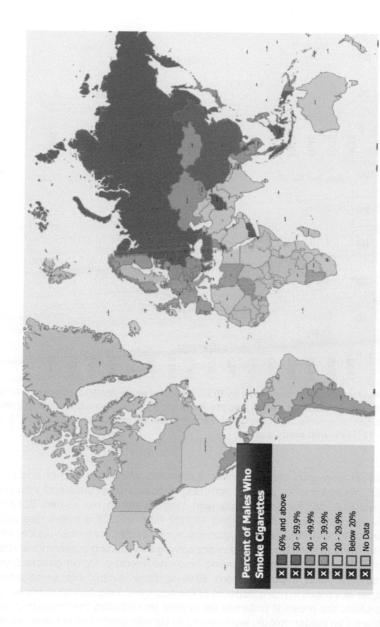

Fig. 4. Smoking rates vary widely throughout the world, with the highest rates among males found in Eastern Europe and Asia. (Image available at: http://tobaccoatlas.org. Accessed March 12, 2011; with permission.)

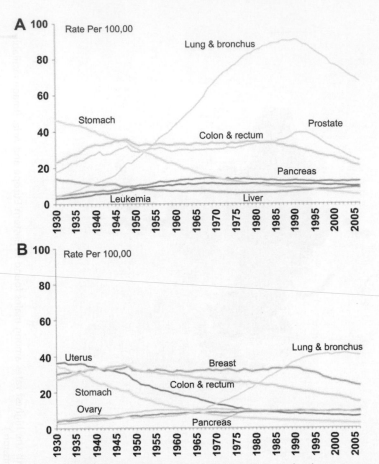

Fig. 5. (*A*) Cancer death rates among men US 1930–2006. (*B*) Cancer death rates among women US 1930–2006. (*From* American Cancer Society Facts and Figures. Available at: http://www.cancer.org/Research/CancerFactsFigures/CancerFactsFigures/cancer-facts-and-figures-2010. Accessed March 12, 2011; with permission.)

diagnosed at an advanced stage, in older individuals who often harbor additional comorbidities, rendering most patients with lung cancer unresectable and incurable. The 5-year survival rate for all patients with lung cancer in the United States is a mere 16%, and this has only changed slightly from a 13% survival rate noted from 1975 to 1977.[5] Over the past 30 years the survival rates for breast cancer have improved from 75% to 90% because of many advances including screening, surgical treatment, and medical treatment including hormonal therapy. Colon cancer 5-year survival rates have also improved from 52% to 66% during this same interim (**Fig. 6**). Despite advances in many aspects of medical care, lung cancer cures remain elusive. Therefore, the greatest potential for impact on reducing the number of lung cancer deaths on an epidemiologic level seems to be with control of risk and prevention rather than advances in treatment of this deadly disease.

The epidemiologic relationship between smoking rates in a population and death rates caused by lung cancer has been extensively analyzed in the Unites States and on a global scale, and fascinating patterns tend to predictably recur from one society

Site	1975-1977	1984-1986	1999-2005
All sites	50	54	68
Breast (female)	75	79	90
Colon	52	59	66
Leukemia	35	42	54
Lung and bronchus	13	13	16
Melanoma	82	87	93
Non-Hodgkin lymphoma	48	53	69
Ovary	37	40	46
Pancreas	3	3	6
Prostate	69	76	100
Rectum	49	57	69
Urinary bladder	74	78	82

Fig. 6. Trends in 5-year relative survival (%) rates, US, 1975–2005. (*From* American Cancer Society Facts and Figures. Available at: http://www.cancer.org/Research/CancerFactsFigures/CancerFactsFigures/cancer-facts-and-figures-2010. Accessed March 12, 2011; with permission.)

to another. Lopez and colleagues[6] noted the rise of the prevalence of cigarette smoking was reflected in the rise in death rate caused by smoking-related illnesses with an approximately 20- to 25-year lag period. The Lopez descriptive model becomes even stronger when gender is taken into account, because smoking rates can vary significantly by gender through time. Overall, it is demonstrated that death rates caused by tobacco-induced illnesses occur at a rate of roughly 50% of the smoking rate given the 20- to 25-year lag (eg, for a population with a 60% smoking rate, 30% of the deaths 20 years later are secondary to smoking). As seen in **Fig. 7**, Stage I represents the initiation where the introduction of cigarettes into a society may initially have low smoking rates, and very low death rates because of smoking. Stage II consists of a rapid rise in the smoking prevalence in men to its peak with a beginning rise in deaths. During this time, smoking in women just starts to rise, but there are few deaths in women. Stage III consists of a decline in smoking in men, with a continued rise in smoking in women. During this time, the deaths in men continue to rise, following the 20- to 25-year lag from the peak in smoking, and the deaths in women also begin to rise. Stage IV consists of a decline in male and female smoking rates, with an eventual decline in death rates. The Lopez model has been applied to many societies, and in general, developing

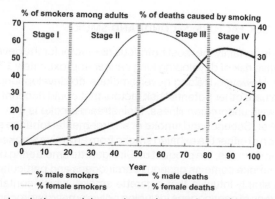

Fig. 7. The Lopez descriptive model associates changes in smoking rates and subsequent changes in death rates caused by smoking-related diseases. (*From* Lopez AD, Collishaw NE, Piha T. A descriptive model of the cigarette epidemic in developed countries. Tobacco Control 1994;3:242–7; with permission.)

nations tend to be represented by Stages I and II, whereas industrialized nations have experienced their peak in smoking rates and deaths, particularly in males, and are in Stages III or IV. This rise and fall of smoking-related deaths closely parallels the rise and fall in lung cancer incidence and mortality rates in the United States. Smoking was relatively uncommon before 1900, which would correlate with Lopez's Stage I. Male smoking in the United States rose from the 1900s and peaked around 1965 (Stage II). After the Surgeon General's report of the link between smoking and cancer, smoking rates in men decreased, yet smoking-related deaths for men continued to rise as seen in Stage III. This eventually led to a peak and decrease in lung cancer deaths in men approximately 20 years later. During this time, the smoking rate for women rose and plateaued. In the late 1990s and beyond, it seems that the death rate for women is just beginning to decrease, marking the Stage IV of Lopez's model. Using this model, future incidence and mortality of lung cancer should continue to fall for men and women in the United States as smoking rates continue to decline. This descriptive model has also been applied to many other societies. Rates of smoking in China and Japan have risen for men, and the smoking-attributable deaths continue to rise in these societies, which represents Stage II of the model. However, such countries as Australia, New Zealand, the United Kingdom, and Sweden have progressed through all phases of the Lopez model and are in Stage IV with declining rates of smoking-related deaths in men and women, which have lagged 20 to 30 years behind declining rates of cigarette use.[6]

The association between rising and falling smoking rates and lung cancer rates is powerful, but even stronger support for tobacco control comes from demonstrating that tobacco control programs lead to decreased lung cancer incidence rates. The predicted fall in lung cancer rates from decreased smoking has been supported by an observational study of the lung cancer incidence in the San Francisco–Oakland area, and its change relative to enactment of the California tobacco control program.[7] In 1988 the California tobacco control program was initiated, and it has demonstrated a significant decrease in cigarette consumption over time with associated decreases in lung cancer and bladder cancer, which has also been strongly linked to cigarette use. Singapore has also clearly demonstrated advantages of tobacco control and now has one of the world's strongest tobacco control policies. From 1978 to 1992, the rates of smoking fell from 42% to 33% and 9.5% to 3% for men and women, respectively, followed by declining rates of smoking-attributed deaths.[6]

ENVIRONMENTAL RISK FACTORS: SECONDHAND SMOKE

Cigarette smoking is certainly the most notorious risk factor for the development of lung cancer, with a relative risk of developing lung cancer approximately 12 to 15 times that of the nonsmoker. However, lifelong never-smokers do develop lung cancer leading researchers to evaluate other potential risk factors that could account for the development of this otherwise uncommon illness. Mainstream smoke is that which is actively drawn in by a smoker. Secondhand smoke or environmental tobacco smoke is defined as passive inhalation of either the exhaled smoke from an active smoker or passive inhalation of "sidestream" smoke, the product of a lit cigarette smoldering but not previously inhaled. Cigarette smoke contains gaseous carcinogens and particulate matter carcinogens ("tar"). It is simply intuitive that cigarette smoke, which contains thousands of chemicals and dozens of carcinogens including polyaromatic hydrocarbons, N-nitrosamines, benzene, arsenic, and acetaldehyde, can lead to the development of lung cancer. No safe level of secondhand smoke has been determined.[8] Certain nonsmokers at increased risk, such as flight attendants from the era when smoking on airplanes was permitted, and bartenders have known secondhand smoke exposure, with elevated levels of carcinogens in their blood,[9] but perhaps the best studied cohort of secondhand smokers is the nonsmoking spouses of men who smoke. Nonsmoking women with husbands who smoke have a relative risk ranging from 1.3 to 2.5 for the development of lung cancer, with higher rates reported in women whose husband were "heavy" smokers (as defined by >20 cigarettes per day) compared with "light" smokers, suggesting a dose-response relationship. An analysis of 37 epidemiologic studies indicated that there was a 24% increased risk (95% confidence interval, 13%–36%) when comparing nonsmoking women who had smoking husbands with nonsmoking women with nonsmoking husbands.[10]

OTHER ENVIRONMENTAL RISK FACTORS

Other sources of air pollution have been implicated in lung cancer risk, but certain factors, such as living in an urban environment, are difficult to define, quantify, and eliminate in the role of secondhand tobacco smoke. One of the earliest occupational risk studies showed that roofers exposed to coal tar fumes had a 50% increased lung cancer risk after 20 years, and 150% increased risk after 40 years, which could not be attributed to smoking status,[11] Inhalation of asbestos is a known risk for development of malignant pleural mesothelioma, and has also been demonstrated as a risk for development of lung cancer. Coal mining and exposure to chromium and nickel have also been demonstrated as risks for development of lung cancer. These are relatively rare environmental carcinogens, affecting a select few who have occupational exposure and risk. A more ubiquitous environmental carcinogen that has been implicated in the development of lung cancer in nonsmokers is exposure to elevated levels of indoor radon-222. A naturally occurring gas, radon is emitted from the earth, often as a degradation product of uranium. It percolates up through the soil, and can become concentrated in indoor structures, particularly underground or those with poor ventilation. Indoor radon exposure accounts for at least half of the background radiation received in the United States, and based on extrapolation from rates in miners, is estimated to be a potential cause of lung cancer for at least 6000 to 36,000 cases per year in the Unites States.[10] Although radon and its decay products, such as polonium-210 and polonium-214, can cause lung cancer in nonsmokers, the combined exposure of radon, its byproducts, and cigarette smoking is believed to have combined effects greater than additive risk and reflect multiplicative risk.[12]

GENETICS AND TOBACCO USE

Much research over the past few decades has focused on behavioral genetics and what role genes may play in tobacco addiction. It is exciting to better understand the complexities of human behaviors, such as the repeated use of tobacco, from research that may identify the possible genes involved. However, as in most human behaviors, repeated tobacco use or tobacco addiction is a combination of genetic composition and the environment. The issue of genetic susceptibility to develop lung cancer adds another layer of complexity. The questions to be teased apart deal with the genetic susceptibilities to tobacco addiction and how these may or may not be the same as the susceptibilities to developing lung cancer. Because tobacco and nicotine addiction is substantially thought to occur within the pathways in the brain, it is reasonable to assume that the same genetic configurations would not influence the development of cancer in the lung. However, it is possible, and is currently being established, that certain genetic characteristics do influence nicotine addiction and the development of lung cancer. Overarching all of the potential influences of genetic susceptibility to either tobacco addiction or lung cancer must remain the most potent susceptibility factor: the tobacco industry and its influence on the human environment.

Exciting recent work by Thomas and colleagues[13] has developed a new methodology to examine a complex biologic "disease," such as tobacco and nicotine addiction. They have established the risk model ontology called "smoking behavior risk ontology." Within this model they have created layered, multiscale modeling to address relationships between genes, environmental factors, and phenotypes of the individuals. Whether an adolescent starts smoking regularly has much to do with the surrounding policies or laws (eg, laws governing availability of youth purchases of tobacco or secondhand smoking restrictions) and parental influences. These environmental factors may strongly overwhelm a genetic predisposition. Similarly, the ability to rapidly metabolize nicotine, which requires more frequent smoking to maintain desired levels of nicotine, influences the ease of cessation and the efficacy of nicotine replacement therapy, which may be impacted by environmental influencers, such as a comorbid diagnosis or insurance coverage of the cost of the pharmacotherapy. Essentially, the smoking behavior risk ontology model assesses complex influencers from the environment and layers them onto known genetic variations. The major genetic variations currently known are discussed next, with the caution that even very "nonsusceptible" genotypes can probably be overwhelmed by environmental influencers.

Nicotine is believed to be the primary chemical causing addiction from tobacco use. Nicotine is known to bind to nicotinic acetylcholine receptors, which occur not only in the central nervous system but throughout other physiologic systems. Nicotinic acetylcholine receptors are comprised of five subunits and encoded in the human by 18 genes. In the brain, the nicotinic acetylcholine receptors most related to nicotine addiction are on dopamine and γ-aminobutyric acid neurons in the ventral tegmental area, which causes dopamine release in the nucleus accumbens.[14] There is known genetic variation in the dopamine receptors and dopamine-mediated neural pathways that register a reward response.[14] Much work is still required to refine the mutations, their associations, and ability to predict appropriate interventions that would increase successful tobacco cessation.

Nicotine is metabolized by the hepatic cytochrome P-450 system, with approximately 80% metabolized by CYP2A6. Much work has demonstrated that polymorphisms in CYP2A6 can control the rate of degradation of nicotine and that slower metabolizers are less likely to become addicted on initiation, smoke fewer cigarettes per day, and have a lower risk of lung cancer.[15–17] In addition, it has been demonstrated that fast metabolizers are more likely to become addicted on initiation, smoke more frequently, and have a higher rate of lung cancer. This information has led to drug development and testing in the hopes to take advantage of this metabolic pathway to assist people with different genetic constructs to quit smoking.[14] None of these drugs have yet past regulatory hurdles.[18]

GENETICS OF LUNG CANCER RISK

This category of lung cancer risk continues to be extensively researched with useable information slowly being validated. Increased risk can be assessed by the probability of being highly addicted to nicotine, as discussed previously. Additionally, genetic risk can be evaluated by the ability to rapidly or efficiently detoxify or eliminate carcinogens. Additionally, the decreased ability to repair DNA after damage from adducts is under some genetic control. The phase I enzymes, such as CYP1A1, the phase II enzymes, such as glutathione S-transferases, and the N-acetyltransferases are probably the most studied for genetic variation that would predict lung cancer susceptibility.

Polymorphisms have been identified in the Phase I (activating) and Phase II (detoxifying) enzymes and can increase or decrease the carcinogenicity of tobacco-derived chemicals. The enzymes with the most research suggesting that they cause an increase in susceptibility are CPY1A1 (MSPI or Ile→Val); CYP2E1; and microsomal epoxide hydrolase (alanine →guanine). Enzymes derived from polymorphisms that suggest decreased susceptibility from tobacco smoke exposure are CYP2A13 or increased susceptibility with GSTM1 null; GSTP1 (Ile→Val); GSTTI; and NAT2 (multiple different transitions). In addition, there may be combinations that amplify the risk, such as a Phase I polymorphism, CYP1A1 MSPI in conjunction with Phase II polymorphism GSTM1null, which leads to an increased risk compared with either polymorphism alone.[1]

Perhaps the most conclusive evidence is from a meta-analysis that demonstrated a 1.4 odds ratio for homozygous GSTM1-null individuals to develop lung cancer.[19] GSTM1-null individuals are also at an increased risk for developing lung cancer from secondhand smoke with an odds ratio of 2.6.[20] Unfortunately, this genetic testing is expensive to perform on a population basis and would be most useful in counseling to prevent people from initiating smoking or to encourage cessation.[14]

Other well-studied genetic characteristics in lung cancer are the mutations in TP53, KRAS, EGFR/EGFR pathway, and more recently described in EML4-ALK.[21] Voluminous research continues to be conducted to determine the best predictor or set of predictors to assess either survival or, increasingly, response to personalized therapy. As the EGFR mutational work has wonderfully demonstrated, identification of specific genetic mutations predicts response to certain chemotherapy treatment plans.[22,23] The discovery of the EML4-ALK mutation with its corresponding prediction of increased response to personalized chemotherapy continues to fuel the excitement to carefully characterize the lung cancer and patient to most specifically and effectively target treatment.[24,25]

Other genes that may be polymorphic and lead to an increased risk of lung cancer are CCND1, TP53, P21, and P73. These genes are involved with cell-cycle control and have been demonstrated to increase the risk of developing lung cancer when exposed to tobacco smoke. The odds ratio for developing lung cancer with any of the polymorphisms in CCND1, TP53, P21, or P73 range from 1.18 to 1.87 (all with lower confidence levels >1) compared with patients who did not have the respective polymorphism. Again, combinations of polymorphisms in these cell-cycle control enzymes and the Phase I and II enzymes would only increase the risk. Interestingly, some of the studies showed variation in the risk dependent on the amount of tobacco smoke exposure, and clearly there are racial and ethnic variations.[1]

The occurrence of lung cancer has a well-recognized familial clustering established in linkage studies. Cancer registries from Utah, Sweden, and Iceland clearly establish the increased risk. Meta-analyses have demonstrated an increased odd ratio of 1.63 (95% confidence interval, 1.31–2.01) if there is a family member who had lung cancer, and this increases substantially as more family members are diagnosed with lung cancer.[26] The patients with lung cancer within this analysis were very significantly more likely to have a history of smoking. Studies have demonstrated an increased familial risk for developing lung cancer without smoking exposure, but the evidence is less clear.

The molecular epidemiology of the genetics of lung cancer susceptibility, specifically in relationship to tobacco smoking, is very complex. The literature is voluminous, often contradictory, and frequently examined in too small of populations to be conclusive. In addition, there are international, racial, or ethnicity differences that may make the interpretation of the molecular epidemiology even more challenging. Models have been developed to predict lung cancer risks that consider multiple risk factors. However, their accuracy as of 2010 remains only moderate.[27] On top of the variety of risk or genetic factors discussed previously, the cigarettes in South Korea are not the same as the cigarettes in the United States, which are different from those in Australia or Canada. Thus, any discussion of the molecular epidemiology of the genetics of lung cancer susceptibility remains preliminary. Smoking history remains the overwhelming predictor of risk for developing lung cancer.

SUMMARY

During the past 100 years, the rise of lung cancer from an otherwise rare disease to the most common cause of cancer death in the United States has been striking. The initial observation of the link between tobacco smoking and development of lung cancer has been demonstrated with voluminous data not merely to be a correlation, but to be a causal relationship, and the decreasing trend in smoking prevalence has been mirrored in declining rates of lung cancer. However, with roughly one in five adults in the United States actively smoking, and millions of exsmokers with decades of prior exposure, lung cancer will continue to be a significant, yet a potentially controllable public health problem. Tobacco control is a key component to reducing the burden of lung cancer on society, but the development of lung cancer is not uniform in all smokers, and it does develop in some lifelong never-smokers. Focusing only on tobacco control simply addresses environmental issues while neglecting the individual patient factors. The development of lung cancer can be better understood by more thoroughly appreciating the complex intertwined relationship of environmental factors and host factors, such as genetic variability, which leads to differences in nicotine metabolism and addiction, and heterogeneity of molecular differences, which lead to variable risks of developing lung cancer. With improvements in the understanding of the environmental and genetic risk that synergistically act to develop lung cancer, high-risk groups may be able to be found that could be impacted by screening, early detection, and individualized treatment.

REFERENCES

1. U.S. Department of Health and Human Services. How tobacco smoke causes disease: the biology and behavioral basis for smoking-attributable disease: a report of the surgeon general. Atlanta (GA): U.S. Department of Health and Human Services, Centers for Disease Control and Prevention, National Center for Chronic Disease Prevention and Health Promotion, Office on Smoking and Health; 2010. p. 225, 246, 294–6.
2. Ochsner A, DeBakey M. Primary pulmonary malignancy; treatment by total pneumonectomy; analysis of 79 collected cases and presentation of 7 personal cases. Surg Gynecol Obstet 1939;68:435–51.
3. McKinnell RG. Epidemiology. In: McKinnell RG, Parchment RE, Perantoni AO, et al, editors. The biological basis of cancer. 2nd edition. New York: Cambridge University Press; 2006. p. 229–30.
4. U.S. Department of Health, Education, and Welfare. Smoking and health: report of the advisory committee to the Surgeon General of the Public Health Service. PHS publication number 1103. U.S. Department of Health, Education, and Welfare; 1964. p. 149–61.
5. Surveillance Epidemiology and End Results: Providing information on cancer statistics to help reduce the burden of this disease on the U.S. population. National Cancer Institute: U.S. National Institutes of Health. Available at: http://seer.cancer.gov/faststats/index.php. Accessed March 12, 2011.

6. Lopez AD, Collishaw NE, Piha T. A descriptive model of the cigarette epidemic in developed countries. Tobacco Control 1994;3:242–7.
7. Barnoya J, Glantz S. Association of the California tobacco control program with declines in lung cancer incidence. Cancer Causes Control 2004;15:689–95.
8. U.S. Department of Health and Human Services. The health consequences of involuntary exposure to tobacco smoke: a report of the Surgeon General. Secondhand smoke what it means to you. U.S. Rockville (MD): Department of Health and Human Services, Center for Disease Control and Prevention, Coordinating Center for Health Promotion, National Center for Chronic Disease Prevention and Health Promotion, Office on Smoking and Health; 2006. p. 11.
9. MacLure M, Katz RBA, Bryant MS, et al. Elevated blood levels of carcinogens in passive smokers. Am J Public Health 1989;79:1381–4.
10. Schottenfield D. The etiology and epidemiology of lung cancer. Principles and Practice of Lung Cancer: the official reference text of the IASLC. 4th edition. Philadelphia: Lippincott Williams and Wilkins; 2010. p. 7–8.
11. Hammond EC, Selikoff IJ, Lawther PL, et al. Inhalation of benzpyrene and cancer in man. Ann N Y Acad Sci 1976;271:116–24.
12. Lubin JH, Boice JD Jr. Lung cancer risk from residential radon: metaanalysis of eight epidemiologic studies. J Natl Cancer Inst 1997;89:49–57.
13. Thomas PD, Mi H, Swan GE, et al, Pharmacogenetics of Nicotine Addiction and Treatment Consortium. A systems biology network model for genetic association studies of nicotine addiction and treatment. Pharmacogenet Genomics 2009;19: 538–51.
14. Lerman CE, Schnoll RA, Munafò MR. Genetics and smoking cessation: improving outcomes in smokers at risk. Am J Prev Med 2007;33(Suppl 6).S398–405.
15. Ray R, Tyndale RF, Lerman C. Nicotine dependence pharmacogenetics: role of genetic variation in nicotine-metabolizing enzymes. J Neurogenet 2009;23(3): 252–61.
16. Benowitz NL, Hukkanen J, Jacob P. Nicotine chemistry, metabolism kinetics and biomarkers. Handb Exp Pharmacol 2009;192:29–60.
17. Johnstone E, Benowitz N, Cargill A, et al. Determinants of the rate of nicotine metabolism and effects on smoking behavior. Clin Pharmacol Ther 2006;80(4): 319–30.
18. Siu EC, Tyndale RF. Non-nicotinic therapies for smoking cessation. Annu Rev Pharmacol Toxicol 2007;47:541–64.
19. McWilliams JE, Sanderson BJ, Harris EL, et al. Glutathione S-Transferase M1 (GSTM1) deficiency and lung cancer risk. Cancer Epidemiol Biomarkers Prev 1995;4:589–94.
20. Bennet WP, Alavanja MC, Biomeke B, et al. Environmental tobacco smoke, genetic susceptibility, and risk of lung cancer in never-smoking women. J Natl Cancer Inst 1999;91(23):2009–14.
21. Soda M, Choi YL, Enomoto M, et al. Identification of the transforming EML4-ALK fusion gene in non-small-cell lung cancer. Nature 2007;448:561–6.
22. Lynch TJ, Bell DW, Sordella R, et al. Activating mutations in the epidermal growth factor receptor underlying responsiveness of non-small-cell lung caner to gefitinib. N Engl J Med 2004;250(21):2129–39.
23. Lee SY, Kim JK, Jin G, et al. Somatic mutations in epidermal growth factor receptor signaling pathway genes in non-small cell lung cancers. J Thorac Oncol 2010;5:1734–40.
24. Gerber DE, Minna JD. ALK inhibition for non-small cell lung cancer: from discovery to therapy in record time. Cancer Cell 2010;18(6):548–51.

25. Brennan P, Hainaut P, Boffetta P. Genetics of lung cancer susceptibility. Lancet Oncol 2011;12(4):399–408.
26. Lissowska J, Foretova L, Dąbek J, et al. Family history and lung cancer risk: international multicentre case-control study in Eastern and Central Europe and meta-analyses. Cancer Causes Control 2010;21:1091–104.
27. D'Amelio AM, Cassidy A, Asomaning K, et al. Comparison of discriminatory power and accuracy of three lung cancer risk models. Br J Cancer 2010;103: 423–9.

Screening for Lung Cancer: Challenges for the Thoracic Surgeon

Brendon M. Stiles, MD, Nasser K. Altorki, MD*

KEYWORDS

• Lung • Cancer • Screening • Surgery

Lung cancer is a global health burden and is among the most common and deadly of all malignancies worldwide. In the United States, lung cancer accounts for more than 25% of all cancer deaths, exceeding deaths from breast, colon, and prostate cancers combined.[1] More than 80% of individuals with lung cancer die of the disease. This is primarily because a large proportion of patients with lung cancer present with locally advanced or metastatic disease. Intuitively, early detection of resectable and potentially curable disease may reduce the overall death rate from lung cancer. However, at the present time, screening for lung cancer is not recommended by most clinical societies and health care agencies in the United States. Most notably, the American Cancer Society and the United States Preventative Services Task Force (USPSTF) do not recommend for or against screening for lung cancer but instead suggest that interested individuals discuss the merits of screening with their physicians. This position is based on the results of 3 randomized trials, conducted in the late 1970s, that examined the value of plain chest radiography (CXR) with or without sputum cytology for lung cancer screening in men who were active or former smokers.[2–4] The 3 trials showed nearly identical lung cancer–related mortality in the screened populations and in the control groups, although arguably the prespecified 50% reduction in mortality may have been overly optimistic.

The introduction of multislice computed tomography (CT) technology has renewed interest in screening for lung cancer given that CT is more sensitive than CXR for the detection of small pulmonary nodules.[5–7] CT-based observational studies have consistently shown that lung cancer is detected in approximately 1% to 2% of high-risk individuals and that most of these cases are early stage disease. These studies generated significant debate about the value of CT screening in reducing lung cancer–related mortality, both on a societal and an individual patient basis. To

Division of Thoracic Surgery, Department of Cardiothoracic Surgery, Weill Cornell Medical College, Suite M404, 525 East 68th Street, New York, NY 10021, USA
* Corresponding author.
E-mail address: nkaltork@med.cornell.edu

Surg Oncol Clin N Am 20 (2011) 619–635
doi:10.1016/j.soc.2011.07.001
1055-3207/11/$ – see front matter © 2011 Elsevier Inc. All rights reserved.

definitively determine the effect of CT screening on disease-related mortality, 2 large randomized trials have been launched including, most prominently, the National Lung Screening Trial (NLST) with 53,000 participants and the Dutch-Belgian randomized lung cancer screening trial (NELSON), which included 15,822 individuals. The National Cancer Institute recently announced that the NLST showed that, after 3 annual screening rounds and 8 years of follow-up, the CT screening arm of the trial was associated with a 20.3% reduction in lung cancer mortality and a 7% reduction in overall mortality compared with CXR screening (http://www.cancer.gov/newscenter/pressreleases/2010/NLSTresultsRelease).

This established mortality benefit seems to be a major step forward in lung cancer screening efforts and may prepare the way for national lung cancer screening programs. This article discusses the history of, and rationale for, lung cancer screening, addresses optimization of screening protocols, and describes our current approach for the evaluation of small pulmonary nodules referred for surgical management.

HISTORY OF LUNG CANCER SCREENING

Interest in screening high-risk patients for lung cancer was sparked when the association between cigarette smoking and lung cancer was first appreciated by Doll and Hill[8] in the 1950s. The first mass screening project was conducted by Brett[9] in London from 1960 to 1964 (1968). Although not a randomized trial, 55,034 men were assigned to undergo either CXR every 6 months for 3 years (the screened group), or a single CXR at the beginning of the study, followed by a repeat CXR at the end of the 3-year period (the unscreened group). At the end of the 3-year period, more lung cancers were detected in the screened group compared with the unscreened group (132 vs 96 cases). In addition, resectability was enhanced in the screened group. Despite these findings, lung cancer–specific mortality was not different between the 2 groups.

In the 1970s, the National Cancer Institute funded 3 randomized trials (**Table 1**) for lung cancer screening using both CXR and sputum cytology.[2–4] Two of these trials (the Johns Hopkins Lung Project and the Memorial Sloan-Kettering Cancer Center [MSKCC] trial) focused on the value of the addition of sputum cytology to annual CXRs. In the MSKCC study, patients were randomized to annual CXR alone or annual CXR plus sputum cytologic assessment every 4 months. The same number of cancers was detected in both groups. No difference was detected in resectability rates or lung cancer–specific mortality. This screening protocol was also used in the Johns Hopkins Lung Project randomized trial, with similar results. In the Mayo Lung Project, patients were randomized to undergo CXR and sputum cytologic assessment every 4 months for 6 years (the screened group), or given the usual recommendation of the Mayo Clinic, namely to undergo both of these examinations annually, but without reminders sent to these individuals (the unscreened group). With more than 10,000 participants, the study was powered to show a 50% reduction in lung cancer–related mortality. After a median follow-up period of 3 years, more lung cancers were detected in the screened group compared with the unscreened group. In addition, the resectability rate in the screened group was significantly higher. Nonetheless, there was no statistically significant difference in the lung cancer–specific mortality between the screened and unscreened populations. Several concerns were raised about the conduct of the study, most notably the significant contamination of the control arm as well as the lack of compliance with the screening protocol in the experimental or screened arm of the trial. For example, more than 50% of individuals in the unscreened group had CXRs performed during the course of the study and

Table 1
Historical lung cancer screening trials involving CXR and sputum sampling

Study Institution/ Location	MSKCC	Johns Hopkins	Mayo	Czechoslovakia
Years of Accrual	1974–1982	1973–1982	1971–1983	1976–1980
Screened Arm				
Sample size	4968	5226	4618	3172
Protocol	Annual CXR; sputum cytology every 4 mo	Annual CXR; sputum cytology every 4 mo	CXR and sputum cytology every 4 mo for 6 y	CXR and sputum cytology every 6 mo for 3 y
Baseline cancers	30	39	Data not available	Data not available
Repeat screen cancers	114	194	206	39
Lung cancer mortality	2.7	3.4	3.2	3.6
Unscreened Arm				
Sample size	5072	5161	4593	3174
Protocol	Annual CXR	Annual CXR	Advised for annual CXR and sputum cytology	CXR and sputum cytology initially and after 3 y
Baseline cancers	23	40	Data not available	Data not available
Repeat screen cancers	121	202	160	27
Lung cancer mortality	2.7	3.8	3.0	2.6

Abbreviation: MSKCC, Memorial Sloan-Kettering Cancer Center.

approximately 25% of participants in the screening group failed to comply with the screening regimen. Furthermore, the trial was significantly underpowered to detect lower, but clinically important, reductions in lung cancer mortality.

A similar screening trial was conducted by Kubik and Polak[10] (see **Table 1**) in the late 1970s in Czechoslovakia, which also focused on the combined effects of CXR and sputum cytologic examination for lung cancer screening (1986). In this trial, participants in the screened group underwent CXR and evaluation of sputum cytology at baseline, then every 6 months for 3 years, whereas those in the unscreened group had only the baseline CXR and sputum cytologic examinations, both of which were repeated at the end of the 3-year period. After the initial screening period, both groups underwent annual CXR and sputum assessment for an additional 3 years. Once again, more lung cancers were diagnosed in the screened group compared with the unscreened group (39 vs 27 cases). However, there was no difference in lung cancer–specific mortality between the 2 groups.

EARLY CT SCREENING TRIALS

In the 1990s, increased resolution and data-acquisition speeds of modern CT scanners rekindled interest in screening for lung cancer. Initial findings from Henschke and colleagues[11] of the Early Lung Cancer Action Project (ELCAP) showed that, in a high-risk population, CT was superior to CXR in detection of lung nodules (1999). Notably, 2.7% of those enrolled in the CT screening program had lung cancer, most of which were stage I (2001). Within the initial ELCAP patient population, 27 screen-diagnosed lung cancers were found at baseline screenings, of which 96% were resectable.[11] A subsequent report by the I-ELCAP group addressed overall curability estimated through 10-year survival rates of patients found to have stage I lung cancer by CT screening.[12] The investigators reported an estimated 88% 10-year survival rate, markedly higher than survival rates predicted by the current staging system or among those presenting as a result of symptoms. Because CT screening leads to early detection of lung cancer and because those lung cancers found as a result of CT screening are curable, they inferred that CT screening leads to a reduction in lung cancer mortality. Several other groups have also evaluated CT screening for lung cancer (**Table 2**). A review by Black and colleagues[16] published in 2007 identified 12 studies, including 2 randomized and 10 single-arm observational studies (2007). Significant variability existed in the study populations and in the definition of a positive finding in each. Nevertheless, the percentage of positive screenings ranged from 5.1% to 51%. From baseline screenings, 1.8% to 18% of positive findings led to a diagnosis of cancer. Most of the tumors were stage I (53%–100%), with a high resectability rate (>78%). Only 1 of the studies reported 5-year survival: 76% for patients with cancer detected at baseline screening and 65% for patients with cancer detected at annual repeat scanning.[28]

In a study published the same year, Bach and colleagues[29] reported the findings from CT screening of 3246 high-risk patients from multiple institutions (2007). The investigators reported a threefold increase in individuals diagnosed with lung cancer and a tenfold increase in patients undergoing lung resection (compared with expected cases). They also found no evidence of a decline in the number of patients with advanced stages of disease or of deaths from lung cancer in the screened groups. The investigators concluded that CT screening may not meaningfully reduce the risk of dying from lung cancer and suggested that CT screening is inherently prone to over-diagnosis, thus exposing patients to unnecessary surgery. The study generated significant controversy given that the follow-up was short (3.9 years) and that at least 1 of the 3 studies did not require the exclusion of symptomatic individuals, possibly undermining the core concept of screening.

RECENT CT SCREENING TRIALS

The NLST enrolled 53,454 smokers and ex-smokers between the ages of 55 and 74 years (**Table 3**). The group compared low-dose CT screening with CXR screening using 3 annual screening rounds with 8 years of follow-up. In the CT screening arm, there were 354 deaths from lung cancer, compared with 442 in the CXR group, translating into a 20.3% reduction in lung cancer–related mortality. In addition, there was a 7% reduction in overall mortality in the CT arm of the trial. This mortality reduction is unprecedented in the history of lung cancer screening and has been greeted with enthusiasm by advocates of CT screening.

Two other recent studies have addressed the magnitude of lung cancer mortality reduction by CT screening using modeling approaches. McMahon and colleagues[30] from the Mayo Clinic used 1520 current or former smokers undergoing CT screening to model predicted cases of lung cancer and deaths, which were compared with a simulated unscreened control arm (2008). The model ultimately simulated 500,000 cases per study arm based on 5 annual screening examinations to generate precise

Table 2
Results of baseline lung cancer screening using CT scans

Study/Year	Number Screened	Positive Screen (%)	Total Lung Cancer (%)	Lung Cancer in Screen Positive Patients (%)	Percent Stage I (for NSCLC)	Percent Resectable (for NSCLC)
ELCAP 2001[6]	1000	23.3	2.7	11.6	88	100
Sone et al,[13] 2001	5483	5.1	0.4	7.9	22	100
Garg et al,[14] 2002	92	33	3.2	10	NR	NR
Tiitola et al,[15] 2002	602	18.4	0.8	4.5	0	20
Sobue et al,[28] 2002	1611	11.5	0.8	7.0	77	92
Nawa et al,[17,18] 2002	7956	6.8	0.45	6.7	86	NR
Pastorino et al,[19,20] 2003	1035	5.9	1.1	18	55	91
Swensen et al,[21,22] 2002, 2003	1520	51	1.7	3.3	69	NR
Diederich et al,[23,24] 2002, 2004	817	43	2.1	4.9	56	100
Gohagan et al,[25] 2004	1586	20.5	1.9	9.2	53	NR
MacRedmond et al,[26] 2004	449	24	0.4	1.8	NR	100
Miller et al,[27] 2004	3598	32	0.61	1.9	NR	NR

Table 3
Mortality results in the NLST (n = 53,000)

	CT Screened Arm	CXR Screened Arm
Screening interval and follow-up	Three annual screenings with 8 y of follow-up	
Number of deaths	354	442
Relative decrease in lung cancer mortality in CT screened group	20.3	
Relative decrease in overall mortality in CT screened group	7	

estimates of mortality. At 6 years of follow-up, the screening arm had an estimated 37% relative increase in lung cancer detection compared with the simulated control arm and a 28% relative reduction in cumulative lung cancer–specific mortality. Although the model included many assumptions, such as lung cancer incidence rates, adherence to the screening protocol, and treatment by established guidelines, the study made a compelling argument for a mortality benefit from CT screening.

Similarly, Foy and colleagues[31] used a lung cancer mortality model developed within the Cancer Intervention and Surveillance Modeling Network (CISNET) to address the potential for mortality reduction by CT screening for lung cancer (2011). The comparison matched members of a CT screening trial (NY-ELCAP) with age, sex, and tobacco exposure–matched control patients from the β-Carotene and Retinol Efficacy Trial (CARET), with well-established lung cancer incidence rates (Goodman and colleagues[32]: 16-from Foy). The simulation was repeated 5000 times to compare expected lung cancer mortality between the 2 groups. Although again subject to inherent assumptions made for the purposes of modeling, the study suggested a 45.6% relative reduction in lung cancer mortality in the group of patients screened with CT. These studies all suggest that CT screening protocols, logically followed by earlier treatment of lung cancer, do provide a mortality benefit.

IMPORTANT STATISTICAL CONCEPTS

Before the report of the NLST, as judged by the morality paradigm, it was argued that lung cancer screening was not beneficial and was potentially harmful. No randomized trial had yet shown a reduction in cancer-specific or overall mortality. However, the efficacy of screening in reducing cancer-specific mortality may be confounded by lead-time, length, and overdiagnosis biases. Although the statistical arguments may be examined from many different vantage points and are sometimes difficult to interpret, they have been well described previously by Strauss[33] (2000). This article highlights some of those important concepts.

In all screening trials, lead time must be distinguished from lead-time bias. The success of any screening program is dependent on a lead time in diagnosis and treatment. In and of itself, this does not present a problem. Bias can arise when short-term survival rates are used to assess the value of screening in populations with and without lead time. Lead-time bias should not affect resectability or, more importantly, curability. In the subpopulations of patients with lung cancer in the older screening trials, there was an increased proportion of 5-year survivors in the screen-detected cases compared with those in the control arms in both the Mayo and Czech studies.[2,10] The survival curves never converged, suggesting that screening did increase the cure rate of patients with cancer. These mature data implies that lead-time bias does not explain differences in survival between those groups. The I-ELCAP investigators' effort to estimate 10-year survival rates, rather than shorter-term rates, was also an attempt to avoid any possible lead-time bias.[12] The I-ELCAP strategy to avoid lead-time bias was to estimate the cure rate, which occurs at the plateau phase of the survival cure, its asymptote, at which point the additional deaths that occur are from competing causes.

Length bias refers to the tendency of screening to lead to the diagnosis of slower-growing cancers more frequently in the baseline round, because these tumors potentially have been present for a considerable amount of time before the screening study. For tumors detected only on repeat rounds of screening, this is less of a concern. However, a review of the Mayo data shows that survival rates were only slightly better in the prevalence cases compared with incidence cases (40% vs 33%), those diagnosed at repeat screening.[33] In the I-ELCAP data, no distinction was made in survival rates between the prevalence and incidence groups.

Similar to the length-bias argument, the overdiagnosis hypothesis is based on the idea that screen-detected cancers may be indolent and perhaps even clinically insignificant. The lung cancer detection rates were higher in the screened groups in both the Mayo and Czech studies. Despite this, mortality for the entire screened cohort in both studies was slightly higher. Similarly, in the more recent CT-based study by Bach and colleagues[29] (2007), there was an increased rate of lung cancer detection (144 cases vs 44.5 expected cases). Despite this increase in detection, there was no decrease in the expected lung cancer mortality. The possibility of overdiagnosis has been used to explain these findings, as well as the excellent projected 10-year survival in the I-ELCAP study. Several authorities suggest that many lung cancers detected by screening would not progress rapidly to the point of clinical detection and would therefore be unlikely to account for a meaningful share of deaths among screened individuals.

There are several arguments against overdiagnosis. The first is based on the known epidemiologic evidence. For example, studies reported by Sobue and colleagues[34] (1992) and by Flehinger and colleagues[35,36] (1992) documented mortalities in excess of 80% for untreated screen-detected lung cancers. The high mortality of screen-detected small tumors argues against their presumed indolent or nonfatal nature. It seems that even the smallest lung cancers are almost always deadly. An analysis by Henschke and colleagues[37] of the Surveillance, Epidemiology and End Results (SEER) database revealed an 87% 8-year fatality rate for untreated 6-mm to 15-mm primary non–small cell lung cancer (NSCLC) (2003). A more recent review of the California Cancer Center registry by Raz and colleagues[38] examined long-term survival in untreated stage I NSCLC. Five-year overall survival was only 6%, with a median survival of 9 months.

More evidence against overdiagnosis may be found from autopsy studies. McFarlane[39] reported that the rate of surprise lung cancer at autopsy was less than 1% and that many of these patients had died of those cancers (1986). Another study found a slightly higher (3.3%) rate of lung cancer at autopsy, but deemed none of the cancers to have been clinically insignificant, because lung cancer was believed to be the direct cause of death in more than half of the cases.[40] Further evidence against overdiagnosis may also be found in the I-ELCAP data. Henschke and colleagues[5,6,12,32,37,41] reported that, for the I-ELCAP screening trial, an expert panel of pulmonary pathologists confirmed that 95% of the patients with stage I cancer had invasive tumors that were morphologically indistinguishable from garden variety lung cancers (2006). In addition, a subgroup of the I-ELCAP screen-detected cancers was analyzed for biomarkers using immunohistochemistry and fluorescence in situ hybridization.[42] The molecular alterations were found to be similar to those found in conventionally diagnosed cancers. All 8 I-ELCAP patients with untreated stage I cancer died within 5 years of screening. In conclusion, the balance of both epidemiologic and pathologic evidence does not seem to make lung cancer a good candidate for overdiagnosis by screening.

Perhaps the most challenging aspect of understanding the issue of overdiagnosis is defining the term itself. The phrase is often used synonymously with pseudodisease, which implies that the disease would progress slowly and would not lead to death before that caused from a competing illness. This definition allows for patients with lung cancer who die of competing (or accidental) causes to be considered as examples of overdiagnosis regardless of tumor stage. This situation is most evident in the Mayo Lung Project, in which the concept of overdiagnosis was first proposed. In that study, there was an excess of early stage lung cancers in the screened group, but no difference in mortality. Therefore, it was concluded that those excess, predominantly early stage, cancers were overdiagnosed. However, when examined critically, they did not fit the profile of indolent cancers. They were on average 2 cm in diameter, not present on the baseline round, had a median growth rate of 101 days, and were nearly all invasive pathologically.[2] Thus, in the screened arm, lung cancers were far more likely to be identified and cannot be described as indolent. The similar disease-specific survival rate between the groups may be explained by the high rate of competing causes of death in the screened group, in which the number of cardiovascular deaths was nearly 4 times the rate of lung cancer deaths.

OTHER APPROACHES TO SCREENING

Conventional, white-light bronchoscopy has a low sensitivity for the detection of pre-invasive lung cancer (carcinoma in situ). According to Lam and colleagues,[43,44] auto-fluorescence bronchoscopy, relying on the difference in autofluorescence spectra between normal and malignant airway epithelia, doubles the detection rate of lung cancer (2000). Normal epithelium fluoresces green, whereas malignant tissue fluoresces brown/red. Importantly, autofluorescence bronchoscopy, or light-induced fluorescent endoscopy (LIFE), may also detect lung cancers that are not visible on CT. In a screening study by McWilliams and colleagues,[45] one-quarter of detected cancers were CT occult and only seen with autofluorescence bronchoscopy (2006). However, using LIFE, it is difficult to distinguish between inflammation and premalignant lesions. As such, many lesions detected with this technique are false-positives, as many as two-thirds in one study.[46] Future work regarding autofluorescence bronchoscopy will entail further refining the fluorescent filters and the design and evaluation of thinner bronchoscopes. A major limitation of this modality is its inability to reach peripheral lesions because of the size of the instruments.

As reviewed by Belinsky,[47] several molecular alterations have been identified in premalignant bronchial lesions and in early lung cancer (2004). These molecular abnormalities may be potentially identified in the sputum or blood of high-risk patients. Sophisticated immunohistochemical and polymerase chain reaction (PCR) sputum analyses are being investigated as adjuncts for sputum cytology. In a retrospective analysis of archived sputum specimens containing moderately atypical cells from the Johns Hopkins Lung Project, 64% of specimens possessing positive immunostaining for the nuclear ribonucleoprotein, hnRNP A2/B1, were from patients who eventually developed lung cancer, whereas 88% with negative staining did not develop cancer.[48] Recent studies have shown aberrant methylation of the p16, MGMT, DAPK, and other genes in sputum specimens of patients with cancer.[49,50] Abnormal methylation of the promoter region of a variety of specific genes may be responsible for the inhibition of gene expression and the subsequent development of cancer. Belinsky and colleagues[49] reported that the risk of lung cancer increases with the number of hypermethylated genes (2006). However, false-positives are common, with aberrant methylation demonstrable in nearly 1 out of 4 long-term smokers without cancer.[50] More recently, Spira and colleagues[51] attempted to document genetic changes in the airways that may be found as clues to early detection (2007). Using a training set (n = 77) and gene-expression profiles on Affymetrix microarrays, they identified an 80-gene biomarker panel that distinguished smokers with and without lung cancer. The panel had an accuracy of 83% (80% sensitive, 84% specific). Combining cytopathology of lower airway cells obtained at bronchoscopy with the biomarker panel yielded a 95% sensitivity and a 95% negative predictive value.

Similarly, molecular diagnostic techniques are under evaluation for the detection of genomic or proteomic signatures in the bloodstream of patients with lung cancer. A recent study identified 26 genes frequently mutated in lung cancer.[52] Such mutated genes may have implications not only for treatment but also for diagnosis. Therefore, many efforts have been made to identify lung cancer–specific biomarkers.[53] Patz and colleagues[20] developed a blood test based on 4 proteins (carcinoembryonic antigen, squamous cell carcinoma antigen, retinol binding protein, and α-1 antitrypsin) for the diagnosis of lung cancer using a training set of 100 patients (2009). In an independent verification set of patients with and without lung cancer, the test had a sensitivity of 77.8% and a specificity of 75.4%. More recently, a multi-institutional group developed a serum proteomic panel of 12 biomarkers from 1326 patients.[54] In their rigorous and well-designed study, the 12-protein panel had an 89% sensitivity and an 83% specificity in a blinded, independent verification set.

Other approaches under evaluation as blood-based detection assays include the evaluation of circulating DNA, messenger and micro-RNA, and the detection of circulating autoantibodies. Although all of these blood-based tests offer promise for lung cancer detection, none have been extensively evaluated or applied to large screening populations. Several obstacles exist to developing a sensitive and specific test for early lung cancer, most importantly the heterogeneity of the disease. As such, whether these techniques will play a role in screening for lung cancer remains to be determined. Currently, there are no adequate standards to evaluate samples, with resulting large disparities among quantitative and qualitative reports. However, the hope is that one day it will be possible to develop accurate blood and sputum tests to facilitate the diagnosis of lung cancer. Such tests will likely be combined with CT screening protocols, either using the biomarker to select patients for screening or to further risk stratify patients found to have nodules on CT screening.

Regardless of the method used to screen patients for lung cancer, controversy about the value of screening will likely continue to exist, much as it does for other cancers including breast and prostate cancer. In 2009, the USPSTF released new recommendations for breast cancer screening that were different from their 2002 recommendations.[55] The Task Force raised the recommended age to begin screening from 40 years to 50 years and recommended stopping screening at 74 years. These recommendations generated significant national controversy. The USPSTF's interpretation of the screening data was subsequently refuted by some investigators who continued to claim a benefit for screening in the age range of 40 to 84 years.[56] Similarly, the value of screening for prostate cancer has also been called into question by the results of 2 disparate landmark studies.[57] The European Randomized Study of Screening for Prostate Cancer reported a statistically significant cancer-specific mortality reduction of 20% favoring prostate-specific antigen-based screening.[58] In contrast, the Prostate, Lung, Colorectal and Ovarian Cancer Screening Trial showed no mortality reduction.[59] Undoubtedly, different structures of competing clinical trials, heterogeneous unscreened populations, and evolving technological advances will also continue to make an absolute interpretation of the data from lung cancer screening trials difficult.

THE SCREENING REGIMEN

Our current screening regimen begins with a low-dose helical CT scan with a-priori definition of what constitutes a positive or negative reading. In its first iteration,[11] ELCAP defined a positive result on baseline as finding 1 to 6 noncalcified nodules. If no nodules, only calcified nodules, or more than 6 nodules were identified, the result was negative and the person was referred to the first annual repeat screening. On the annual repeat scan, a positive result is defined as the presence of any growing non-calcified nodule, including new nodules.[5,6] If the initial test is positive, a well-defined diagnostic algorithm is followed until a diagnosis of cancer is established. If the CT result is negative or the diagnostic algorithm does not lead to a diagnosis of malignancy, the person is referred to the next routinely scheduled screening round.

As technology improved and more knowledge was gained about the performance of the algorithm, the definition of a positive result as well as the resulting choice of additional tests was updated. Helical CT scanning has rapidly advanced since the initiation of the I-ELCAP project. Using modern multislice scanners, images of less than 1-mm slice thickness can be obtained in a single breath hold. Because resolution markedly improves with thinner slices, many more nodules are being detected. However, most of these nodules are less than 5.0 mm in diameter. The current I-ELCAP definition of positive result on baseline is 1 or more noncalcified solid or part-solid nodules 5.0 mm or larger or a nonsolid nodule 8.0 mm or larger (I-ELCAP Web site). Using this updated definition, the percentage of positive results on the baseline low-dose screening is reduced to less than 15% without any increase in the false-negative rate. The definition of positive results on annual repeat screening has remained unchanged. Positive results continue to occur in less than 6% of these screening studies.

There have also been changes in the diagnostic workup, including changes in time intervals for follow-up scans, the use of biopsy as a possible alternative without documenting growth (only when the nodule is $\geq$15 mm at baseline), the use of antibiotics, and the use of positron emission tomography (PET)/CT scans. As technologic innovations continue, the definition of positive results of baseline and annual repeat screening and the algorithm of diagnostic workup will need to be further updated.

MANAGEMENT OF THE SCREEN-DETECTED NODULE

No matter how the current debate on screening unfolds or how the technology evolves, thoracic surgeons will continue to be asked to evaluate individuals with either screen-detected or incidentally discovered small pulmonary nodules. The management of these patients presents several challenges. It is important to understand the likelihood of malignancy in relationship to nodule size. Most nodules found by screening or on incidental studies are not cancer. A large proportion of these nodules are less than 5 mm on the baseline round of screening and therefore do not constitute a positive result. Even for larger nodules, it is important to reassure patients that a positive CT scan does not mean that they have cancer. In the I-ELCAP data, 11.6% of patients with positive baseline CT scans were found to have cancer.[12]

Several factors may influence the probability of cancer in a pulmonary nodule. Of these factors, nodule size is the most critical. In the initial ELCAP publication, the rate of malignant disease was 1% in nodules less than or equal to 5 mm, 24% in those

6 to 10 mm, 33% in those 11 to 20 mm, and 80% for those greater than 20 mm.[11] Change in size is also an important factor to consider, because nodules that show growth are considered to be active. Time to follow-up CT scanning is in part dependent on the initial size of the nodule (because documentation of growth in small nodules is more challenging) and on whether the nodules were initially detected on the baseline or repeat round. The time to follow-up is typically shorter on the repeat round, because cancers found on repeat screening are typically faster growing. Sophisticated three-dimensional software packages are available to more accurately assess doubling times.

Several factors other than size play a role in the probability of malignancy. Patients with numerous small nodules (>6) are generally believed to be at low risk for malignancy and more likely to have inflammatory lung disease. The consistency of the nodule also affects the probability of cancer. According to data from the initial ELCAP group, part-solid nodules have a higher rate of malignancy (63%) than nonsolid nodules (18%), whereas solid nodules have the lowest malignancy rate (7%).[41] Patients with part-solid or nonsolid nodules predominantly had bronchioloalveolar carcinoma or adenocarcinoma with bronchioloalveolar features. Other factors to consider are patient age, smoking history, occupational history, and endemic rates of granulomatous disease.

Our general algorithm for radiographic follow-up is well documented. A specific protocol is available on the I-ELCAP Web site. For nodules less than 5 mm in diameter or for nonsolid nodules less than 8 mm found on baseline CT, we recommend repeat CT in 1 year. For nodules 5 to 15 mm in diameter (8–15 mm for nonsolid nodules), we obtain a repeat CT scan in 3 months to assess for growth or resolution. For nodules found on annual repeat screening, those less than 3 mm in diameter should have another CT in 6 months, whereas those greater than 3 mm and less than 5 mm should have CT follow-up within 3 months. For those larger than 5 mm, a course of antibiotics and repeat in 1 month is an additional option. In the I-ELCAP patient population, an initial course of antibiotics of 7 to 10 days resulted in partial or complete resolution of 29% of nodules on baseline screening and 74% of nodules on repeat screening.[60] In all instances, nodule growth should prompt careful consideration of a biopsy or closer follow-up. PET scans may be an additional diagnostic option for screen-detected nodules, particularly for patients with nodules greater than 1 cm in diameter. Veronesi and colleagues[61] reported the sensitivity and specificity of PET for screen-detected lung nodules to be 89% and 93% respectively (2007). Median nodule size was 14 mm for their cohort of patients. Even for nodules less than 10 mm, sensitivity and specificity were 83% and 100%. As part of their diagnostic strategy, the investigators suggested lowering the positive maximum standardized uptake value cutoff for smaller nodules to 1.5.

Once the possibility of cancer exists, it is imperative to establish an accurate tissue diagnosis. When a nodule is deemed to be suspicious for malignancy, either based on baseline characteristics, positive PET scan findings, or the demonstration of growth, we typically proceed to fine-needle aspiration (FNA), even for nodules less than 10 mm in size. FNA performed at high-volume centers can be accurate, with a sensitivity of 82% and a diagnostic accuracy of 88% overall, although the yield decreases with nodules less than 8 mm.[62] Accuracy of FNA may be higher with larger nodules, particularly those larger than 1.5 cm; however, these are typically larger than the nodules detected by CT screening. FNA may result in 4 possible outcomes: malignant, specific benign, nonspecific benign, and nondiagnostic. For malignant and specific benign nodules, the treatment course is typically obvious. However, those patients with nonspecific benign and nondiagnostic results require further workup. A review of 74 cases of FNA with either nonspecific benign or nondiagnostic findings showed an eventual malignancy rate of almost 18%.[63] Such nonspecific diagnoses may include atypical cells or inflammation. For lesions greater than 1.5 cm, the diagnosis rate of FNA exceeds 93%.

We typically repeat CT scans at short intervals (within 3 months), with or without a course of antibiotics, and gradually increase the interval to the subsequent scan so that nodule stability can be ascertained. Volumetric analysis with serial CT scans can also be performed to assess nodule growth with time and to infer malignancy. However, such techniques are not universally available, are costly, and potentially delay treatment in patients in whom there may be significant concern for malignancy. Further growth necessitates repeat FNA or surgical biopsy, depending on clinical suspicion and surgical risk.

In institutions in which CT-guided FNA is not routinely performed, there should be a higher reliance on more invasive diagnostic techniques for suspicious nodules, such as bronchoscopic biopsy or surgical biopsy, either by open thoracotomy or via video-assisted thoracoscopic surgery (VATS). Bronchoscopic biopsy is an option for establishing tissue diagnosis, although the yield for flexible bronchoscopy has historically been low, especially in small peripheral nodules. Newer techniques, including endobronchial ultrasound (EBUS) and electromagnetic navigation (EMN), have been reported to increase the diagnostic yield of transbronchial biopsy to more than 60%, even for small, peripheral lesions.[64,65]

When surgical biopsy is necessary, VATS is believed to decrease postoperative morbidity compared with open thoracotomy, but occasionally has difficulty palpating and visualizing the small lesions that are often found on screening studies. Several techniques are available to localize and excise small pulmonary nodules using a mini-mally invasive approach.[38,66–73] Preoperative marking with methylene blue, wire hooks, and metallic coils have all been described. Reported complications are rare, but include marker dislodgement, pneumothorax, intrapulmonary hemorrhage, and air embolism. Recently, Sortini and colleagues[74] and other investigators also reported good results with ultrasound localization (2002), although this method is strongly oper-ator dependent. Other groups have described a VATS radiotracer localization tech-nique, with a success rate of 92% for nodules with a median size of 8 mm.[75] The technique can be applied to all pleural surfaces, including interlobar regions with complete fissures, and enables rapid and predictable intraoperative localization. The procedure uses readily available technical components with minimal additional cost. Regardless of the method used to localize small nodules, VATS resection typi-cally can be performed with low morbidity, short hospital stays, and excellent diag-nostic accuracy.

Such a tailored approach should lead to a higher likelihood of a cancer diagnosis following invasive workups. Evidence for increased refinement of management approaches exists in the literature. For example, in the initial report on the NLST trial, reported in 2004, 20% of CT screening subjects had a lesion suspicious for cancer, of which 56% had invasive workups that resulted in a lung cancer diagnosis. More recently, by more narrowly defining their diagnostic algorithm, the NY-ELCAP reported a much lower (14%) incidence of suspicious nodules, of which 93% of invasive workups confirmed lung cancer.[76] In the NELSON trial, with an even stricter definition of suspicious nodules based on defining volume doubling times, only 2.6% of subjects tested positive by CT screening.[30] Of these, 41% were found to have lung cancer and the false-negative rate was only 0.3%. Improved diagnostic workups such as these should decrease invasive workups for benign disease and ultimately contribute to a more favorable mortality reduction benefit.

ONGOING STUDIES AND SUMMARY

Before the release of the NLST data, the USPSTF reviewed the results of 6 RCTs for lung cancer screening and found that none of them showed a benefit. In addition, they reviewed 5 case-controlled studies and found that all of them showed a benefit. Each of these studies was rated on a 3-point scale of good, fair, or poor. Not a single one of these studies was given a good rating. As a result of their inability to balance the benefits and harms from screening, they gave lung cancer screening an I recommendation. Namely, The USPSTF concludes that the evidence is insufficient to recommend for or against screening asymptomatic persons for lung cancer with low-dose computerized tomography (LDCT), CXR, sputum cytology, or a combination of these tests. Thus at this time, there is still no definitive guideline regarding the practice of screening for lung cancer.

It has been proposed that ongoing studies will help to answer the questions of whether screening for lung cancer is cost effective, whether it improves cure rates of lung cancer, and whether screening for lung cancer saves lives. The data from the NLST must be published and further evaluated before definitive conclusions can be made, but the mortality benefits evident in this study are likely to change the recommendations of major task forces and societies. Also to be reported are the results of the Prostate, Lung, Colorectal and Ovarian (PLCO) Cancer Screening Trial, begun in 1993. The PLCO trial is a complex, multicenter trial sponsored by the National Cancer Institute with a target accrual of 148,000 subjects.[77] The PLCO trial has an 89% power to detect a 10% reduction in lung cancer–specific mortality. Patients were randomized to undergo an annual CXR for 3 (smokers) or 2 (nonsmokers) years versus routine medical care (unscreened group). Although accrual began in 1994 and was completed in 2001, the results have yet to be reported. The technology of film-based CXR used in this study has been routinely replaced by digital CXR. In addition, CXR has already been shown to be inferior to CT scans for the detection of nodules, which will certainly lessen the impact of the results of the study. Other major trials still accruing include the Dutch-Belgian Randomized Lung Cancer Screening (NELSON) study, the Milan Multicentric Italian Lung Detection (MILD) trial, and the United Kingdom Lung Cancer Screening Trial (UKLS). It is hoped that these trials can further define mortality reductions from CT screening programs, the number of screening rounds needed, and the optimal screening interval.

Lung cancer continues to be a deadly disease. The goal of screening programs is to detect tumors in earlier, curable stages, consequently reducing disease-specific mortality. The issue of screening has great relevance to thoracic surgeons, who should play a leading role in the debate about screening and its consequences, which is especially important because screening protocols may generate a tenfold increase in the number of patients presenting for surgical resection.[29] The burden is on thoracic surgeons to guide and treat these patients safely and responsibly, with low morbidity and mortality of potential diagnostic or therapeutic interventions.

REFERENCES

1. Jemal A, Siegel R, Xu J, et al. Cancer statistics, 2010. CA Cancer J Clin 2010; 60(5):277–300.
2. Fontana RS, Sanderson DR, Taylor, et al. Early lung cancer detection: results of the initial (prevalence) radiologic and cytologic screening in the Mayo Clinic study. Am Rev Respir Dis 1984;130(4):561–5.
3. Melamed MR, Flehinger BJ, Zaman MB, et al. Screening for early lung cancer. Results of the Memorial Sloan-Kettering study in New York. Chest 1984;86(1):44–53.

4. Tockman M. Survival and mortality from lung cancer in a screened population: the John Hopkins study. Chest 1986;89:325s.

5. Henschke CI, McCauley DI, Yankelevitz DF, et al. Early lung cancer action project: a summary of the findings on baseline screening. Oncologist 2001; 6(2):147–52.

6. Henschke CI, Naidich DP, Yankelevitz DF, et al. Early lung cancer action project: initial findings on repeat screenings. Cancer 2001;92(1):153–9.

7. Sone S, Takashima S, Li F, et al. Mass screening for lung cancer with mobile spiral computed tomography scanner. Lancet 1998;351(9111):1242–5.

8. Doll R, Hill AB. Smoking and carcinoma of the lung. Preliminary report. Br Med J 1950;2(4682):739–48.

9. Brett GZ. The value of lung cancer detection by six-monthly chest radiographs. Thorax 1968;4:414–20.

10. Kubík A, Polák J. Lung cancer detection. Results of a randomized prospective study in Czechoslovakia. Cancer 1986;57(12):2427–37.

11. Henschke CI, McCauley DI, Yankelevitz DF, et al. Early Lung Cancer Action Project: overall design and findings from baseline screening. Lancet 1999; 354(9173):99–105.

12. Henschke CI, Yankelevitz DF, Libby DM, et al. Survival of patients with stage I lung cancer detected on CT screening. N Engl J Med 2006;355(17):1763–71.

13. Sone S, Li F, Yang ZG, et al. Results of three-year mass screening programme for lung cancer using mobile low-dose spiral computed tomography scanner. Br J Cancer 2001;84(1):25–32.

14. Garg K, Keith RL, Byers T, et al. Randomized controlled trial with low-dose spiral CT for lung cancer screening: feasibility study and preliminary results. Radiology 2002;225(2):506–10.

15. Tiitola M, Kivisaari L, Huuskonen MS, et al. Computed tomography screening for lung cancer in asbestos-exposed workers. Lung Cancer 2002;35(1):17–22.

16. Black C, de Verteuil R, Walker S, et al. Population screening for lung cancer using computed tomography, is there evidence of clinical effectiveness? A systematic review of the literature. Thorax 2007;62(2):131–8.

17. Nawa T, Nakagawa T, Kusano S, et al. Lung cancer screening using low-dose spiral CT: results of baseline and 1-year follow-up studies. Chest 2002;122(1): 15–20.

18. Nishii K, Ueoka H, Kiura K, et al. A case-control study of lung cancer screening in Okayama Prefecture, Japan. Lung Cancer 2001;34(3):325–32.

19. Pastorino U, Bellomi M, Landoni C, et al. Early lung-cancer detection with spiral CT and positron emission tomography in heavy smokers: 2-year results. Lancet 2003;362(9384):593–7.

20. Patz EF Jr, Campa MJ, Gottlin EB, et al. Panel of serum biomarkers for the diagnosis of lung cancer. J Clin Oncol 2007;25(35):5578–83.

21. Swensen SJ, Jett JR, Hartman TE, et al. Lung cancer screening with CT: Mayo Clinic experience. Radiology 2003;226(3):756–61.

22. Swensen SJ, Jett JR, Sloan JA, et al. Screening for lung cancer with low-dose spiral computed tomography. Am J Respir Crit Care Med 2002;165(4):508–13.

23. Diederich S, Thomas M, Semik M, et al. Screening for early lung cancer with low-dose spiral computed tomography: results of annual follow-up examinations in asymptomatic smokers. Eur Radiol 2004;14(4):691–702.

24. Diederich S, Wormanns D, Semik M, et al. Screening for early lung cancer with low-dose spiral CT: prevalence in 817 asymptomatic smokers. Radiology 2002; 222(3):773–81.

25. Gohagan J, Marcus P, Fagerstrom R, et al. Writing Committee, Lung Screening Study Research Group. Baseline findings of a randomized feasibility trial of lung cancer screening with spiral CT scan vs chest radiograph: the Lung Screening Study of the National Cancer Institute. Chest 2004;126(1):114–21.
26. MacRedmond R, Logan PM, Lee M, et al. Screening for lung cancer using low dose CT scanning. Thorax 2004;59(3):237–41.
27. Miller A, Markowitz S, Manowitz A, et al. Lung cancer screening using low-dose high-resolution CT scanning in a high-risk workforce: 3500 nuclear fuel workers in three US states. Chest 2004;125(Suppl 5):15.
28. Sobue T, Moriyama N, Kaneko M, et al. Screening for lung cancer with low-dose helical computed tomography: anti-lung cancer association project. J Clin Oncol 2002;20(4):911–20.
29. Bach PB, Jett JR, Pastorino U, et al. Computed tomography screening and lung cancer outcomes. JAMA 2007;297(9):953–61.
30. McMahon PM, Kong CY, Johnson BE, et al. Estimating long-term effectiveness of lung cancer screening in the Mayo CT screening study. Radiology 2008;248(1): 278–87.
31. Foy M, Yip R, Chen X, et al. Modeling the mortality reduction due to computed tomography screening for lung cancer. Cancer 2011;117(12):2703–8.
32. Goodman GE, Thornquist MD, Balmes J, et al. The Beta-Carotene and Retinol Efficacy Trial: incidence of lung cancer and cardiovascular disease mortality during 6-year follow-up after stopping beta-carotene and retinol supplements. J Natl Cancer Inst 2004;96:1743–50.
33. Strauss GM. Randomized population trials and screening for lung cancer: breaking the cure barrier. Cancer 2000;89(Suppl 11):2399–421.
34. Sobue T, Suzuki T, Naruke T. A case-control study for evaluating lung-cancer screening in Japan. Japanese Lung-Cancer-Screening Research Group. Int J Cancer 1992;50(2):230–7.
35. Flehinger BJ, Kimmel M, Melamed MR. The effect of surgical treatment on survival from early lung cancer. Implications for screening. Chest 1992;101(4): 1013–8.
36. Flieder DB, Port JL, Korst RJ, et al. Tumor size is a determinant of stage distribution in t1 non-small cell lung cancer. Chest 2005;128(4):2304–8.
37. Henschke CI, Wisnivesky JP, Yankelevitz DF, et al. Small stage I cancers of the lung: genuineness and curability. Lung Cancer 2003;39(3):327–30.
38. Raz DJ, Zell JA, Ou SH, et al. Natural history of stage I non-small cell lung cancer: implications for early detection. Chest 2007;132(1):193–9.
39. McFarlane MJ, Feinstein AR, Wells CK. Clinical features of lung cancers discovered as a postmortem "surprise". Chest 1986;90(4):520–3.
40. Burton EC, Troxclair DA, Newman WP 3rd. Autopsy diagnoses of malignant neoplasms: how often are clinical diagnoses incorrect? JAMA 1998;280(14):1245–8.
41. Henschke CI, Yankelevitz DF, Mirtcheva R, et al. ELCAP Group. CT screening for lung cancer: frequency and significance of part-solid and nonsolid nodules. AJR Am J Roentgenol 2002;178(5):1053–7.
42. Pajares MJ, Zudaire I, Lozano MD, et al. Molecular profiling of computed tomography screen-detected lung nodules shows multiple malignant features. Cancer Epidemiol Biomarkers Prev 2006;15(2):373–80.
43. Lam S, MacAulay C, leRiche JC, et al. Detection and localization of early lung cancer by fluorescence bronchoscopy. Cancer 2000;89(Suppl 11):2468–73.
44. Libby DM, Smith JP, Altorki NK, et al. Managing the small pulmonary nodule discovered by CT. Chest 2004;125(4):1522–9 Review.

45. McWilliams AM, Mayo JR, Ahn MI, et al. Lung cancer screening using multi-slice thin-section computed tomography and autofluorescence bronchoscopy. J Thorac Oncol 2006;1(1):61–8.
46. Ikeda N, Hayashi A, Iwasaki K, et al. Comprehensive diagnostic bronchoscopy of central type early stage lung cancer. Lung Cancer 2007;56(3):295–302.
47. Belinsky SA. Gene-promoter hypermethylation as a biomarker in lung cancer. Nat Rev Cancer 2004;4(9):707–17.
48. Tockman MS, Gupta PK, Myers JD, et al. Sensitive and specific monoclonal antibody recognition of human lung cancer antigen on preserved sputum cells: a new approach to early lung cancer detection. J Clin Oncol 1988;6(11):1685–93.
49. Belinsky SA, Liechty KC, Gentry FD, et al. Promoter hypermethylation of multiple in sputum precedes lung cancer incidence in a high-risk cohort. Cancer Res 2006;66(6):3338–44.
50. Palmisano WA, Divine KK, Saccomanno G, et al. Predicting lung cancer by detecting aberrant promoter methylation in sputum. Cancer Res 2000;60(21):5954–8.
51. Spira A, Beane JE, Shah V, et al. Airway epithelial gene expression in the diagnostic evaluation of smokers with suspect lung cancer. Nat Med 2007;13(3):361–6.
52. Ding L, Getz G, Wheeler DA, et al. Somatic mutations affect key pathways in lung adenocarcinoma. Nature 2008;455(7216):1069–75.
53. Brower V. Biomarker studies abound for early detection of lung cancer. J Natl Cancer Inst 2009;101(1):11–3.
54. Ostroff RM, Bigbee WL, Franklin W, et al. Unlocking biomarker discovery: large scale application of aptamer proteomic technology for early detection of lung cancer. PLoS One 2010;5(12):e15003.
55. U.S. Preventive Services Task Force. Screening for breast cancer: U.S. Preventive Services Task Force recommendation statement. Ann Intern Med 2009;151:716–26.
56. Hendrick RE, Helvie MA. United States Preventive Services Task Force screening mammography recommendations: science ignored. AJR Am J Roentgenol 2011;196:W112–6.
57. Eckersberger E, Finkelstein J, Sadri H, et al. Screening for prostate cancer: a review of the ERSPC and PLCO trials. Rev Urol 2009;11(3):127–33.
58. Schroder FH, Hugosson J, Roobol MJ, et al. Screening and prostate-cancer mortality in a randomized European study. N Engl J Med 2009;360:1320–8.
59. Andriole GL, Crawford ED, Grubb RL 3rd, et al. Mortality results from a randomized prostate-cancer screening trial. N Engl J Med 2009;360:1310–9.
60. Libby DM, Wu N, Lee IJ, et al. CT screening for lung cancer: the value of short-term CT follow-up. Chest 2006;129(4):1039–42.
61. Veronesi G, Bellomi M, Veronesi U, et al. Role of positron emission tomography scanning in the management of lung nodules detected at baseline computed tomography screening. Ann Thorac Surg 2007;84(3):959–65 [discussion: 965–6].
62. Wallace MJ, Krishnamurthy S, Broemeling LD, et al. CT-guided percutaneous fine-needle aspiration biopsy of small (< or = 1-cm) pulmonary lesions. Radiology 2002;225(3):823–8.
63. Savage C, Walser EM, Schnadig V, et al. Transthoracic image-guided biopsy of lung nodules: when is benign really benign? J Vasc Interv Radiol 2004;15(2 Pt 1):161–4.
64. Gildea TR, Mazzone PJ, Karnak D, et al. Electromagnetic navigation diagnostic bronchoscopy: a prospective study. Am J Respir Crit Care Med 2006;174(9):982–9.

65. Kurimoto N, Miyazawa T, Okimasa S, et al. Endobronchial ultrasonography using a guide sheath increases the ability to diagnose peripheral pulmonary lesions endoscopically. Chest 2004;126(3):959–65.
66. Chella A, Lucchi M, Ambrogi MC, et al. A pilot study of the role of TC-99 radionuclide in localization of pulmonary nodular lesions for thoracoscopic resection. Eur J Cardiothorac Surg 2000;18(1):17–21.
67. Eichfeld U, Dietrich A, Ott R, et al. Video-assisted thoracoscopic surgery for pulmonary nodules after computed tomography-guided marking with a spiral wire. Ann Thorac Surg 2005;79(1):313–6 [discussion: 316–7].
68. Partik BL, Leung AN, Müller MR, et al. Using a dedicated lung-marker system for localization of pulmonary nodules before thoracoscopic surgery. AJR Am J Roentgenol 2003;180(3):805–9.
69. Powell TI, Jangra D, Clifton JC, et al. Peripheral lung nodules: fluoroscopically guided video-assisted thoracoscopic resection after computed tomography-guided localization using platinum microcoils. Ann Surg 2004;240(3):481–8 [discussion: 488–9].
70. Rose G, Hamilton PJ, Colwell L, et al. A randomised controlled trial of anti-smoking advice: 10-year results. J Epidemiol Community Health 1982;36(2): 102–8.
71. Sagawa M, Tsubono Y, Saito Y, et al. A case-control study for evaluating the efficacy of mass screening program for lung cancer in Miyagi Prefecture, Japan. Cancer 2001;92(3):588–94.
72. Santambrogio R, Montorsi M, Bianchi P, et al. Intraoperative ultrasound during thoracoscopic procedures for solitary pulmonary nodules. Ann Thorac Surg 1999;68(1):218–22.
73. Torre M, Ferraroli GM, Vanzulli A, et al. A new safe and stable spiral wire needle for thoracoscopic resection of lung nodules. Chest 2004;125(6):2289–93.
74. Sortini A, Carrella G, Sortini D, et al. Single pulmonary nodules: localization with intrathoracoscopic ultrasound – a prospective study. Eur J Cardiothorac Surg 2002;22(3):440–2.
75. Stiles BM, Altes TA, Jones DR, et al. Clinical experience with radiotracer-guided thoracoscopic biopsy of small, indeterminate lung nodules. Ann Thorac Surg 2006;82(4):1191–6 [discussion: 1196–7].
76. Carter D, Vazquez M, Flieder DB, et al, ELCAP, NY-ELCAP. Comparison of pathologic findings of baseline and annual repeat cancers diagnosed on CT screening. Lung Cancer 2007;56(2):193–9.
77. Gohagan JK, Prorok PC, Hayes RB, et al, Prostate, Lung, Colorectal and Ovarian Cancer Screening Trial Project Team. The Prostate, Lung, Colorectal and Ovarian (PLCO) Cancer Screening Trial of the National Cancer Institute: history, organization, and status. Control Clin Trials 2000;21(Suppl 6):251S–72S.

The Changing Pathology of Lung Cancer

Zhen Fan, MD[a],*, Richard Schraeder, MD[b]

KEYWORDS

• Lung • Cancer • Pathology • Classification • Therapy

Lung cancer classification and prognosis have evolved with increasing knowledge of the biology of the disease and advances in therapy. The distinction of the histologic cell type of lung cancer is important for treatment and prognosis. Traditionally, the role of the pathologist has been to distinguish small cell lung carcinoma (SCLC) from non–small cell lung carcinomas (NSCLC). However, with current therapies, the subclassification of NSCLCs, especially the distinction of adenocarcinoma from squamous cell carcinoma (SCC), has become important. The use of uniform terminology and diagnostic criteria enables accurate and reproducible diagnosis. This article discusses the current classification of NSCLCs and lung neuroendocrine tumors (NET) based on histopathologic and immunohistochemical findings and the clinical implications for oncologic therapy.

NON–SMALL CELL LUNG CARCINOMAS

NSCLCs account for 75% to 85% of all lung cancers in the United States.[1,2] There are three main types of NSCLC: (1) SCC, (2) adenocarcinoma, and (3) large cell carcinoma. Most patients present with advanced-stage disease at diagnosis, often necessitating medical treatment.[1–3] The histologic type of NSCLC is important for selection of therapy. For example, premetrexed is more active in combination with cisplatin in the treatment of advanced adenocarcinoma and large-cell carcinoma of the lung than in the treatment of SCC.[4] Another therapeutic agent, bevacizumab (Avastin), a vascular endothelial growth factor monoclonal antibody, is approved in combination with cystotoxic chemotherapy in the treatment of adenocarcinoma, but not SCC because of concern for life-threatening bleeding.[5] Subclassification of NSCLC is

The authors have nothing to disclose.

[a] Department of Pathology, St Joseph Pathology Associates, St Joseph Medical Center, 7601 Osler Drive, Towson, MD 21204, USA

[b] Department of Medicine, St Joseph Cancer Institute, St Joseph Medical Center, 7501 Osler Drive, Towson, MD 21204, USA

* Corresponding author.

E-mail address: zhenfan@catholichealth.net

Surg Oncol Clin N Am 20 (2011) 637–653

doi:10.1016/j.soc.2011.07.004

thus necessary when possible and is aided by the use of immunohistochemical and mucin stains. In some cases, however, a specific cell type still cannot be identified because of poor differentiation or limited sampling; these tumors should be referred to as "NSCLC, not further classified."

SQUAMOUS CELL CARCINOMA

Although most lung cancers are known to be associated with cigarette smoking, the association is strongest for SCC, followed by small cell carcinoma and adenocarcinoma.[6] SCCs predominantly occur in the large central airways but may also be seen in the small peripheral airways.[6,7] Disease progression has been documented to occur in the airway epithelium in a step-wise fashion from dysplasia to carcinoma in situ to invasive carcinoma.[8] Microscopically, these tumors show evidence of squamous differentiation in the form of intercellular bridges and keratinization (**Fig. 1**). Invasive SCC is graded as well-, moderately, or poorly differentiated based on the degree of resemblance to normal squamous epithelium. Poorly differentiated SCC may be difficult to distinguish from poorly differentiated adenocarcinoma, small cell carcinoma, or large cell carcinoma by morphology. In such cases, immunohistochemistry can be helpful to establish a diagnosis of SCC (**Table 1**). Histologic variants of SCC include papillary, clear cell, small cell, basaloid, and alveolar space-filling type.[6] The alveolar space-filling pattern, which has been described in peripheral SCC, seems to be a favorable prognostic indicator.[7,9] The stage of disease and performance status at diagnosis, however, remain the most important prognostic indicators for survival.[6] Stage for stage, the survival rate for SCC is better than for adenocarcinoma.[6,10]

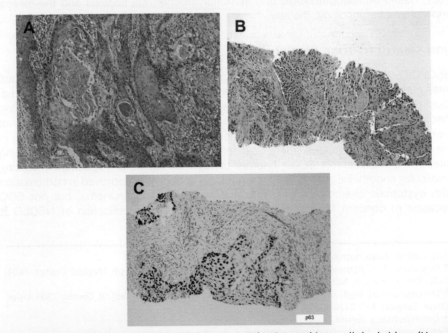

Fig. 1. (*A*) Well-differentiated SCC with keratin production and intercellular bridges (Hematoxylin-Eosin (H&E), original magnification ×100). (*B*) Moderately to poorly differentiated SCC. (*C*) p63 immunostaining of moderately to poorly differentiated SCC (H&E, original magnification ×100).

Table 1
Typical immunohistochemical profiles of NSCLC

	Adenocarcinoma	Squamous Carcinoma	Large Cell Carcinoma	Lung Neuroendocrine Tumors[a]
Thyroid transcription factor-1	+	–	±	+[b]
P63	–	+	–	–
CK5/6 or34BE12	–	+	–	–
Neuroendocrine markers[c]	–	–	–	+

[a] Includes lung carcinoids, SCLC, and large cell neuroendocrine carcinoma.
[b] Thyroid transcription factor-1 positivity is specific for lung origin for carcinoids but not for SCLC or large cell neuroendocrine carcinoma.
[c] Neuroendocrine markers include synaptophysin, chromogranin, and CD56.

ADENOCARCINOMA

In recent decades, lung adenocarcinoma has surpassed SCC as the dominant histologic subtype of lung cancer for men and women in North America, likely because of changes in smoking habits and a true increased incidence of adenocarcinomas.[11–15] Worldwide, adenocarcinoma is the most common histologic type in women, nonsmokers, and Asians.[3,11,15] Adenocarcinomas may show variable patterns of lung involvement. They commonly occur as peripheral solitary masses but can also arise in the central airways or present as lobar consolidation, diffuse bilateral disease, or rarely pleural thickening mimicking malignant mesothelioma.[6] Microscopically, adenocarcinomas show glandular differentiation or mucin production (**Fig. 2**). The main growth patterns are acinar, papillary; bronchioloalveolar (lepidic); and solid with mucin.[6] Most lung adenocarcinomas show a mixture of these patterns.[6,16] The recognition of solid adenocarcinoma with mucin requires detection of cytoplasmic mucin by a mucin stain. Because focal mucin can be seen in squamous cell and large

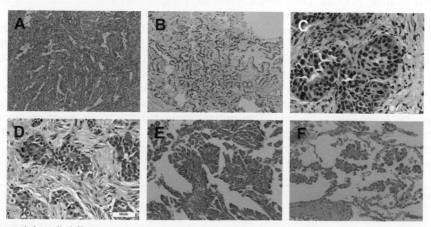

Fig. 2. (*A*) Well-differentiated adenocarcinoma, acinar-pattern (H&E, original magnification ×100). (*B*) Thyroid transcription factor-1 immunostaining (H&E, original magnification ×100). (*C*) Adenocarcinoma, solid-pattern (H&E, original magnification ×200). (*D*) Mucicarmine stain highlighting intracytoplasmic mucin in solid-pattern adenocarcinoma (H&E, original magnification ×200). (*E*) Adenocarcinoma, papillary-pattern with central fibrovascular cores. (*F*) Adenocarcinoma, micropapillary-pattern without fibrovascular cores (H&E, original magnification ×100).

cell carcinomas, the World Health Organization (WHO) classification requires detection of mucin in at least five tumor cells in each of two high-power fields (HPF) for the diagnosis of solid adenocarcinoma with mucin (see **Fig. 2C, D**).[6] Similar to SCCs, lung adenocarcinomas are graded as well-, moderately-, or poorly differentiated. The use of immunohistochemical and mucin stains can help to distinguish lung adenocarcinoma from poorly differentiated SCC and metastases to lung (see **Table 1; Table 2**). Rare histologic variants of lung adenocarcinoma include fetal; mucinous (colloid); mucinous cystadenocarcinoma; signet ring-cell; and clear cell carcinoma.[6] A micropapillary pattern, characterized by papillary tufts without fibrovascular cores, is associated with aggressive behavior and poor prognosis, particularly for early stage disease (see **Fig. 2F**).[17–21] Although not currently part of the WHO classification (2004), micropapillary adenocarcinoma is proposed as a distinct subtype of lung adenocarcinoma in the new international multidisciplinary classification.[22]

A number of recent articles suggest that lung adenocarcinomas with mixed histology should be classified according to their predominant histologic pattern with mention of minor histologic patterns, because these subtypes may have distinct clinical behavior and molecular associations.[3,22,23] For example, bronchioloalveolar, papillary, and micropapillary subtypes have been found to be more likely than other subtypes to be associated with the epidermal growth factor receptor (EGFR) mutations. However, the solid subtype tends to lack EGFR mutation and is also associated with adverse prognosis.

BRONCHIOLOALVEOLAR CARCINOMA

Bronchioloalveolar carcinoma (BAC) is a subtype of lung adenocarcinoma and is defined by the WHO classification as an adenocarcinoma with bronchioloalveolar pattern and no evidence of stromal, vascular, or pleural invasion.[6] Thus, strictly defined, BACs are rare, but the BAC (lepidic) pattern is commonly seen at the periphery of mixed-pattern adenocarcinomas. A diagnosis of BAC cannot be established on small biopsies, because complete sampling of the tumor on resected specimens is needed to exclude invasion.

BACs disproportionally affect nonsmokers, women, and Asians. They can present as a peripheral solitary mass, multiple nodules, or a diffuse infiltrate (pneumonic pattern) simulating lobar pneumonia.[6,24] Multiple lobes and bilateral lungs can be involved. Microscopically, BACs are classified as nonmucinous and mucinous (**Fig. 3**).[6] Nonmucinous BAC is composed of a proliferation of cuboidal neoplastic cells growing along intact alveolar walls, whereas the mucinous-type is lined by tall columnar mucinous epithelium. The nonmucinous-type is more common, more frequently solitary, and frequently harbors EGFR mutations.[25] In contrast, the mucinous-type more commonly presents with pseudopneumonic infiltrates and is associated with KRAS rather than EGFR mutations. Mucinous BACs tend to have

Table 2 Typical CK7 and CK20 immunoprofiles of tumors of different sites		
	CK 7	CK20
NSCLC, breast carcinoma, gynecologic tract carcinoma	+	−
Colonic adenocarcinoma	−	+
Prostatic, renal cell, and hepatocellular carcinoma	−	−
Pancreatic adenocarcinoma, urothelial carcinoma, mucinous ovarian, and mucinous bronchoaveolar lung carcinoma	+	+

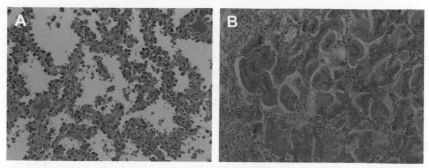

Fig. 3. (A) Nonmucinous BAC showing intact alveolar wall lined by a proliferation of cuboidal neoplastic cells. (B) Mucinous BAC (H&E, original magnification ×100).

a worse prognosis than the nonmucinous-type; however, the clinical pattern and stage are the most important prognostic factors for survival.[26,27] Pneumonic pattern is associated with worse survival than solitary or multifocal disease. The 5-year survival is greater than 80% for stages I and II and approximately 60% for higher-stage disease.[27] Despite the tendency for intrathoracic recurrence and spread, the behavior of BAC is more indolent than that of conventional adenocarcinoma.[24] It should be noted that previous studies on BACs may have included cases that are actually invasive adenocarcinomas with predominant bronchioloalvoelar pattern.

Studies have shown that patients with solitary adenocarcinoma with either pure lepidic growth (pure BAC) or predominantly lepidic growth with less than 5 mm invasion (minimally invasive adenocarcinoma) have 100% survival after complete resection.[16,28,29] Based on these findings, the new international multidisciplinary classification proposes the new concepts of adenocarcinoma in situ (for BAC) and minimally invasive adenocarcinoma (for predominant BAC pattern with <5 mm invasion).[22] These new concepts are, however, not part of the current WHO classification.

BAC is distinguished from atypical adenomatous hyperplasia (AAH) by size: AAH is less than 0.5 cm.[6] BAC and AAH are, otherwise, histologically similar and their distinction may not be possible on small biopsies. AAH is a frequent incidental finding in lung resections for adenocarcinomas and is recognized as a putative precursor of adenocarcinoma.[8,30–33]

LARGE CELL CARCINOMA

Large cell carcinoma is defined in the WHO classification as an undifferentiated non–small cell carcinoma lacking cytologic and architectural features of small cell carcinoma and showing no glandular or squamous differentiation.[6] Large cell carcinoma accounts for approximately 9% of all lung cancers.[11] These tumors tend to occur in the peripheral lung and tend to be large (>5 cm) and bulky.[6] Microscopically, large cell carcinomas are comprised of large cells with round to irregular nuclei with vesicular chromatin, prominent nucleoli, and variably distinct cytoplasmic borders. The tumor cells are arranged in aggregates or sheets with frequent tumor necrosis. This diagnosis should be reserved for resected specimens wherein one can exclude squamous or glandular differentiation. Variant types of large cell carcinoma include large cell neuroendocrine carcinoma (LCNEC), combined LCNEC, basaloid carcinoma, lymphoepithelioma-like carcinoma, clear cell carcinoma, and large cell carcinoma with rhabdoid phenotype.[6] LCNEC is recognized as a distinct entity and is discussed separately in the section on lung NET.

Basaloid variant of large cell carcinoma, rhabdoid phenotype, LCNEC, and combined LCNEC all have worse prognosis than classic large cell carcinoma.[6,34,35] Rhabdoid phenotype has been described not only in large cell carcinoma but also in sarcomatoid carcinoma and adenocarcinoma and is associated with aggressive behavior in all these tumors.[35] Lymphoepithelioma-like carcinomas, described mostly in Chinese patients, tend to present in early stage and have better prognosis than conventional NSCLC.[36,37] These tumors are associated with Epstein-Barr virus infection in Asians but not in whites.[38]

OTHER NSCLC TYPES

Adenosquamous carcinomas represent less than 5% of all lung cancers.[39–44] These tumors show components of both SCC and adenocarcinoma with each comprising at least 10% of the tumor.[6] Most are located in the lung periphery. The behavior is more aggressive than either adenocarcinoma or SCC.

Sarcomatoid carcinomas account for approximately 1% of lung cancers.[6] These tumors are defined by the WHO as a group of poorly differentiated non–small cell carcinomas that contain a component of sarcoma or sarcoma-like differentiation.[6] This category includes tumors that have been variously termed pleomorphic carcinoma, spindle cell carcinoma, giant cell carcinoma, carcinosarcoma, and pulmonary blastoma. These tumors are thought to represent epithelial neoplasms that have undergone divergent sarcomatous differentiation.[45,46] Although sarcomatoid features may be seen on a needle biopsy or cytology specimen, a diagnosis of sarcomatoid carcinoma may not be possible until after complete evaluation of the tumor on a resected specimen. The use of immunohistochemical stains, such as cytokeratins and EMA, can help identify the epithelial component of these tumors. Most cases of sarcomatoid carcinoma are in men with a history of heavy smoking. The upper lobes are preferentially involved.[6] The pattern of metastasis is similar to NSCLC, but the behavior is more aggressive than conventional NSCLC.[6]

Salivary gland type tumors of the lung represent less than 1% of all lung cancers.[6] Subtypes include mucoepidermoid carcinoma, adenoid cystic carcinoma, acinic cell carcinoma, and epithelial-myoepithelial carcinoma. These tumors tend to arise in the central airways. No predilection for gender or association with cigarette smoking or other risk factors has been found. The behaviors of these tumors are dependent on the grade and stage.

LUNG NETs

In the current WHO classification, lung NETs are placed into four categories: (1) typical carcinoid (TC), (2) atypical carcinoid (AC), (3) SCLC, and (4) LCNEC (**Table 3**).[6] A three-tiered grading system is also applicable: low grade (= TC); intermediate grade (= AC); and high grade (= LCNEC and SCLC). Microscopically, these tumors all exhibit varying degrees of neuroendocrine morphology in the form of organoid nests, palisading, trabecular growth, and rosette-like structures (**Fig. 4**). The main distinguishing features for the different NET types are mitotic activity and the presence or absence of necrosis.

Lung NETs represent 20% to 25% of all primary lung tumors.[47,48] SCLC is the most common (20%), followed by LCNEC (1%–3%), TC (2%), and AC (0.2%).[6,47–49] There has been an unexplained increase in the incidence of carcinoid tumors in the United States in recent decades.[47] Lung is by far the most common site of origin for small cell carcinomas, and it is the second most common site of origin for carcinoid tumors, after the tubular gastrointestinal tract.[47,48]

Table 3
Summary of diagnostic criteria for lung neuroendocrine tumors (2004 WHO)

	Typical Carcinoid	Atypical Carcinoid	Small Cell Carcinoma	Large Cell Neuroendocrine Carcinoma
Morphology	Well-differentiated NE morphology[a] 0.5 cm or larger	Well-differentiated NE morphology[a]	Cells with finely granular chromatin, absent nucleoli, and scant cytoplasm	NE morphology,[a] cytologic features of NSCLC, and positive immunohistochemical staining for NE markers[b]
Grade	Low	Intermediate	High	High
Mitotic count per 10 HPFs[c]	<2	2–10	>10	>10
Necrosis	Absent	Present (often punctate)	Extensive	Extensive

Abbreviations: HPFs, high-power fields; NE, neuroendocrine.
[a] NE morphology refers to organoid nesting, rosettes, palisading, or trabecular pattern.
[b] NE markers include synaptophysin, chromogranin, and CD56.
[c] 10 HPFs = 2 mm².

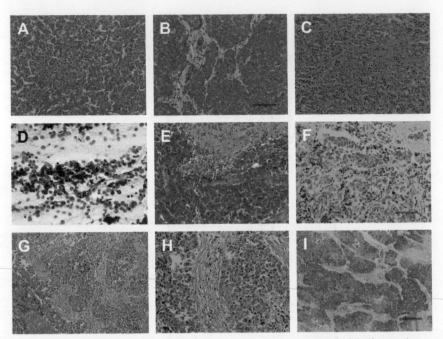

Fig. 4. (*A*) Typical carcinoid (TC) (H&E, original magnification ×100). (*B*) Chromo/synaptophysin immunostaining of TC (H&E, original magnification ×100). (*C*) Atypical carcinoid with focal central necrosis (H&E, original magnification ×100). (*D*) SCLC, cytologic smear showing nuclei with fine chromatin pattern without nucleolus and scant cytoplasm (Papnicolou, original magnification ×200). (*E*) SCLC, tissue section of tumor with necrosis (H&E, original magnification ×200). (*F*) Chromogranin immunostaining of SCLC with dot-like pattern (H&E, original magnification ×200). (*G*) Large cell neuroendocrine carcinoma (LCNEC), low-power neuroendocrine morphology with necrosis (H&E, original magnification ×100). (*H*) LCNEC, high power showing NSCLC nuclear features with prominent nucleoli, vesicular chromatin, and cytoplasmic borders (H&E, original magnification ×200). (*I*) Synatophysin immunostaining of LCNEC (H&E, original magnification ×100).

The clinical setting of lung carcinoid tumors (TC and AC) differs from those of high-grade NETs (SCLC and LCNEC). TC and AC tumors present at a younger age (mean, 45–50 years) and show no gender predilection.[6,48,50] In addition, TC tumors show no relationship to cigarette smoking.[51] In contrast, high-grade NETs occur in older patients (60–65 years); are strongly associated with smoking; and are more common in men.[6] Carcinoid syndrome is infrequent in lung carcinoids, whereas paraneoplastic syndrome is frequent in SCLC.[6,50] Lung carcinoids occur in 5% of patients with multiple neuroendocrine neoplasia 1, but no such association is seen with high-grade NETs.[47,52,53]

The TNM staging system is applicable for all lung NETs, because TNM stage has been shown to have prognostic value for these tumors. Lung NETs are included in the 7th edition of the AJCC cancer staging manual and are staged in the same fashion as NSCLCs.[54–56] For SCLC, the traditional clinical concept of limited (restricted to one radiation portal [ie, one hemithorax with hilar, mediastinal, and supraclavicular nodes and ipsilateral effusions]) versus extensive (contralateral or distant disease) disease is still considered by some to be clinically useful.[6]

TYPICAL CARCINOID

Most TCs are centrally located.[48] These tumors show well-differentiated neuroendo-crine morphology consisting of growth in organoid nests, trabeculae, and rosettes (see **Fig. 4**A). The tumor cells are uniform with coarsely granular "salt and pepper" nuclei and indistinct nucleoli. Mitotic activity is very low (up to 1 per 10 HPFs) and tumor necrosis is not seen.[6]

TC is a low-grade malignancy. At presentation, regional lymph node metastasis is present in 10% to 15% of patients.[48,50] Distant metastases occur rarely, with a tendency to involve bone and liver. The 5- and 10-year survival rates are 87% to 100% and 82% to 87%, respectively.[47,51,57-60] The survival is excellent even in patients with regional nodal metastasis.[61]

TC is distinguished from carcinoid tumorlet by size (tumorlets are <0.5 cm).[6] Carci-noid tumorlet is, in turn, distinguished from neuroendocrine hyperplasia by extension beyond the basement membrane of the respiratory epithelia.[48] Carcinoid tumorlet is a common incidental finding in lung as an isolated lesion.[48] Less commonly, diffuse NE cell hyperplasia and multiple tumorlets can be found in the following settings: in chronic lung injury with fibrosis or inflammation, adjacent to carcinoid tumors, and as diffuse idiopathic neuroendocrine cell hyperplasia with or without airway fibrosis.[48,61-64] Although uncommon, diffuse idiopathic neuroendocrine cell hyper-plasia is recognized as a precursor for carcinoid tumors.[8]

ATYPICAL CARCINOID

Both TC and AC tumors show well-differentiated neuroendocrine morphology, but AC has a higher mitotic activity (2–10 per 10 HPFs) or necrosis (see **Fig. 4**C).[6] The distinc-tion of AC and TC is generally deferred to the resected specimen.[6,48]

AC is significantly more aggressive than TC. At presentation, 30% to 50% of patients have nodal metastasis, and approximately 20% have distant metas-tasis.[6,48,51] The 5- and 10-year survival rates are approximately 60% and 40%, respectively.[6,47,65]

SMALL CELL LUNG CARCINOMA

SCLC is defined in the WHO classification as a high-grade neuroendocrine carcinoma with greater than 10 mitotic figures per 10 HPFs and extensive necrosis.[6] The defining cytologic features include finely granular nuclei without distinct nucleoli, scant cyto-plasm, and indistinct cell borders (see **Fig. 4**D, E). Nuclear molding and crush artifact are also common. SCLC may be difficult to distinguish from basaloid SCC, lymphoma, or "small blue cell" tumors by morphology. Immunohistochemistry (discussed later) is helpful in resolving the differential diagnoses.

SCLC is highly aggressive with a 5-year survival of less than 5%.[47] Most patients have metastatic disease at the time of diagnosis. Common sites of metastasis include contralateral lung, skin, distant nodes, brain, liver, adrenals, and bone.[6] SCLC is generally considered a nonsurgical disease, although it is highly sensitive to radiation and chemotherapy, in contrast to carcinoid tumors, which are typically resistant to standard cytotoxic chemotherapy and radiation. Patients with low-stage disease may, however, benefit from surgical resection.[65,66]

The current WHO recognizes two types of SCLC: pure and combined.[6] In a study of 100 surgical cases of SCLC, 28% were combined and 72% were pure.[67] Combined SCLC has a component of NSCLC, which most frequently is LCNEC, followed by adenocarcinoma and SCC. Because scattered large cells with nucleoli are allowed in pure SCLC, more than 10% large cell component is needed for designation as combined SCLC-LC.[6,67] By contrast, any amount of adenocarcinoma or SCC is considered combined SCLC. Because of sampling and tumor heterogeneity, a NSCLC component may be underrecognized on a biopsy or cytology specimen at the time of the initial diagnosis of SCLC. In an autopsy study, 13% of patients initially diagnosed with and treated for SCLC were subsequently found to have a NSCLC component at death.[68] Although some studies suggest less treatment response and shorter survival in patients with combined SCLC compared with pure SCLC, others find no survival difference in the two groups.[67–69]

LARGE CELL NEUROENDOCRINE CARCINOMA

LCNEC is defined in the current WHO classification as a high-grade carcinoma with neuroendocrine morphology but with cytologic features of NSCLC and positive immunohistochemical staining for at least one neuroendocrine marker (see **Fig. 4**G–I).[6] The high-grade features refer to greater than 10 mitoses per 10 HPFs and extensive necrosis. The neuroendocrine morphology refers to growth pattern as organoid nests, palisading, rosettes, or trabeculae. NSCLC cytologic features refer to prominent nucleoli, vesicular chromatin, abundant cytoplasm, and distinct cell borders. Immunohistochemically, LCNECs show staining for at least one neuroendocrine marker: synaptophysin, chromogranin, or CD56. Similar to SCLC, LCNEC may be pure or combined with NSCLC.

The diagnosis of LCNEC can be challenging because of its overlapping features with SCLC, AC, and NSCLC. This may be particularly difficult on a frozen section, cytology specimen, or small biopsy. The distinction of LCNEC from SCLC primarily rests on the nuclear features. LCNEC exhibits prominent nucleoli and distinct cell borders, whereas these features are absent in SCLC. In practice, this distinction can be difficult. In reproducibility studies of lung NETs, the most common disagreements occurred between the diagnosis of LCNEC and SCLC.[70,71] Compared with LCNEC, AC has less obviously high-grade features (lower mitotic count and less extensive necrosis); less distinct nucleoli; and less pleomorphism. LCNEC is distinguished from NSCLC by low-power neuroendocrine appearance and staining for at least one neuroendocrine marker. On cytology specimens, however, LCNEC is commonly interpreted as "NSCLC not otherwise specified."[48] Approximately 10% to 20% of NSCLC show some immunohistochemical staining for neuroendocrine markers but without neuroendocrine morphology. These tumors are referred to as "NSCLC with neuroendocrine differentiation," the clinical significance of which remains controversial.[6,48]

LCNEC is considered a highly aggressive disease, but the survival rates vary (15%–57%).[47,49] The wide range of survival rates may reflect the challenges in diagnostic reproducibility and lack of consensus on the clinical management of LCNEC. Currently, however, the National Comprehensive Cancer Network guidelines recommend treating LCNEC along the NSCLC treatment paradigm.

IMMUNOHISTOCHEMISTRY

Immunohistochemistry is useful in distinguishing SCC from adenocarcinoma when the histologic features are ambiguous, particularly on small biopsies or cytology specimens (see **Table 1**). A frequently used panel includes thyroid transcription factor-1 (TTF-1), p63, and CK5/6. 34BE12, another high molecular weight cytokeratin that is similar to CK5/6. Most lung adenocarcinomas are positive for TTF-1 but negative for p63 and CK5/6. The converse (TTF-1–/p63+/CK5/6+) is typical for SCC (see **Fig. 1**C). Outside of thyroid and with few exceptions, TTF-1 is specific for lung adenocarcinomas. It is positive in approximately 75% of all lung adenocarcinomas (see **Fig. 2**B).[72] An exception is mucinous tumors of the lung, especially mucinous BAC, which are typically TTF-1 negative.[73] Additional markers, such as CK7 and CK20, are also frequently used in the workup of lung tumors, mainly in differentiating primary lung adenocarcinoma from a metastasis from another site, especially when TTF-1 is negative (see **Table 2**). Although not specific for lung origin or histologic type, the CK7+/CK20– immunoprofile is typical of lung adenocarcinoma; other CK7/CK20 profiles would raise the possibility of a metastasis from another site (eg, CK7–/CK20+ suggests colonic origin and CK7–/CK20– raises the possibilities of renal cell, prostatic, or hepatocellular carcinoma). CK7+/CK20+ immunoprofile is uncommon in NSCLC, but it is common in mucinous BAC.[74]

For lung NETs, the most frequently used markers of neuroendocrine differentiation are chromogranin A, synaptophysin, and CD56.[75] Carcinoid tumors show strong and diffuse positivity for at least one of the neuroendocrine markers (see **Fig. 4**B). TTF-1 is positive in 30% to 50% of lung carcinoids.[76–79] Among well-differentiated NETs, TTF-1 expression is specific for lung.[78,79] In contrast, intestinal carcinoid tumors, particularly midgut derived, frequently express CDX2 but not TTF-1. In high-grade NETs, however, TTF-1 expression is not specific for lung.[76]

Most SCLCs show staining for neuroendocrine markers and cytokeratins, often with a dot-like staining pattern. A small percentage of SCLCs are negative for all three neuroendocrine markers.[6,48,80] In the absence of positive neuroendocrine markers, it is important to exclude lymphoma; basaloid SCC; and "small blue cell" tumors, such as Ewing sarcoma. For example, expression of leukocyte common antigen supports lymphoma, expression of CK5/6 supports basaloid SCC, and expression of CD99 supports Ewing sarcoma. Approximately 90% of SCLCs are TTF-1 positive, but TTF-1 is also positive in extrapulmonary small cell carcinomas.[76,77]

The diagnosis of LCNEC requires one positive neuroendocrine marker (synaptophysin, chromogranin A, or CD56) (see **Fig. 4**I). Neuron-specific enolase is not included as a marker of neuroendocrine differentiation in the WHO definition of LCNEC because of its lack of specificity.[6] LCNECs are also frequently positive for TTF-1, but TTF-1 also stains extrapulmonary LCNECs.[76]

The proliferation rate marker Ki67 is useful in distinguishing carcinoid tumors from high-grade NETs, particularly on small biopsies.[48] The Ki67 proliferation rate is generally less than 20% for carcinoids, but it is much higher for high-grade NETs. A diagnosis of SCLC should be questioned if the proliferation rate is less than 25%, because the proliferation rate for SLCL is typically 60% to 100%.[48,81]

THERAPY

Cancer treatment is heading in the direction of personalized medical therapy and targeted therapy based on an individual's tumor molecular profile. The oncology community is slowly moving away from standard cytotoxic chemotherapy and toward targeted therapy. The targeted therapeutic agents erlotinib (Tarceva) and gefitinib are oral, small-molecule tyrosine kinase inhibitors (TKI) of EGFR. Although EGFR expression in lung cancer alone has been an unreliable predictor of response to oral TKIs, EGFR mutations are associated with higher response rates to erlotinib and gefitinib.[82,83] In the general lung cancer population, the frequency of EGFR mutations is approximately 20% to 25%.[82] These mutations are most frequently found in female patients, nonsmokers, Asians, and patients with adenocarcinoma. The most common activating mutations of EGFR are deletions in exon 19 and the L858R point mutation in exon 21, both of which predict improved response to erlotinib or getifinib. However, certain EGFR mutations, in particular T790M in exon 20, are associated with resistance to oral TKIs.[84] Currently, the National Comprehensive Cancer Network guidelines recommend EGFR mutation testing in adenocarcinoma, large cell carcinoma, and NSCLC not otherwise specified, and the use of erlotinib in the treatment of tumors positive for EGFR mutations. The guideline also indicates that KRAS mutations in NSCLCs are associated with intrinsic TKI resistance, thus KRAS gene sequencing could be useful in the selection of patients against TKI therapy.

An exciting new potential target in the treatment of NSCLC is the echinoderm microtubule-associated protein-like 4 and anaplastic lymphoma kinase fusion oncogene. Although this mutation is estimated to be present in approximately 4% of NSCLC patients, the oral TKI crizotinib has recently been reported to have high response rates in ALK fusion-positive patients.[85] Most ALK fusion-positive cases are found in adenocarcinomas. Another mutation, excision repair cross-complementation group 1 protein, found to occur in SCC and adenocarcinoma, suggests resistance to platinum-based therapy.[86] These different molecular profiles illustrate that unlike chronic myelogenous leukemia where the BCR-ABL1 translocation is the major molecular abnormality seen in nearly all patients, the molecular pathways associated with NSCLC are very heterogeneous. This heterogeneity highlights the importance of histology and molecular profiling in the optimal, personalized therapy of an individual NSCLC patient.

SUMMARY

Tissue diagnosis, together with cancer stage, is of paramount importance in determining an oncology patient's treatment plan. In lung cancer classification, NSCLCs are further subclassified as SCC, adenocarcinoma, or large cell carcinoma, whereas lung NETs are subclassified as TC, AC, SCLC, and LCNEC. Treatment paradigms are no longer based only on the pathologic distinction between NSCLC and SCLC. Tumor histologic cell type and mutation profiles are increasingly important in personalizing lung cancer treatment. Effective communication between the treating physician and pathologist plays a valuable role for optimizing individualized patient management.

ACKNOWLEDGMENTS

The authors thank Drs David Brinker, James Eagan, and Theresa Nicol for manuscript review and Yvonne Campbell for secretarial assistance.

REFERENCES

1. Rossi A, Maione P, Bareschino MA, et al. The emerging role of histology in the choice of first-line treatment of advanced non-small cell lung cancer: implication in the clinical decision-making. Curr Med Chem 2010;17(11):1030–8.
2. Molina JR, Yang P, Cassivi SD, et al. Non-small cell lung cancer; epidemiology, risk factors, treatment, and survivorship. Mayo Clin Proc 2008;83(5):584–94.
3. Cagle PT, Allen TC, Dacic S, et al. Revolution in lung cancer: new challenges for the surgical pathologist. Arch Pathol Lab Med 2011;135:110–6.
4. Scagliotti GV, Parikh P, von Pawel J, et al. Phase III study comparing cisplatin plus gemcitabine with cisplatin plus pemetrexed in chemotherapy-naïve patients with advanced-stage non-small-cell lung cancer. J Clin Oncol 2008;26(21):3543–51.

5. Sandler A, Gray R, Perry MC. Paclitaxel-carboplatin alone or with bevacizumab for non-small-cell lung cancer. N Engl J Med 2006;355(24):2542–50.
6. Travis WD, Brambilla E, Muller-Hermelink HK, et al. Pathology and genetics of tumours of the lung, pleura, thymus and heart. In: World Health Organization classification of tumours, vol. 10. Lyon (France): IARC Press; 2004. p.12–77.
7. Funai K, Yokose T, Ishii G, et al. Clinicopathologic characteristics of peripheral squamous cell carcinoma of the lung. Am J Surg Pathol 2003;27:978–84.
8. Lantuejoul S, Salameire D, Salon C, et al. Pulmonary preneoplasia-sequential molecular carcinogenetic events. Histopathology 2009;54(1):43–54.
9. Watanabe Y, Yokose T, Sakuma Y, et al. Alveolar space filling ratio as a favorable prognostic factor in small peripheral squamous cell carcinoma of the lung. Lung Cancer 2011;73(2):217–21.
10. Chansky K, Sculier JP, Crowley JJ, et al. The International Association for the Study of Lung Cancer Staging Project: prognostic factors and pathologic TNM stage in surgically managed non-small cell lung cancer. J Thorac Oncol 2009; 4(7):792–801.
11. Parkin DM, Whelan SL, Ferlay J, et al. Cancer incidence in five continents. IARC Scientific Publications No. 155, vol. 8. Lyon (France): IARCPress; 2002.
12. Colby TV, Koss M, Travis WD. Tumors of the lower respiratory tract. 3rd edition. Washington: Armed Forces Institute of Pathology; 1995.
13. Wahbah M, Boroumand N, Castro C, et al. Changing trends in the distribution of the histologic types of lung cancer: a review of 4,439 cases. Ann Diagn Pathol 2007;11(2):89–96.
14. Travis WD, Travis LB, Devesa SS. Lung cancer. Cancer 1995;75(Suppl 1): 191–202.
15. Charloux A, Quoix E, Wolkove N, et al. The increasing incidence of lung adenocarcinoma: reality or artifact? A review of the epidemiology of lung adenocarcinoma. Int J Epidemiol 1997;26(1):14–23.
16. Teraski H, Niki T, Matsuno Y, et al. Lung adenocarcinoma with mixed bronchiolo-alveolar and invasive components: clinicopathological features, subclassification by extent of invasive foci, and immunohistochemical characterization. Am J Surg Pathol 2003;27:937–51.
17. Maeda R, Isowa N, Onuma H, et al. Lung adenocarcinomas with micropapillary components. Gen Thorac Cardiovasc Surg 2009;57(10):534–9.
18. Kamiya K, Hayashi Y, Douguchi J, et al. Histopathological features and prognostic significance of the micropapillary pattern in lung adenocarcinoma. Mod Pathol 2008;21(8):992–1001.
19. Sanchez-Mora N, Presmanes MC, Monroy V, et al. Micropapillary lung adenocarcinoma: a distinctive histologic subtype with prognostic significance. Case series. Hum Pathol 2008;39(3):324–30.
20. Tsutsumida H, Nomoto M, Goto M, et al. A micropapillary pattern is predictive of a poor prognosis in lung adenocarcinoma, and reduced surfactant apoprotein A expression in the micropapillary pattern is an excellent indicator of a poor prognosis. Mod Pathol 2007;20(6):638–47.
21. Miyoshi T, Satoh Y, Okumura S, et al. Early-stage lung adenocarcinomas with a micropapillary pattern, a distinct pathologic marker for a significantly poor prognosis. Am J Surg Pathol 2003;27(1):101–9.
22. Travis WD, Brambilla E, Noguchi M, et al. International association for the study of lung cancer/American Thoracic Society/European Respiratory Society international multidisciplinary classification of lung adenocarcinoma. J Thorac Oncol 2011;6(2):244–85.

23. Motoi N, Szoke J, Riely G, et al. Lung adenocarcinoma: modification of the 2004 WHO mixed subtype to include the major histologic subtype suggests correlations between papillary and micropapillary adenocarcinoma subtypes, EGFR mutations and gene expression analysis. Am J Surg Pathol 2008;32(6):810–24.

24. Raz DJ, He B, Rosell R, et al. Bronchioloalveolar carcinoma: a review. Clin Lung Cancer 2006;7(5):313–22.

25. Garfield DH, Cadranel J, West HL. Bronchioloalveolar carcinoma: the case for two diseases. Clin Lung Cancer 2008;9(1):24–9.

26. Manning JT, Spjut HJ, Tschen JA. Bronchioloalveolar carcinoma: the significance of two histopathologic types. Cancer 1984;54:525–34.

27. Ebright MI, Zakowski MF, Martin J, et al. Clinical pattern and pathologic stage but not histologic features predict outcome for bronchioloalveolar carcinoma. Ann Thorac Surg 2002;74:1640–7.

28. Travis WD, Garg K, Franklin WA, et al. Bronchioloalveolar carcinoma and lung adenocarcinoma: the clinical importance and research relevance of the 2004 World Health Organization pathologic criteria. J Thorac Oncol 2006;1(Suppl 9): S13–9.

29. Sakuri H, Dobashi Y, Mizutani E, et al. Bronchioloalveolar carcinoma of the lung 3 centimeters or less in diameter: a prognostic assessment. Ann Thorac Surg 2004; 78(5):1728–33.

30. Morandi L, Asioli S, Cavazza A, et al. Genetic relationship among atypical adenomatous hyperplasia, bronchioloalveolar carcinoma, and adenocarcinoma of the lung. Lung Cancer 2007;56:35–42.

31. Koga T, Hashimoto S, Sugio K, et al. Lung adenocarcinoma with bronchioloalveolar component is frequently associated with foci of high-grade atypical adenomatous hyperplasia. Am J Clin Pathol 2002;117:464–70.

32. Chapman AD, Kerr KM. The association between atypical adenomatous hyperplasia and primary lung cancer. Br J Cancer 2000;83:632–6.

33. Mori M, Rao SK, Popper HH, et al. Atypical adenomatous hyperplasia of the lung: a probable forerunner in the development of adenocarcinoma of the lung. Mod Pathol 2001;14(2):72–84.

34. Moro D, Brichon PY, Brambilla E, et al. Basaloid bronchial carcinoma. A histologic group with a poor prognosis. Cancer 1994;73:2734–9.

35. Tamboli P, Toprani TH, Amin MB, et al. Carcinoma of lung with rhabdoid features. Hum Pathol 2004;35(1):8–13.

36. Han AJ, Xiong M, Gu YY, et al. Lymphoepithelioma-like carcinoma of the lung with a better prognosis: a clinicopathologic study of 32 cases. Am J Clin Pathol 2001; 115:841–50.

37. Chan JK, Hui PK, Tsang WY, et al. Primary lymphoepithelioma-like carcinoma of the lung. A clinicopathologic study of 11 cases. Cancer 1995;76:413–22.

38. Castro CY, Ostrowski ML, Barrios R, et al. Relationship between Epstein-Barr virus and lymphoepithelioma-like carcinoma of the lung: a clinicopathologic study of 6 cases and review of the literature. Hum Pathol 2001;32(8):863–72.

39. Nakagawa K, Yasumitsu T, Fukuhara K, et al. Poor prognosis after lung resection for patients with adenosquamous carcinoma of the lung. Ann Thorac Surg 2003; 75:1740–4.

40. Hsia JY, Chen CY, Hsu CP, et al. Adenosquamous carcinoma of the lung. Surgical results compared with squamous cell and adenocarcinoma. Scand Cardiovasc J 1999;33:29–32.

41. Ben Y, Yu H, Wang Z, et al. Adenosquamous lung carcinoma: clinical characteristics, surgical treatment and prognosis. Chin Med Sci J 2000;15(4):238–40.

42. Naunheim KS, Taylor JR, Skosey C, et al. Adenosquamous lung carcinoma: clinical characteristics, treatment, and prognosis. Ann Thorac Surg 1987;44:462–6.
43. Fitzgibbons PL, Kern WH. Adenosquamous carcinoma of the lung: a clinical and pathologic study of seven cases. Hum Pathol 1985;16:463–6.
44. Hofmann HS, Knolle J, Neef H. The adenosquamous lung carcinoma: clinical and pathological characteristics. J Cardiovasc Surg 1994;35:543–7.
45. Nakajima M, Kasai T, Hashimoto H, et al. Sarcomatoid carcinoma of the lung: a clinicopathologic study of 37 cases. Cancer 1999;86(4):608–16.
46. Ro JY, Chen JL, Lee JS, et al. Sarcomatoid carcinoma of the lung. Immunohistochemical and ultrastructural studies of 14 cases. Cancer 1992;69(2):376–86.
47. Gustafsson BI, Kidd M, Chan A, et al. Bronchopulmonary neuroendocrine tumors. Cancer 2008;113(1):5–21.
48. Rekhtman N. Neuroendocrine tumors of the lung: an update. Arch Pathol Lab Med 2010;134:1628–38.
49. Takei H, Asamura H, Maeshima A, et al. Large cell neuroendocrine carcinoma of the lung: a clinicopathologic study of eighty-seven cases. J Thorac Cardiovasc Surg 2002;124:285–92.
50. McCaughan BC, Martini N, Bains MS. Bronchial carcinoids: review of 124 cases. J Thorac Cardiovasc Surg 1985;89(1):8–17.
51. Fink G, Krelbaum T, Yellin A, et al. Pulmonary carcinoid: presentation, diagnosis, and outcome in 142 cases in Israel and review of 640 cases from the literature. Chest 2001;119(6):1647–51.
52. Sachithanandan N, Harle RA, Burgess JR. Bronchopulmonary carcinoid in multiple endocrine neoplasia type 1. Cancer 2005;103(3):509–15.
53. Debelenko LV, Swalwell JI, Kelley MJ, et al. MEN1 gene mutation analysis of high-grade neuroendocrine lung carcinoma. Genes Chromosomes Cancer 2000;28: 58–65.
54. Vallieres E, Shepherd FA, Crowley J, et al. The IASLC Lung Cancer Staging Project: proposals regarding the relevance of TNM in the pathologic staging of small cell lung cancer in the forthcoming (seventh) edition of the TNM classification for lung cancer. J Thorac Oncol 2009;4(9):1049–59.
55. Shepherd FA, Crowley J, Van Houtte P, et al. The International Association for the Study of Lung Cancer lung cancer staging project: proposals regarding the clinical staging of small cell lung cancer in the forthcoming (seventh) edition of the tumor, node, metastasis classification for lung cancer. J Thorac Oncol 2007; 2(12):1067–77.
56. Travis WD, Giroux DJ, Chansky K, et al. The IASLC lung cancer staging project: proposals for the inclusion of broncho-pulmonary carcinoid tumors in the forthcoming (seventh) edition of the TNM classification for lung cancer. J Thorac Oncol 2008;3(11):1213–23.
57. Travis WD, Rush W, Flieder DB, et al. Survival analysis of 200 pulmonary neuroendocrine tumors with clarification of criteria of atypical carcinoid and its separation from typical carcinoid. Am J Surg Pathol 1988;22(8):934–44.
58. Mezzetti M, Raveglia F, Panigalli T, et al. Assessment of outcomes in typical and atypical carcinoids according to latest WHO classification. Ann Thorac Surg 2003;76(6):1838–42.
59. Morandi U, Casali C, Rossi G. Bronchial typical carcinoid tumors. Semin Thorac Cardiovasc Surg 2006;18(3):191–8.
60. Thomas CF Jr, Tazelaar HD, Jett JR. Typical and atypical pulmonary carcinoids: outcome in patients presenting with regional lymph node involvement. Chest 2001;119(4):1143–50.

61. Miller RR, Muller NL. Neuroendocrine cell hyperplasia and obliterative bronchiolitis in patients with peripheral carcinoid tumors. Am J Surg Pathol 1995;19(6): 653–8.
62. Travis WD, Colby TV, Corrin B, et al. WHO Histological Classification of tumours. Histological typing of lung and pleural tumours. 3rd edition. Berlin (Germany): Springer-Verlag; 1999.
63. Rizvi SM, Goodwill J, Lim E, et al. The frequency of neuroendocrine cell hyperplasia in patients with pulmonary neuroendocrine tumours and non-neuroendocrine cell carcinomas. Histopathology 2009;55(3):332–7.
64. Beasley MB, Thunnissen FB, Brambilla E, et al. Pulmonary atypical carcinoid: predictors of survival in 106 cases. Hum Pathol 2000;31(10):1255–65.
65. Wick MR, Leslie KO, Ritter JH, et al. Neuroendocrine neoplasms of the lung. In: Practical pulmonary pathology: a diagnostic approach. Churchill Livingstone (Philadelphia): Elsevier; 2005. p. 424–48.
66. Lim E, Belcher E, Yap YK, et al. The role of surgery in the treatment of limited disease small cell lung cancer: time to reevaluate. J Thorac Oncol 2008;3(11): 1267–71.
67. Nicholson SA, Beasley MB, Brambilla E, et al. Small cell lung carcinoma (SCLS): a clinicopathologic study of 100 cases with surgical specimens. Am J Surg Pathol 2002;26:1184–97.
68. Sehested M, Hirsch FR, Osterlind K, et al. Morphologic variations of small cell lung cancer. A histopathologic study of pretreatment and posttreatment specimens in 104 patients. Cancer 1986;57(4):804–7.
69. Radice PA, Matthews MJ, Ihde DC, et al. The clinical behavior of "mixed" small cell/large cell bronchogenic carcinoma compared to "pure" small cell subtypes. Cancer 1982;50(12):2894–902.
70. den Bakker MA, Willemsen S, Grünberg K, et al. Small cell carcinoma of the lung and large cell neuroendocrine carcinoma interobserver variability. Histopathology 2010;56(3):356–63.
71. Travis WD, Gal AA, Colby TV, et al. Reproducibility of neuroendocrine lung tumor classification. Hum Pathol 1998;29(3):272–9.
72. Zamecnik J, Kodet R. Value of thyroid transcription factor-1 and surfactant apoprotein A in the differential diagnosis of pulmonary carcinomas: a study of 109 cases. Virchows Arch 2002;400:353–61.
73. Lau SK, Desrochers MJ, Luthringer DJ. Expression on thyroid transcription factor-1, cytokeratin 7, and cytokeratin 20 in bronchioloalveolar carcinomas: an immunohistochemical evaluation of 67 cases. Mod Pathol 2002;15:538–42.
74. Shah RN, Badve S, Papreddy K, et al. Expression of cytokeratin 20 in mucinous bronchioalveolar carcinoma. Hum Pathol 2002;33(9):915–20.
75. Kaufmann O, Georgi T, Dietel M. Utility of 123C3 monoclonal antibody against CD56 (NCAM) for the diagnosis of small cell carcinomas on paraffin sections. Hum Pathol 1997;28(12):1373–8.
76. Kaufmann O, Dietel M. Expression of thyroid transcription factor-1 in pulmonary and extrapulmonary small cell carcinomas and other neuroendocrine carcinomas of various primary sites. Histopathology 2000;36:415–20.
77. Folpe AL, Gown AM, Lamps LW, et al. Thyroid transcription factor-1: immunohistochemical evaluation in pulmonary neuroendocrine tumors. Mod Pathol 1999;12: 5–8.
78. Lin X, Saad RS, Luckasevic TM, et al. Diagnostic value of CDX-2 and TTF-1 expressions in separating metastatic neuroendocrine neoplasms of unknown origin. Appl Immunohistochem Mol Morphol 2007;15(4):407–14.

79. Srivastava A, Hornick JL. Immunohistochemical staining for CDX-2, PDX-1, NESP-55, and TTF-1 can help distinguish gastrointestinal carcinoid tumors from pancreatic endocrine and pulmonary carcinoid tumors. Am J Surg Pathol 2009; 33(4):626–32.
80. Guinee DB Jr, Fishback NF, Koss MN, et al. The spectrum of immunohistochemical staining of small-cell lung carcinoma in specimens from transbronchial and open-lung biopsies. Am J Clin Pathol 1994;102(4):406–14.
81. Aslan DL, Gulbahce HE, Pambuccian SE, et al. Ki-67 immunoreactivity in the differential diagnosis of pulmonary neuroendocrine neoplasms in specimens with extensive crush artifact. Am J Clin Pathol 2005;123(6):874–8.
82. Tsao MS, Sakurada A, Cutz JC, et al. Erlotinib in lung cancer: molecular and clinical predictors of outcome. N Engl J Med 2005;353(2):133–44.
83. Maemondo M, Inove A, Kobayashi K, et al. Gefitinib or chemotherapy for non-small-cell lung cancer with mutated EGFR. N Engl J Med 2010;362(25):2380–8.
84. Cataldo VD, Gibbons DL, Perez-Soler R, et al. Treatment of non-small-cell lung cancer with erlotinib or gefitinib. N Engl J Med 2011;364(10):947–55.
85. Kwak EL, Banq YJ, Camidge DR, et al. Anaplastic Lymphoma Kinase Inhibition in non-small-cell lung cancer. N Engl J Med 2010;363(18):1603–703.
86. Olaussen KA, Dunant A, Fouret P, et al. DNA Repair by ERCC1 in Non-small-cell lung cancer and cisplatin-based adjuvant therapy. N Engl J Med 2006;355(10): 983–91.

Updated Staging System for Lung Cancer

Peter Goldstraw, MB, FRCS[a,b,c],*

KEYWORDS

- Staging • Lung cancer • TNM classification
- Prognostic factors

Among the many prognostic factors identified in Lung Cancer,[1] the anatomic extent of disease, as described by the tumor-node-metastasis (TNM) classification, has the longest history and remains the most important. Devised by Pierre Denoix,[2] a surgical oncologist at the Institut Gustave-Roussy in Paris and reported in a series of articles between 1943 and 1952, the first international attempt to unify the classification of malignant tumors using this nomenclature was published by the International Union Against Cancer (UICC) in 1968.[3] Thereafter, the initiative passed to the American Joint Committee on Cancer Staging and End Results Reporting (AJC), now the American Joint Committee on Cancer (AJCC), whose Task Force on Lung Cancer, headed by Mountain and colleagues,[4] produced the first data-driven recommendations for change in 1974. Their proposals were derived from a database of 2155 cases of lung cancer, of which 1712 were cases of non–small cell lung cancer (NSCLC), diagnosed at least 4 years before analysis. Practically all of the T descriptors in use today were introduced in that report, including the use of a 3-cm cutoff point for size; the impact on T category of invasion of the chest wall, diaphragm, and mediastinum; the bronchoscopic criteria of T category; and those based on the extent of atelectasis or obstructive pneumonitis. These proposals were incorporated in to the second edition of the UICC *TNM Classification of Malignant Tumors* published in 1975[5] and the first publication by the AJC in 1977.[6] Dr Clifton Mountain developed his own database at the MD Anderson Cancer Center in Houston and the reiterative analysis of this developing source informed all future editions of the TNM classification for lung cancer up to and including the sixth edition published in 2002.[7,8] However, in the intervening

Financial disclosure: The author has nothing to disclose.

[a] Academic Department of Thoracic Surgery, Royal Brompton Hospital, Sydney Street, London SW3 6NP, UK

[b] National Heart and Lung Institute, Imperial College, London, UK

[c] International Association for the Study of Lung Cancer, Aurora, CO, USA

* Academic Department of Thoracic Surgery, Royal Brompton Hospital, Sydney Street, London SW3 6NP, UK.

E-mail address: p.goldstraw@rbht.nhs.uk

years, the process of revision was increasingly considered to be unsatisfactory. The international staging system had been based on data from a single institution, leading to doubts as to whether it was appropriate for global implementation. No external validation had ever been applied, and, even at the last analysis in 1997,[9] the database consisted of slightly more than 5000 cases, too few to validate the large number of descriptors within the TNM classification. The cases were predominately surgical candidates, and TNM staging was increasingly thought to be irrelevant by those treating the bulkier tumors treated by nonsurgical modalities.

In response to these concerns, in 1998 the International Association for the Study of Lung Cancer (IASLC) was convinced that it should develop a role in future revisions and established its Lung Cancer Staging Project.[10] It developed an international database in collaboration with Cancer Research and Biostatistics (CRAB), a not-for-profit organization based in Seattle (OR). Forty-six data sources in more than 20 countries around the globe donated more than 100,000 cases. After an initial sift, 81,495 cases have adequate data to be included in an analysis: 68,463 cases of NSCLC and 13,032 cases of small cell lung cancer (SCLC). The recommendations for the seventh edition of *TNM* were based on analysis of the NSCLC cases. Of those receiving active therapy, approximately half had undergone surgery as part of their treatment, around one-third had received chemotherapy, one-quarter radiotherapy, and there were many cases treated by bimodality and multimodality treatment. The analysis of this huge number of cases was conducted by CRAB and supervised by several subcommittees tasked with formulating recommendations on the T,[11] N,[12] and M[13] descriptors and the role of TNM in SCLC.[14,15] All such recommendations were overseen by a validation and methodology subcommittee who established strict criteria for internal and external validation.[16] Once the T, N, and M descriptors had been defined, the resultant TNM stage groups were established using recursive partitioning and amalgamation statistical methods.[17] The recommendations of the IASLC were submitted to the UICC and AJCC and, after internal review, were accepted without change for the seventh edition of *TNM for lung cancer* enacted in January 2011.[18,19]

The changes to the T and M descriptors in the 7th edition are shown in **Box 1**.

Fig. 1 shows the T and M descriptors as they were in the sixth edition and as they are now classified in the seventh edition, with the resultant changes to the stage groupings.

The full list of T, N, and M descriptors in the seventh edition is given in **Box 2**.

The resultant stage groupings in the seventh edition of *TNM* are presented in **Table 1**.

ADDITIONAL RECOMMENDATIONS

The TNM classification has traditionally applied to all carcinomas of the lung, including SCLC. However, the TNM classification has only been applied to those unusually localized cases of SCLC suitable for surgical treatment, oncologists preferring the simpler, binary division into limited disease and extensive disease. The IASLC Staging Committee, having formulated its recommendations for the seventh edition of TNM from an analysis of the 68,463 cases of NSCLC, studied the usefulness of the TNM classification in the 13,032 cases of SCLC in the database, the largest database of this cell type in the literature. TNM stage details, using the sixth edition of TNM, were available on 8088 patients; 3430 cM0 cases had full clinical TNM data and 4530 were classified as cM1. The analysis of these cases confirmed the value of TNM in the clinical staging of SCLC,[14] a finding that remained relevant for the smaller number of cases suitable for reclassification according to the seventh edition. The SCLC cases in the database contained 349 cases that had undergone complete

---

Box 1
Changes recommended to the T and M descriptors in the 6th edition of TNM for Lung Cancer by analysis of the IASLC Data base

The changes to T and M descriptors in the seventh edition of TNM were:

1. A new cutpoint of 2 cm was created dividing T1 tumors into T1a $\leq$2 cm and T1b tumors >2 cm but $\leq$3 cm.

2. A new cutpoint of 5 cm was created dividing T2 tumors into T2a >3 cm but $\leq$5 cm and T2b tumors >5 cm but $\leq$7 cm.

3. A new cutpoint of 7 cm was created and tumors >7 cm are now classified as T3, size for the first time becoming a T3 descriptor.

4. Tumors associated with additional tumor nodules in the same lobe as the primary are reclassified as T3.

5. Tumors associated with additional tumor nodules in other ipsilateral lobe(s) are reclassified as T4.

6. Tumors associated with additional tumor nodules in the contralateral lung remain M1 but are reclassified as M1a.

7. Tumors associated with malignant pleural/pericardial effusion or pleural/pericardial nodules are reclassified as M1a.

8. Tumors associated with distant metastases are reclassified as M1b.

Reproduced from Sobin L, Gospodarowicz M, Wittekind C, editors. TNM classification of malignant tumors. 7th edition. Oxford (UK): Blackwell Publishing Ltd; 2010; with permission of UICC.

---

surgical resection and thus had pathologic TNM staging information, including 218 cases in which there was also cTNM data. Analysis of these cases confirmed the usefulness of TNM in the pathologic classification of SCLC.[15] Therefore, the use of TNM for SCLC cases is strongly encouraged in the seventh edition of *TNM*, especially for stratification in trials of chemotherapy/radiotherapy in limited disease and for those cases treated by surgery.

T and M Descriptors		N0	N1	N2	N3
6th Edition	7th Ed	Stage	Stage	Stage	Stage
T1 (<= 2 cm)	T1a	IA	IIA	IIIA	IIIB
T1 (> 2 – 3 cm)	T1b	IA	IIA	IIIA	IIIB
T2(> 3 – 5 cm)	T2a	IB	IIA IIB	IIIA	IIIB
T2 (> 5 – 7 cm)	T2b	IIA IB	IIB	IIIA	IIIB
T2 (> 7 cm)		IIB IB	IIIA IIB	IIIA	IIIB
T3 invasion	T3	IIB	IIIA	IIIA	IIIB
T4 (same lobe nodules)		IIB IIIB	IIIA IIIB	IIIA IIIB	IIIB
T4 (extension)	T4	IIIA IIIB	IIIA IIIB	IIIB	IIIB
M1 (ipsilateral lung)		IIIA IV	IIIA IV	IIIB IV	IIIB IV
T4 (pleural effusion)		IV IIIB	IV IIIB	IV IIIB	IV IIIB
M1 (contralateral lung)	M1a	IV	IV	IV	IV
M1 (distant)	M1b	IV	IV	IV	IV

Fig. 1. The changes to the T and M descriptors and resultant stage groupings in the seventh edition of *TNM for Lung Cancer*. The left column shows the T and M descriptors as they were in the sixth edition of *TNM*, the next column shows their designation in the seventh edition. The other 4 columns show the stage grouping in the seventh edition for these descriptors when associated with N0, N1, N2, and N3 disease. Where a stage grouping has changed from the sixth to the seventh edition, that box is highlighted in blue and the stage according to the sixth edition is in red, and that in the seventh edition is in larger font and black.

Box 2
The T, N, and M descriptors and stage groupings from the seventh edition of TNM for Lung Cancer

T – Primary Tumour

TX Primary tumour cannot be assessed, *or* tumour proven by the presence of malignant cells in sputum or bronchial washings but not visualized by imaging or bronchoscopy

T0 No evidence of primary tumour

Tis Carcinoma in situ

T1 Tumour 3 cm or less in greatest dimension, surrounded by lung or visceral pleura, without bronchoscopic evidence of invasion more proximal than the lobar bronchus (i.e., not in the main bronchus)

  T1a Tumour 2 cm or less in greatest dimension[a]
  T1b Tumour more than 2 cm but not more than 3 cm in greatest dimension

T2 Tumour more than 3 cm but not more than 7 cm; or tumour with *any* of the following features[b]:

- Involves main bronchus, 2 cm or more distal to the carina
- Invades visceral pleura
- Associated with atelectasis or obstructive pneumonitis that extends to the hilar region but does not involve the entire lung

  T2a Tumour more than 3 cm but not more than 5 cm in greatest dimension
  T2b Tumour more than 5 cm but not more than 7 cm in greatest dimension

T3 Tumour more than 7 cm or one that directly invades any of the following: chest wall (including superior sulcus tumours), diaphragm, phrenic nerve, mediastinal pleura, parietal pericardium; *or* tumour in the main bronchus less than 2 cm distal to the carina[a] but without involvement of the carina; *or* associated atelectasis or obstructive pneumonitis of the entire lung or separate tumour nodule(s) in the same lobe as the primary.

T4 Tumour of any size that invades any of the following: mediastinum, heart, great vessels, trachea, recurrent laryngeal nerve, oesophagus, vertebral body, carina; separate tumour nodule(s) in a different ipsilateral lobe to that of the primary.

N–Regional Lymph Nodes

NX Regional lymph nodes cannot be assessed

N0 No regional lymph node metastasis

N1 Metastasis in ipsilateral peribronchial and/or ipsilateral hilar lymph nodes and intrapulmonary nodes, including involvement by direct extension

N2 Metastasis in ipsilateral mediastinal and/or subcarinal lymph node(s)

N3 Metastasis in contralateral mediastinal, contralateral hilar, ipsilateral or contralateral scalene, or supraclavicular lymph node(s)

M–Distant Metastasis

M0 No distant metastasis

M1 Distant metastasis

  M1a Separate tumour nodule(s) in a contralateral lobe; tumour with pleural nodules or malignant pleural or pericardial effusion[c]
  M1b Distant metastasis

[a] The uncommon superficial spreading tumour of any size with its invasive component limited to the bronchial wall, which may extend proximal to the main bronchus, is also classified as T1a.
[b] T2 tumours with these features are classified T2a if 5 cm or less or if size cannot be determined, and T2b if greater than 5 cm but not larger than 7 cms.
[c] Most pleural (pericardial) effusions with lung cancer are due to tumour. In a few patients, however, multiple microscopical examinations of pleural (pericardial) fluid are negative for tumour, and the fluid is non-bloody and is not an exudate. Where these elements and clinical judgment dictate that the effusion is not related to the tumour, the effusion should be excluded as a staging element and the patient should be classified as M0.

Table 1
Stage groupings in the seventh edition of *TNM*

Occult Carcinoma	TX	N0	M0
Stage 0	Tis	N0	M0
Stage IA	T1a, b	N0	M0
Stage IB	T2a	N0	M0
Stage IIA	T2b	N0	M0
	T1a, b	N1	M0
	T2a	N1	M0
Stage IIB	T2b	N1	M0
	T3	N0	M0
Stage IIIA	T1a, b, T2a, b	N2	M0
	T3	N1, N2	M0
	T4	N0, N1	M0
Stage IIIB	T4	N2	M0
	Any T	N3	M0
Stage IV	Any T	Any N	M1

Carcinoid tumors were not previously included in the TNM classification. The IASLC database contained 513 cases of carcinoid tumors and was combined with 1619 cases from the Surveillance Epidemiology and End Results (SEER) database for a similar period, of which 1437 had been treated surgically. Analysis of these cases has shown that TNM has prognostic power in this tumor type.[20] As a result, carcinoid tumors of the lung and tracheobronchial tree are now, for the first time, included in the seventh edition of *TNM*.

The subcommittee analyzing the N descriptors was hampered by a lack of uniformity in the nomenclature of the regional lymph nodes. The IASLC Staging Project sought international agreement on a new nodal chart that, for the first time, has reconciled the Japanese Naruke and US Mountain/Dressler nodal charts and allowed the development of agreed definitions for the anatomic boundaries of each nodal station.[21] The UICC and AJCC have now recognized this chart and the associated definitions as the "recommended means of describing regional lymph node involvement for lung cancer" (**Fig. 2**). This development has allowed for the reintroduction of a minimum number of lymph nodes to be removed and examined histologically before assigning a pN category. The seventh edition recommends that "6 nodes/nodal stations should be removed/sampled for histologic examination. These should include 3 nodes/stations from the mediastinum, one of which should be sub-carinal node #7, and 3 nodes/stations from the hilum or other N1 locations."

Visceral pleural invasion has been a T2 descriptor since the early 1980s. However, there was no agreed definition of this feature. The pathologists within our committee reviewed the available literature and developed a precise definition of visceral pleural invasion as "invasion beyond the elastic layer, including invasion to the visceral pleural surface."[22] The use of elastic stains is recommended when this feature is not clear on routine histology (**Fig. 3**).

PROPOSALS FOR TESTING

The TNM classification allows for proposals for new classification to be trialed for a period to assess whether they should be incorporated into future editions. The

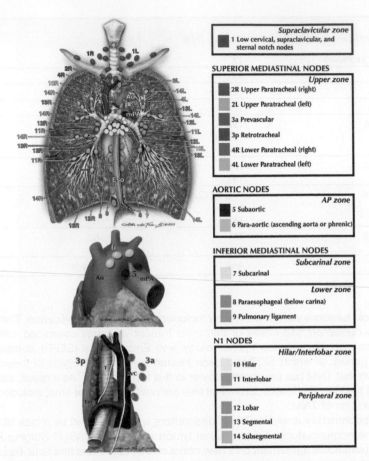

Fig. 2. The IASLC International Nodal Chart showing each nodal station. The box shows how these could be grouped using the new concept of nodal zones. This chart is now the recommended means of describing regional lymph node involvement for lung cancers. (*Courtesy of* the International Association for the Study of Lung Cancer. Copyright © 2008 Aletta Ann Frazier, MD; with permission.)

IASLC Staging Project developed several such proposals. It is hoped that clinicians, radiologists, and pathologists will collect data on these features to allow future analysis, such as:

1. Imaging evidence of lymphangitis carcinomatosis is usually a contraindication to surgical treatment. The L category, which is used to assess lymphatic invasion, is therefore not applicable. The radiological extent of lymphangitis is believed to be of prognostic importance. An exploratory analysis of this feature is proposed using a cLy category in which cLy0 indicates that radiological evidence of lymphangitis is absent, cLy1 indicates lymphangitis is present and confined to the area around the primary tumor, cLy2 indicates lymphangitis at a distance from the primary tumor but confined to the lobe of the primary, cLy3 indicates lymphangitis in other ipsilateral lobes, and cLy4 indicates lymphangitis affecting the contralateral lung.

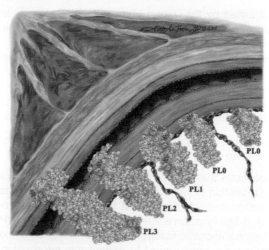

Fig. 3. The definition of visceral pleural invasion in the seventh edition of *TNM*. The pleural lavage (PL) subcategories have been proposed for testing. PL1 and PL2 are classified as visceral pleural invasion defined as invasion beyond the elastic layer including invasion to the visceral pleural surface. (*Courtesy of* the International Association for the Study of Lung Cancer. Copyright © 2008 Aletta Ann Frazier, MD; with permission.)

2. Concerns have been expressed that the definition of complete resection conferring R0 status is too imprecise. The category Uncertain Resection has been proposed[23] for testing. There is extant a category R1(is) that is applicable when the requirements for R0 have been met, but in situ carcinoma is found at the bronchial resection margin. Similarly, category R1(cy+) is appropriate when the requirements for R0 have been met, but pleural lavage cytology (PLC) is positive for malignant cells visceral invasion. The wider use of these descriptors is encouraged to facilitate data collection and to assess the prognostic impact of these features following resection. A new category, R0(un), is proposed to document those other features that are within the proposed category of Uncertain Resection, that is, no macroscopic or microscopic evidence of residual disease but any of the following reservations applies:
   a. Nodal assessment has been based on less than the number of nodes/stations recommended for complete resection.
   b. The highest mediastinal node removed/sampled is positive.
3. A recent meta-analysis[24] has confirmed that PLC, undertaken immediately on thoracotomy and shown to be positive for cancer cells, has an adverse and independent prognostic impact following complete resection. Such patients may be candidates for adjuvant chemotherapy. Surgeons and pathologists are encouraged to undertake this simple addition to intraoperative staging and collect data on PLC-positive and PLC-negative cases. Where the resection fulfills all of the requirements for classification as a complete resection, R0, but PLC has been performed and is positive, the resection should be classified as R1(cy+).
4. A standardized definition of visceral pleural invasion (VPI) has been incorporated into the seventh edition of *TNM* and recommendations included on the use of elastic stains in the determination of VPI. It is important that data be collected using this definition so that the usefulness of this pT2 descriptor can be assessed more accurately in future revisions. A subclassification has been proposed based

on a system published by the Japan Lung Cancer Society[25] and by Hammar[26] (see **Fig. 3**). It is proposed that the pleural lavage (PL) category be used to describe the pathologic extent of pleural invasion:

a. PL0 tumor within the subpleural lung parenchyma or invades superficially into the pleural connective tissue beneath the elastic layer[a]

b. PL1 tumor invades beyond the elastic layer

c. PL2 tumor invades to the pleural surface

d. PL3 tumor invades into any component of the parietal pleura.

It is recommended that pathologists prospectively collect data based on these subcategories to facilitate future revisions of *TNM*.

5. There are suggestions that the depth of chest wall invasion may influence prognosis following resection of lung cancer. A subclassification has been proposed, based on the histopathologic findings of the resection specimen, dividing such pT3 tumors into pT3a if invasion is limited to the parietal pleura (PL 3), pT3b if invasion involves the endothoracic fascia, and pT3c if invasion involves the rib or soft tissue. Pathologists are encouraged to collect this information prospectively to facilitate analysis and future revisions.

6. The IASLC Nodal Chart has been adopted as the new international chart for the documentation of nodal stations at clinical or pathologic staging where detailed assessment of nodes has been made, usually by invasive techniques or at thoracotomy (see **Fig. 2**). The concept of nodal zones has been suggested as a simpler, more utilitarian system for clinical staging where surgical exploration of lymph nodes has not been performed.[21] An exploratory analysis suggested that nodal extent could be grouped into 3 categories with differing prognoses: (1) involvement of a single N1 zone, designated as N1a, (2) involvement of more than 1 N1 zone, designated as N1b, or a single N2 zone, designated N2a, and (3) involvement of more than 1 N2 zone, designated N2b. It is suggested that radiologists, clinicians, and oncologists use the classification prospectively, where more detailed data on nodal stations is not available, to assess the usefulness of such a classification for future revision.

7. The designation of additional tumor nodules of similar histologic appearance in the lung(s) has been reclassified in the seventh edition of *TNM*. The UICC cannot determine that this is valid for cases in which multiple deposits are encountered, and prospective data collection is necessary to fully validate this reclassification. It is recommended that radiologists, oncologists, surgeons, and pathologists document in their clinical and pathologic staging the number of nodules in the lobe of the primary, other ipsilateral lobes, and the contralateral lung, and the diameter of the largest deposit in each location. When found in the lobe of the primary, T3 disease, the size of the closest nodule from the primary tumor, and its distance from the primary tumor should also be documented.

8. All cases in which there is metastatic spread to distant organs are classified as M1b disease. However, there are clear differences in prognosis based on tumor burden and the critical nature of some organ sites. Such differences influence the choice of treatment and the intent of treatment by all modalities of care. Selected patients with isolated metastases to a single organ may benefit from surgical treatment. Clinicians, oncologists, and surgeons are encouraged to fully document the extent

---

[a] In the *TNM* seventh edition, PL0 is not regarded as a T descriptor and the T category should be assigned on other features. PL1 or PL2 indicate VPI that is, T2a. PL3 indicates invasion of the parietal pleura, that is, T3.

of disease in M1b cases, collecting data on all of the sites of (suspected) metastatic disease and whether such organs contain single or multiple deposits.

9. Carcinoid tumors are included within the seventh edition of *TNM*. This inclusion validates its use by surgeons and pathologists for several decades. However, further details are needed to assess the prognostic impact of certain features in carcinoid tumors[20]; Typical versus atypical features, T size cutpoints, the prognostic impact of multiple deposits, and whether these are associated with the syndrome of diffuse idiopathic neuroendocrine cell hyperplasia (DIPNECH). In addition, in carcinoid tumors, in which long-term survival can be expected even when associated with multiple tumor nodules or nodal disease, it is important to collect data on disease-specific survival.

10. The IASLC Staging Project studied the impact of those prognostic factors, in addition to the anatomic extent of disease, for which data were available in the international database. For cases of NSCLC when prognostic factors were analyzed by clinical stage,[27] using the seventh edition, histology cell type was a significant prognostic factor for survival only in patients with stage IIIA, whereas performance status (PS), sex, and age were significant in all stages, but with a lower limit for age in advanced stages. In advanced disease, stage IIIB or IV, in which there were data on at least 1 laboratory test (calcium, albumin, sodium, hemoglobin, and white blood cell count), an analysis compared the prognostic power of each laboratory test against age, gender, and PS. The laboratory variables in advanced NSCLC were strong prognostic factors in a magnitude similar to PS, whereas age and gender were weaker. In patients for whom data were available in all 5 laboratory tests, a multivariate model identified PS and white blood count as strong significant prognostic factors, followed by calcium, albumin, and age. For surgically managed, pathologically staged I to IIIA NSCLC,[28] age, sex, and, to a lesser degree, certain cell types, in addition to pTNM stage, are all prognostic factors. Stage remains the most important factor, followed by age, and, in early stage cases, sex.

11. In lung cancer, molecular markers have been shown to be useful as predictive markers of response to chemotherapeutic agents. However, although there have been many articles on the prognostic capabilities of these markers in lung cancer, these have been limited to univariate analyses. International validation using multivariate analyses in prospective studies is still required.

12. Positron emission tomography (PET) scanning using [^{18}F]fluorodeoxyglucose is now widely used and has had an impact on the accuracy of clinical staging and referrals for surgical treatment. A meta-analysis, undertaken by the European Lung Cancer Working Party for the IASLC Lung Cancer Staging Project, has shown that PET features, such as the maximum value of the standardized uptake value (SUVmax) in the primary tumor before treatment, is an independent prognostic factor.[29] Nuclear medicine specialists, clinicians, and oncologists are encouraged to document the use of PET in clinical staging of lung cancer, and to record features such as SUVmax in the primary and any nodal and/or metastatic sites.

The IASLC, in a further departure from previous practice, has developed a range of educational materials that represent the first such site-specific products in lung cancer. The *IASLC Staging Handbook in Thoracic Oncology*[30] contains all of the basic information in a compact pocket book format, whereas the *IASLC Staging Manual in Thoracic Oncology*[31] includes more detail, additional background material, and extensive color illustrations. These illustrations depict the nodal stations of the IASLC nodal map with the accompanying definitions for each nodal station and a computed tomography atlas of images in axial, coronal, and sagittal views. There are also figures illustrating the new T, N, and M descriptors and the subclassification of VPI. Further details of these products are available from the IASLC Web site (www.iaslc.org).

Despite the enormous number of cases submitted to the IASLC international database, there were some descriptors in previous editions that could not be validated, partly because much of the data had been collected primarily for other purposes. Hence, although there were data on the stage in all cases, data on the individual T, N, and M categories in most cases, and data on individual descriptors in some, we had data on all of the features that could lead to a particular descriptor being assigned in very few cases. For some descriptors, such as VPI or nodal station, the lack of a uniform definition hindered collation of data from different institutions in different counties. Data on some of the descriptors were sparse and, although we suspected that this was because these descriptors had little clinical usefulness, we lacked the data to prove this. For these reasons, the next phase of the IASLC Staging Project is to incorporate prospective data,[32] which will also allow us to correct the geographic and treatment-related biases in the retrospective database. In addition, the IASLC has joined with colleagues in the International Mesothelioma Interest Group (IMIG) and the International Thymic Malignancies Interest Group (ITMIG) to expand the scope of our proposals for the eighth edition of *TNM* to include mesothelioma and thymic tumors. Any institution that wishes to contribute to this project need only email information@crab.org with IASLC Staging Project in the subject line to establish a dialog with our data center.

SUMMARY

The anatomic extent of disease, as reflected by the TNM classification, has stood the test of time and remains an important prognostic factor in most tumor sites. In lung cancer, it is still the most important prognostic factor in most clinical scenarios. The changes developed for the seventh edition have aligned stage with prognosis more accurately than had ever been possible previously. The challenge for the future is to combine TNM with other prognostic factors to develop a composite prognostic index. In lung cancer, this will undoubtedly include molecular markers but international validation and agreement on those that have prognostic value are awaited.

REFERENCES

1. Brundage MD, Mackillop WJ. Lung cancer. In: Gospodarowicz MK, O'Sullivan B, Sobin LH, editors. Prognostic factors in cancer. 3rd edition. Hoboken (NJ): Wiley-Liss; 2006. p. 159–63.
2. Denoix PF. The TNM staging system. Bull Inst Nat Hyg (Paris) 1952;7:743.
3. UICC. TNM classification of malignant tumours. 1st edition. Geneva (Switzerland): UICC; 1968.
4. Mountain CF, Carr DT, Anderson WA. A system for the clinical staging of lung cancer. Am J Roentgenol Radium Ther Nucl Med 1974;120:130–8.
5. UICC. TNM classification of malignant tumours. 2nd edition. Geneva (Switzerland): UICC; 1975.
6. American Joint Committee on Cancer Staging and End Results Reporting. AJC Cancer Staging Manual. 1st edition. Philadelphia: Lippincott-Raven; 1977.
7. American Joint Committee on Cancer. AJCC cancer staging manual. 6th edition. New York: Springer; 2002.
8. UICC International Union Against Cancer. TNM classification of malignant tumours. 6th edition. New York: Wiley-Liss; 2002.

9. Mountain CF. Revisions in the international system for staging lung cancer. Chest 1997;111:1710–7.

10. Goldstraw P. The International Staging Committee of the IASLC: its origins and purpose. Lung Cancer 2002;37:345–8.

11. Rami-Porta R, Ball D, Crowley JJ, et al. The IASLC Lung Cancer Staging Project: proposals for the revision of the T descriptors in the forthcoming (seventh) edition of the TNM Classification for Lung Cancer. J Thorac Oncol 2007;2:593–602.

12. Rusch VR, Crowley JJ, Giroux DJ, et al. The IASLC Lung Cancer Staging Project: proposals for revision of the N descriptors in the forthcoming (seventh) edition of the TNM Classification for Lung Cancer. J Thorac Oncol 2007;2:603–12.

13. Postmus PE, Brambilla E, Chansky K, et al. The IASLC Lung Cancer Staging Project: proposals for revision of the M descriptors in the forthcoming (seventh) edition of the TNM Classification for Lung Cancer. J Thorac Oncol 2007;2: 686–93.

14. Shepherd FA, Crowley J, Van Houtte P, et al. The IASLC Lung Cancer Staging Project: proposals regarding the clinical staging of small-cell lung cancer in the forthcoming (seventh) edition of the TNM Classification for Lung Cancer. J Thorac Oncol 2007;2:1067–77.

15. Vallieres E, Shepherd FA, Crowley J, et al. The IASLC Lung Cancer Staging Project: proposals regarding the relevance of TNM in the pathological staging of small-cell Lung cancer in the forthcoming (seventh) edition of the TNM Classification for Lung Cancer. J Thorac Oncol 2009;4:1049–59.

16. Groome PA, Bolejack V, Crowley JJ, et al. The IASLC Lung Cancer Staging Project: validation of the proposals for revision of the T, N and M descriptors and consequent stage groupings in the forthcoming (seventh) TNM Classification for Lung Cancer. J Thorac Oncol 2007;2:694–705.

17. Goldstraw P, Crowley JJ, Chansky K, et al. The IASLC Lung Cancer Staging Project: proposals for revision of the stage groupings in the forthcoming (seventh) edition of the TNM Classification for Lung Cancer. J Thorac Oncol 2007;2:706–14.

18. AJCC cancer staging Manual. In: Edge SB, Byrd DR, Compton CC, et al, editors. 7th edition. New York: Springer; 2009. chapters 25, 26.

19. TNM classification of malignant tumours. In: Sobin LH, Gospodarowicz MK and Wittekind, editors. Goldstraw P and Groome P, chapter editors. 7th edition. Oxford (UK): Blackwell Publishing; 2010. p. 138–50.

20. Travis WD, Giroux DJ, Chansky K, et al. The IASLC Lung Cancer Staging Project: proposals for the inclusion of carcinoid tumours in the forthcoming (seventh) edition of the TNM Classification for Lung Cancer. J Thorac Oncol 2008;3: 1213–23.

21. Rusch V, Asamura H, Watanabe H, et al. The IASLC Lung Cancer Staging Project: a proposal for a new international node map in the forthcoming seventh edition of the TNM Classification for Lung Cancer. J Thorac Oncol 2009;4:568–77.

22. Travis WD, Brambilla E, Rami-Porta R, et al. Visceral pleural invasion: pathologic criteria and use of elastic stains: proposals for the 7th edition of the TNM Classification for Lung Cancer. J Thorac Oncol 2008;3:1384–90.

23. Rami-Porta R, Wittekind C, Goldstraw P. Complete resection in lung cancer surgery: proposed definition. Lung Cancer 2005;49:25–33.

24. International Pleural Lavage Cytology Collaborators. Impact of positive pleural lavage cytology on survival in patients undergoing lung resection for non-small cell lung cancer: an international individual patient data meta-analysis. J Thorac Cardiovasc Surg 2010;139:1441–6.

25. Japan Lung Cancer Society. In: Classification of lung cancer: first English edition. 1st edition. Tokyo: Kanehara and Co Ltd; 2000. p. 38.
26. Hammar SP. Common tumors. In: Dail DH, Hammar SP, editors. Pulmonary pathology. 2nd edition. New York: Springer-Verlag; 1994. p. 1138.
27. Sculier JP, Chansky K, Crowley JJ, et al, IASLC International Staging Project. The impact of additional prognostic factors on survival and their relationship with the Anatomical Extent of Disease as expressed by the 6th edition of the TNM Classification of Malignant Tumours and the proposals for the 7th edition. J Thorac Oncol 2008;3:457–66.
28. Chansky K, Sculier JP, Crowley JJ, et al. The International Association for the Study of Lung Cancer Staging Project: prognostic factors and pathological TNM stage in surgically managed non-small cell lung cancer. J Thorac Oncol 2009;4:792–801.
29. Berghmans T, Dusart M, Paesmans M, et al. Primary tumour standardized uptake value (SUV max) measured on fluorodeoxyglucose emission tomography (PDG-PET) is of prognostic value for survival in non-small cell lung cancer (NSCLC): a systematic review and meta-analysis (MA) by the European Lung Cancer Working Party for the IASLC Lung Cancer Staging Project. J Thorac Oncol 2008;3:6–12.
30. Goldstraw P. IASLC staging handbook in thoracic oncology. 1st edition. Orange Park (FL): Editorial Rx Press; 2009.
31. Goldstraw P. IASLC staging manual in thoracic oncology. 1st edition. Orange Park (FL): Editorial Rx Press; 2009.
32. Giroux DJ, Rami-Porta R, Chansky K, et al. The IASLC Lung Cancer Staging Project: data elements for the prospective project. J Thorac Oncol 2009;4:679–83.

Diagnostic Workup of Lung Cancer

David J. Sugarbaker, MD*, Marcelo C. DaSilva, MD

KEYWORDS

- Lung cancer • Non–small cell lung cancer
- Small cell lung cancer • Imaging • Staging • Treatment

Lung cancer is the most frequent cause of mortality worldwide. According to recent estimates, 222,520 new cases of lung cancer (non–small cell and small cell combined) were diagnosed and 157,300 lung cancer–related deaths occurred in 2010 in the United States alone.[1] The two major histologic types of lung cancer are small cell lung cancer (SCLC) and non–small cell lung cancer (NSCLC). SCLC (oat cell) is the more aggressive cancer, with median survival of 2 to 4 months without treatment. However, it is usually responsive to systemic chemotherapy, with median survival rates of 18 to 36 months. Less prevalent than NSCLC, SCLC accounts for only 20% of all new lung cancers per year. In contrast, NSCLC accounts for 80% of all new lung cancers annually and is amenable to surgical excision in select patients. NSCLC includes three major subtypes: squamous cell carcinoma (30%–40%), adenocarcinoma (25%–30%), and large cell lung carcinoma (<10%). The diagnosis and management of lung cancer requires a multidisciplinary approach. The method of diagnosis of suspected lung cancer depends on the pathologic type, the size and location of the primary tumor, the presence of metastasis, and the overall clinical status of the patient.[2]

DIAGNOSIS

Patients with lung cancer usually present with an abnormal finding on a routine chest radiograph, such as a nodule or effusion. This study is generally followed by a contrast-enhanced chest CT scan, which should include examination of the liver and adrenal glands along with mediastinal lymph node stations. The overall accuracy of CT in mediastinal staging for lung cancer is only 0.75 to 0.80, with 20% to 40% false-negative and 18% to 23% false-positive results.[3] Although integrated PET-CT scanning is more sensitive and specific, yielding up to 98% correct tumor staging compared with final histologic staging,[4] it is not as widely available as CT.

A lymph node is considered malignant when its shortest axis is at least 10 mm.[3] The four most common sites of lung cancer metastases (stage IV disease) are brain, bone, liver, and adrenal glands. Consequently, head CT, brain MRI, and bone scans are

Division of Thoracic Surgery, Brigham and Women's Hospital, 75 Francis Street, Boston, MA 02115-6195, USA
* Corresponding author.
E-mail address: dsugarbaker@partners.org

Surg Oncol Clin N Am 20 (2011) 667–679
doi:10.1016/j.soc.2011.08.003
1055-3207/11/$ – see front matter © 2011 Published by Elsevier Inc.

surgonc.theclinics.com

often part of the metastatic evaluation. In the absence of central nervous system or bony symptoms in patients presenting with small tumors, the incidence of a true-positive finding is less than 10%. If disease in these sites is excluded, the cancer is confined to the chest (stages I–IIIB).

Positron emission tomography (PET) relies on the uptake and concentration of 2,3-fluorodeoxyglucose (FDG) in lung cancer cells. It is more sensitive and specific (approximately 90% sensitive and specific) for mediastinal nodal metastases compared with CT. PET scan is also fairly sensitive in detecting distant metastatic disease throughout the body exclusive of the brain. PET has an overall sensitivity of 96% (range, 83%–100%), specificity of 79% (range, 52%–100%), and accuracy of 91% (range, 86%–100%).[5] False-negative results can occur with lesions smaller than 1 cm because a critical mass of metabolically active malignant cells is required for PET diagnosis. Lowe and colleagues[6] found a sensitivity of only 80% in lesions smaller than 1.5 cm, compared with 92% in larger lesions.

False-negatives can also occur in tumors with low metabolism, such as carcinoid tumors. False-positive FDG uptake, particularly in pulmonary nodules or mediastinal lymph nodes, is seen in inflammatory conditions such as bacterial pneumonia, pyogenic abscesses, and aspergillosis, and in granulomatous diseases, such as tuberculosis, sarcoidosis, histoplasmosis, Wegener granulomatosis, and coal miner's lung. Guidelines for obtaining PET scan are shown in **Box 1**.

Approximately 70% of lung cancers are diagnosed and staged through small biopsies or cytology rather than using surgical resection specimens, with increasing numbers of transbronchial needle aspirations (TBNA), endobronchial ultrasound–guided needle aspirations (EBUS/TBNA), and esophageal ultrasound–guided needle aspirations being performed each year.[7] Patients with suspected lung cancer who present with a pleural effusion should undergo thoracentesis first to differentiate between a malignant versus paramalignant effusion. When three separate pleural fluid specimens with malignant pleural disease are submitted to an experienced cytologist, a positive diagnosis can be expected in approximately 80% of patients,[8] whereas percutaneous closed pleural biopsy is reported to be diagnostic for malignancy in approximately 50% of patients.[9] Thoracoscopic biopsy of the pleura is safe and can provide a definitive diagnosis with a high degree of accuracy and minimal risk to the patient. In most instances it is performed as an outpatient procedure.[10,11] The reported sensitivity rate for thoracoscopic biopsy ranges between 0.80 and 0.99, the specificity rate ranges between 0.93 and 1, and the negative predictive value ranges between 0.93 and 0.96.[10,12–14] False-negative results are more common with mesothelioma than with primary lung carcinoma.[12] In the case of a small (<3 cm) solitary peripheral lung lesion suspicious for lung cancer, the diagnostic dilemma generally centers on whether to obtain a biopsy specimen to confirm the diagnosis before surgical resection. In the presence of a high index of suspicion for lung cancer, an excisional wedge biopsy performed via video-assisted thoracic surgery has a much higher sensitivity than transthoracic needle aspiration (TTNA) and is the most definitive method of establishing a diagnosis. The diagnostic workup of lung cancer has evolved into a multidisciplinary approach. Patients suspected of having lung cancer require a histologic diagnosis and disease staging before appropriate treatment can be established. In addition, the development and clinical application of so-called targeted therapies require an increasing number of molecular investigations, such as gene amplification or mutation analysis, capable of scutinizing cancer at the nucleic acid level.

The histopathologic typing of lung tumors is performed according to the WHO criteria, but several specific antibodies are useful in establishing or eliminating diagnoses of primary lung cancers. A few examples of proved and reliable markers are

> **Box 1**
> **Suggested recommendations related to FDG-PET in the evaluation of indeterminate lung lesions**
>
> FDG-PET imaging is recommended in patients with low to moderate pretest probability of malignancy (5%–60%) and an indeterminate solitary primary nodule (SPN) greater than 8 to 10 mm in diameter.
>
> FDG-PET is not recommended to characterize the SPN in patients with high pretest probability of malignancy (>60%) or with SPNs less than 8 to 10 mm in diameter.
>
> In patients with an indeterminate SPN greater than 8 to 10 mm in diameter who are candidates for curative treatment, observation with serial CT scans is an acceptable management strategy under the following circumstances:
>
> 1. When the clinical probability of malignancy is very low (<5%)
>
> 2. When clinical probability is low (<30%–40%) and the lesion is not hypermetabolic on FDG-PET or does not enhance greater than 15 Hounsfield units (HU) on dynamic contrast CT
>
> 3. When needle biopsy is nondiagnostic and the lesion is not hypermetabolic on FDG-PET
>
> 4. When a fully informed patient prefers this nonaggressive approach
>
> In patients with an indeterminate SPN greater than 8 to 10 mm in diameter who are candidates for curative treatment, a transthoracic needle biopsy or bronchoscopy is appropriate under the following circumstances:
>
> 1. When clinical pretest probability and findings on imaging tests are discordant; for example, when the pretest probability of malignancy is high and the lesion is not hypermetabolic on FDG-PET
>
> 2. When a benign diagnosis that requires specific medical treatment is suspected
>
> 3. When a fully informed patient desires proof of a malignancy before surgery, especially when the risk for surgical complications is high
>
> In surgical candidates with an indeterminate SPN greater than 8 to 10 mm in diameter, surgical diagnosis is preferred under most circumstances, including the following:
>
> 1. When the clinical probability of malignancy is moderate to high (>60%)
>
> 2. When the nodule is hypermetabolic on FDG-PET imaging
>
> 3. When a fully informed patient prefers to undergo a definitive diagnostic procedure

available for a few common malignant tumor groups; *large cell neuroendocrine carcinoma* (chromogranin+, synaptophysin+, NCAM/CD56+, TTF-+/−, CK7+, CK high/lowMW+/−, AE1/AE3), SCLC (TTF-1+, CD56 or other neuroendocrine marker+, CK+, CK lowMW+, AE1/AE3, CK highMW-, LCA-, MIB-1/Ki-67 >50%), *typical carcinoid* (neuroendocrine marker+, TTF-1-, CK7, MIB1/Ki67<, <2 mitoses/2sqmm (10HPF), and atypical carcinoid (neuroendocrine marker+, TTF-1+/−, CK7+, MIB-1/Ki-67>, 2–10 mitoses/2sqmm and necroses). It also depends on the *type* of lung cancer, the *size* and *location* of the primary tumor, the *presence of metastasis*, the radiographic appearance of the lesion, and the *overall clinical status of the patient*.

SCLC

Bulky lymphadenopathy and direct mediastinal invasion are often associated with SCLC. A hilar mass is a particular characteristic of SCLC and is seen in approximately 78% of cases.[15,16] SCLC may present with paraneoplastic syndromes, namely syndrome of inappropriate antidiuretic hormone, ectopic adrenocorticotropic hormone production, and Lambert-Eaton syndrome.[17] SCLC can be diagnosed through sputum cytology, thoracentesis, fine-needle aspiration (FNA) of a supraclavicular node or metastatic site, and bronchoscopy with or without TBNA of mediastinal nodes or a submucosal process. When SCLC is diagnosed in a biopsy-proven specimen of the primary lesion, the next step is staging. One must determine whether the cancer is localized to the hemithorax or if extensive disease is present. Routine staging of SCLC includes a CT scan of the chest and abdomen or one of the chest with cuts through the entire liver and adrenal glands; a CT scan or MRI scan of the brain; and a bone scan.

NSCLC

In patients suspected of having NSCLC, the method for diagnosis is usually dictated by the presumed stage of the disease. Patients with metastatic NSCLC (stage IV disease) usually present with constitutional symptoms (eg, fatigue, weight loss), organ-specific symptoms (eg, bone pain, neurologic symptoms), or abnormal laboratory findings (eg, anemia, elevated alkaline phosphatase levels, elevated liver enzyme levels). In many of these patients, FNA or a needle biopsy of a site of metastasis represents the most efficient way to diagnose and confirm the stage of the disease. In some cases, however, the metastatic site may be technically difficult to biopsy. If metastatic disease can be predicted with a high degree of accuracy based on radiographic findings (eg, multiple brain, liver, bone lesions), using whatever method is easiest for the patient (eg, sputum cytology, bronchoscopy, TTNA) to diagnose the primary lung lesion may be more efficient. This decision must be made after weighing the technical considerations involved in each approach and the reliability of diagnosing an extrathoracic lesion as a site of metastasis based on radiographic appearances alone. A joint decision among the surgeon, radiologist, pulmonologist, and medical or radiation oncologist is the desirable approach.

NSCLC can present with extensive infiltration of the mediastinum, which is defined as a mass that infiltrates and encases the mediastinal structures, with no visible discrete mediastinal lymph nodes. In these patients, the method that has the most favorable risk/benefit ratio should be used for diagnosis. Bronchoscopy with TBNA for cytologic or histologic examination of mediastinal lymph nodes has been shown to be a safe procedure.[18-21] Technical aspects that are frequently emphasized as important to a high success rate include accurate preparation of the specimen, rapid on-site evaluation by a cytopathologist, and use of the larger 19-gauge needles, which provide better tissue samples for histologic evaluation.[22,23] The overall sensitivity of TBNA is 0.76 and the specificity is 0.96.[14-22,24-26] The negative predictive value of TBNA is not high enough (0.71) to obviate the need for further confirmation of negative results. Mediastinoscopy is warranted in patients with nondiagnostic results.

TTNA (CT-guided) of mediastinal masses can also be performed safely if needed.[27] The role of TTNA in patients with extensive mediastinal disease (defined as such extensive mediastinal tumor growth that discrete lymph nodes can no longer be discerned) is usually to confirm the presence of SCLC or NSCLC; these patients are not surgical candidates because of the extent of mediastinal disease.

Finally, two major areas of interaction between specialties drive the need for a multidisciplinary approach to lung cancer diagnosis: staging and treatment. An international multidisciplinary classification was sponsored by the International Association for the Study of Lung Cancer, American Thoracic Society, and European Respiratory Society.[7] The terms *bronchioloalveolar cell carcinoma* (BAC) and *mixed subtype adenocarcinoma* were eliminated. The new classification of adenocarcinoma of the lung reflects the recent progress in molecular biology and oncology, such as the discovery of epidermal growth factor receptor (EGFR) mutation and its prediction of response to EGFR tyrosine kinase inhibitors (TKIs) in adenocarcinoma[28-31]; the requirement to exclude a squamous cell carcinoma diagnosis to determine eligibility for treatment with pemetrexed[32-35] or bevacizumab[36,37]; the emergence of radiologic–pathologic correlations between ground-glass opacity and solid or mixed opacities seen on CT and BAC versus invasive lung cancer[38-41] in patient prognosis; and improved preoperative assessment for choice of timing and type of surgical intervention.[38-45]

For resection specimens, new concepts have been introduced, such as adenocarcinoma in situ (AIS) and minimally invasive adenocarcinoma (MIA) for small solitary adenocarcinomas with either pure lepidic growth (AIS) or predominant lepidic growth with less than 5 mm invasion (MIA). These categories define patients who, if they undergo complete resection, will have 100% or near 100% disease-specific survival, respectively (further detail is provided in the article on pathology by Drs Fan and Schraeder elsewhere in this issue).

STAGING
Staging: NSCLC

The seventh edition of the lung cancer stage classification system was adopted in the United States on January 1, 2010.[46] The Union Internationale Contre le Cancer and the American Joint Committee on Cancer are the organizations that periodically review, refine, and define the stage classification systems. The TNM stage classification system was developed to enable classification of tumor extension (TX–4), nodal involvement (NX–3), and distant metastatic spread (M0–1a,b). The most recent (7th) international lung cancer staging system is shown in **Table 1**. The two most common types of stage assessment are clinical staging (determined using all the information available before any treatment) and pathologic staging (determined after resection). Clinical stage is denoted by the prefix "c" and pathologic stage by the prefix "p."

Differences between the 6th and the 7th edition include the deletion of category MX (ie, cannot be assessed or proved), because clinical staging is always available. The *T* descriptor definitions maintain a size threshold of 3 cm as the cut point between a T1 and T2 tumor. However, significant new cut points have been identified at 2, 5, and 7 cm. Tumors larger than 7 cm are classified as T3, because they have a survival rate similar to other T3 tumors characterized by invasion or central location. No survival differences were shown between cT1a, cT1b, and cT2a, although this probably was the result of patient numbers too small to yield statistically significant values.

Another modification of the 7th edition relates to additional tumor nodules. Patients with additional satellite nodules in the same lobe as the primary tumor have survival rates similar to those with T3 disease and are now classified as T3$_{Satell}$, whereas previously they were classified as T4. Survival for patients with T3$_{Satell}$ disease is statistically significantly better than survival of those with T4. Patients with an ipsilateral nodule in a different lobe are classified as having stage T4$_{Ipsi Nod}$ or simply T4, whereas they were previously classified as having stage M1. Patients with pleural dissemination now are classified as having stage M1a, because their prognosis is statistically significantly worse than those with T4 disease.

The *N* descriptor categorization (ie, N0, N1, N2, and N3) has not changed. No survival differences were found between patients with involvement of only peripheral (N1) nodes versus hilar (N2) nodes, and no survival differences were seen based on which N2 nodal stations were involved. In examining the effect of skip metastases (involvement of an N2 station without any N1 stations), survival in patients with right upper lobe tumors and N2-positive nodes, with or without N1 nodes, was not altered, although a small difference was seen among these patients when the tumor was in the left upper lobe.[47] The number of involved nodal zones does seem to have prognostic impact. Patients with single-zone N1 or N2 involvement have better survival than those

Table 1
Comparison between the 6th and the 7th edition of the lung cancer stage classification system

		6th Edition	7th Edition
T	TX	Primary tumor cannot be assessed, or evidence of malignant cells in sputum or bronchial lavage fluid but no visualization of tumor on imaging or bronchoscopy	Primary tumor cannot be assessed, or evidence of malignant cells in sputum or bronchial lavage fluid but no visualization of tumor on No evidence of primary tumor imaging or bronchoscopy
	T0	No evidence of primary tumor	No evidence of primary tumor
	Tis	Carcinoma in situ	Carcinoma in situ
	T1	Tumor ≤3 cm greatest diameter, surrounded by lung tissue or visceral pleura, no bronchoscopic evidence of invasion proximal to the lobar bronchus (ie, main bronchi are free)	Tumor ≤3 cm greatest diameter, surrounded by lung tissue or visceral pleura, no bronchoscopic evidence of infiltration proximal to the lobar bronchus (ie, main bronchi are free)
	T1a		Tumor ≤2 cm greatest diameter
	T1b		Tumor >2 cm but ≤3 cm greatest diameter
	T2	Tumor >3 cm or tumor with one of the following features: invasion of the main bronchus, ≥2 cm distal to the carina invasion of the visceral pleura associated atelectasis or obstructive pneumonia extending as far as the hilus but not involving the whole lung	Tumor >3 cm but ≤7 cm with one of the following features: invasion of the main bronchus, ≥2 cm distal to the carina invasion of the visceral pleura Associated atelectasis or obstructive pneumonia extending as far as the hilus but not involving the whole lung
	T2a		Tumor >3 cm but ≤5 cm greatest diameter
	T2b		Tumor >5 cm but ≤7 cm greatest diameter
	T3	Tumor of any size with direct invasion of one of the following structures: chest wall (including tumors of the superior sulcus) diaphragm phrenic nerve mediastinal pleura parietal pericardium or tumor in the main bronchus <2 cm distal to the carina, without or without associated a telectasis or obstructive pneumonia of the whole lung	Tumor >7 cm or any tumor with direct invasion of one of the following structures: chest wall (including tumors of the superior sulcus) diaphragm phrenic nerve mediastinal pleura parietal pericardium or tumor in the main bronchus <2 cm distal to the carina, without involvement of the carina and without associated atelectasis or obstructive pneumonia of the whole lung or satellite tumor nodule(s) in the same lobe

T4	Tumor of any size invading one of the following structures: mediastinum heart great vessels trachea recurrent laryngeal nerve esophagus vertebral body carina or separate tumor nodule(s) in the same lobe or tumor with malignant pleural effusion or pericardial effusion	**T3$_{Satell}$**	Separate tumor nodule(s) in the same lobe (used to be T4)
		T4 or	Tumor of any size invading one of the following structures: mediastinum heart great vessels trachea recurrent laryngeal nerve esophagus vertebral body carina
		T4$_{psi\ Nod}$	Separate tumor nodule(s) in another ipsilateral lobe (used to be M1)
N	**NX** Regional lymph nodes could not be evaluated	**NX**	Regional lymph nodes could not be evaluated
	N0 No regional lymph node metastases	**N0**	No regional lymph node metastases
	N1 Metastasis/metastases in the ipsilateral peribronchial and/or ipsilateral hilar lymph nodes and intrapulmonary lymph nodes, including involvement by direct extension of the primary tumor	**N1**	Metastasis/metastases in the ipsilateral peribronchial and/or ipsilateral hilar lymph nodes and intrapulmonary lymph nodes, including involvement by direct extension of the primary tumor
	N2 Metastasis/metastases in the ipsilateral mediastinal and/or subcarinal lymph nodes	**N2**	Metastasis/metastases in the ipsilateral mediastinal and/or subcarinal lymph nodes
	N3 Metastasis/metastases in the contralateral mediastinal, contralateral hilar, ipsilateral or contralateral scalene or supraclavicular lymph nodes	**N3**	Metastasis/metastases in the contralateral mediastinal, contralateral hilar, ipsilateral or contralateral scalene or supraclavicular lymph nodes
M	**MX** Distant metastases could not be evaluated		
	M0 No distant metastases	**M0**	No distant metastases
	M1 Distant metastases, including separate tumor nodules in another pulmonary lobe	**M1a**	Separate tumor nodule(s) in a contralateral lobe; tumor with pleural nodes or malignant pleural (or pericardial) effusion (used to be T4)
		M1b	Distant metastases

Data from Hammerschmidt S, Wirtz H. Lung cancer: current diagnosis and treatment. Dtsch Arztebl Int 2009;106(49):809–20.

with multizone N1 or N2 involvement (5-year survival rate of 48% vs 35% [P<.09] and 34% vs 20% [P<.001] respectively). Finally, the cohorts remaining in the M descriptor were separated into two distinct prognostic groups. M1a is reserved for patients with either pleural dissemination or contralateral pulmonary nodules. The M1b subgroup is reserved for those with distant metastases.

The revised TNM classification with stage grouping is shown in **Table 2**. For stages I through IIB, surgical therapy is generally offered as monotherapy, occasionally followed by chemotherapy. Stage IIIA (positive ipsilateral tracheal or subcarinal nodes) is best treated preoperatively with chemotherapy or chemoradiation followed by resection in responders. Several small, randomized trials suggest a doubling of the 5-year survival rate with this strategy. Patients with residual disease have a very poor 5-year survival prognosis. Resection of tumors with contralateral paratracheal positive nodes (stage IIIB) is controversial, with a worse 5-year survival prognosis than stage IIIA disease. Surgical resection for patients with stage IV disease is generally not indicated except in the few who may have isolated and treatable brain or adrenal metastases.

One of the greatest challenges clinicians face today is the effective use of advancing clinical and molecular knowledge to positively impact patient treatment. Therapeutic targets have been identified in only 20% of patients with NSCLC with activated *EGFR* mutations; 75% of these patients are candidates for TKI-targeted therapy. The frequency for primary resistance against EGFR-TKI is more than 80%. Targeted therapies in specific patient populations may reduce the need for chemotherapy and allow clinicians to tailor treatment to individual patients. Targeted cancer therapies may be used alone, in combination with other targeted therapies, or with other lung cancer treatments, such as chemotherapy, radiation therapy, and interventional pulmonology. Thus, finally patients might benefit distinctly from a multidisciplinary approach to their disease, with an increased response/survival rate and improved quality of life. Although results have been encouraging, much work remains.

PREOPERATIVE EVALUATION
Estimation of Pulmonary Reserve

Most patients who undergo surgical resection are current or former smokers. They may present with chronic pulmonary insufficiency and poor physiologic reserve.

Table 2
Stage groups according to TNM descriptor and subgroups

T/M	Subgroups	N0	N1	N2	N3
T1	T1a	IA	IIA	IIIA	IIIB
	T1b	IA	IIA	IIIA	IIIB
T2	T2a	IB	IIA	IIIA	IIIB
	T2b	IIA	IIB	IIIA	IIIB
T3	T3>7	IIB	IIIA	IIIA	IIIB
	T3$_{Inv}$	IIB	IIIA	IIIA	IIIB
	T3$_{Satell}$	IIB	IIIA	IIIA	IIIB
T4	T4$_{Inv}$	IIIA	IIIA	IIIB	
	T4$_{Ipsi Nod}$	IIIA	IIIA	IIIB	
				IIIB	
				IIIB	
M1	M1a$_{Contr Nod}$	IV	IV	IV	IV
	M1a$_{Pl Dissem}$	IV	IV	IV	IV
	M1b	IV	IV	IV	IV

Preoperative assessment of pulmonary physiology and reserve and cardiac function is paramount for a successful operation. Cessation of smoking at least 2 weeks (preferably 6 weeks) before resection aids in the perioperative control of secretions and the avoidance of pneumonia. A thorough physical examination; medical history; social history, including tobacco smoking and exposure to arsenic and asbestos; list of medications; a posteroanterior and lateral chest radiograph, CT scan, PET-CT scan, MRI, and pulmonary function tests are part of the preoperative assessment (**Fig. 1**).

Risk assessment is a complex process, and whether the patient is able to tolerate a pneumonectomy, lobectomy, or limited resection (segmental or wedge resection) is determined based on his or her physiologic reserve. Clinicians should make an effort to determine the individual patient's resectability and operability. Resectability depends directly on the amount of pulmonary reserve of the patient and is linked to the amount of lung tissue and tumor that can be safely removed without the patient developing respiratory insufficiency. Operability refers to the ability of a patient to survive the proposed operation and the associated perioperative complications. Therefore, operability depends mostly on the patient's comorbid conditions. However, neither operability of an individual patient nor resectability of a tumor should influence the decision regarding the effect of a complete resection on survival.

Pulmonary function testing comprises four elements of evaluation: (1) pulmonary spirometry, (2) pulmonary hemodynamic response testing, (3) exercise testing, and (4) quantitative ventilation/perfusion scan (V/Q). Pulmonary spirometry is affected by height, age, weight, sex, race, and posture, and arterial oxygenation and diffusion capacity. Although pulmonary spirometry and arterial oxygenation may aid to predict mortality, they are not good predictors of postoperative complications. Diffusion capacity of the lung for carbon oxide (DL_{co}) is a more sensitive predictor of postoperative complications. DL_{co} measures the partial pressure difference between inspired and expired carbon monoxide. It relies on the strong affinity and large absorption capacity of erythrocytes for carbon monoxide and thus shows gas uptake by the capillaries that is less dependent on cardiac output. Thus DL_{co} value is decreased in patients with emphysema, chronic pulmonary hypertension, and interstitial lung disease. DL_{co} is an important and independent predictor of postoperative complications after major lung resection, even in patients without chronic obstructive pulmonary disease.

V/Q scan is useful for predicting postoperative lung function. A calculated (predicted) postoperative forced expiratory volume in 1 second ($ppoFEV_1$) of less than 40% is associated with a 50% mortality rate. The absolute minimum $ppoFEV_1$ in patients undergoing lobectomy is 800 mL. Pulmonary hemodynamic response testing includes the measurement of pulmonary artery pressure and pulmonary vascular resistance. Systolic pulmonary artery pressure greater than 35 mm Hg is associated with a 10-fold decrease in survival rate, and pulmonary vascular resistance greater than 190 $(dyn^*sec)/cm^5$ is associated with a 90% mortality rate.

Maximum exercise testing is concerned with the amount of arterial desaturation that occurs during exercise. Patients with a maximum oxygen consumption (Vo_2max) of less than 15 mL/kg/min are considered high risk, whereas those with a Vo_2max of 16 to 20 mL/kg/min could probably undergo surgery.

Postoperative pulmonary function is calculated by obtaining preoperative pulmonary function tests and measuring forced expiratory volume in 1 second and DL_{co}. Postoperative lung function is estimated by the following equation:

$$\% \ ppoFEV_1 = \% \ \text{preoperative } FEV_1 - (\text{preoperative } FEV_1 \times \text{number of segments to be removed}/18), \text{ with 18 as the total number of segments in the normal lung.}$$

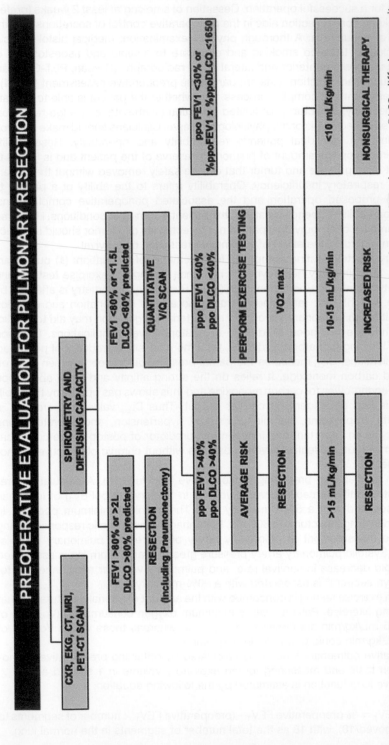

Fig. 1. Preoperative evaluation algorithm for pulmonary resection. CT, computerized tomography scan; CXR, chest x-ray; DLCO, diffusing capacity of the lung for carbon dioxide; EKG, electrocardiogram; FEV1, forced expiratory volume in 1 second; MRI, magnetic resonance imaging; PET, positron emission tomography; ppoDLCO, predicted postoperative DLCO; ppoFev1, predicted postoperative FEV1.

The ppoFEV$_1$ and DL$_{co}$ should be greater than 35% predicted according to age, height, and sex. Exceptions are patients with obstructed bronchi or nonfunctioning areas of lung who could tolerate removal of that portion of lung. Patients with otherwise unacceptably poor lung function may tolerate lung resection if there are concomitant lung volume reduction benefits (usually from upper lobe lesions). Quantitative ventilation and perfusion scanning and cardiopulmonary exercise testing can help clarify uncertain situations. Patients with predicted postoperative$\dot{V}o_2$(oxygen consumption) maximum greater than 12 mL/kg/m^2 can generally tolerate anatomic resection, whereas those with predicted values less than 10 mL/kg/m^2 are at very high risk.

SUMMARY

The diagnostic workup of lung cancer has evolved over the past several years with the introduction of new clinical technologies such as PET-CT scan, transbronchial needle biopsy (TBNA), EBUS/TBNA, EUS CT-guided biopsy, and VATS biopsy, which improve our ability to accurately stage disease. A multidisciplinary team should be involved in deciding which diagnostic method to use, usually progressing from the least invasive to most invasive modality with the highest diagnostic yield. As the staging system continues to be refined, so will the treatment options for lung cancer. Once the diagnostic workup is completed, operability and resectability are determined during the preoperative evaluation by assessing the physiologic reserve of the individual patient. Finally, the role of targeted therapies, though promising, remains to be determined. Only time will show whether these new treatments will prove effective for patients with lung cancer.

REFERENCES

1. Jemal A, Siegel R, Xu J, et al. Cancer statistics, 2010. CA Cancer J Clin 2010;60: 277–300.
2. Rivera MP, Mehta AC. Initial diagnosis of lung cancer: ACCP evidence-based clinical practice guidelines (2nd edition). Chest 2007;132:131S–48S.
3. Kramer H, Groen HJ. Current concepts in the mediastinal lymph node staging of nonsmall cell lung cancer. Ann Surg 2003;238:180–8.
4. Lardinois D, Weder W, Hany TF, et al. Staging of non-small-cell lung cancer with integrated positron-emission tomography and computed tomography. N Engl J Med 2003;348:2500–7.
5. Schrevens L, Lorent N, Dooms C, et al. The role of PET scan in diagnosis, staging, and management of non-small cell lung cancer. Oncologist 2004;9:633–43.
6. Lowe VJ, Fletcher JW, Gobar L, et al. Prospective investigation of positron emission tomography in lung nodules. J Clin Oncol 1998;16:1075–84.
7. Travis WD, Brambilla E, Noguchi M, et al. International Association for the Study of Lung Cancer/American Thoracic Society/European Respiratory Society International Multidisciplinary Classification of Lung Adenocarcinoma. J Thorac Oncol 2011;6:244–85.
8. Johnston WW. The malignant pleural effusion. A review of cytopathologic diagnoses of 584 specimens from 472 consecutive patients. Cancer 1985;56:905–9.
9. Prakash UB, Reiman HM. Comparison of needle biopsy with cytologic analysis for the evaluation of pleural effusion: analysis of 414 cases. Mayo Clin Proc 1985;60:158–64.
10. Boutin C, Viallat JR, Cargnino P, et al. Thoracoscopy in malignant pleural effusions. Am Rev Respir Dis 1981;124:588–92.

11. Rusch VW, Mountain C. Thoracoscopy under regional anesthesia for the diagnosis and management of pleural disease. Am J Surg 1987;154:274–8.
12. Menzies R, Charbonneau M. Thoracoscopy for the diagnosis of pleural disease. Ann Intern Med 1991;114:271–6.
13. Page RD, Jeffrey RR, Donnelly RJ. Thoracoscopy: a review of 121 consecutive surgical procedures. Ann Thorac Surg 1989;48:66–8.
14. Harris RJ, Kavuru MS, Mehta AC, et al. The impact of thoracoscopy on the management of pleural disease. Chest 1995;107:845–52.
15. Forster BB, Muller NL, Miller RR, et al. Neuroendocrine carcinomas of the lung: clinical, radiologic, and pathologic correlation. Radiology 1989;170:441–5.
16. Pearlberg JL, Sandler MA, Lewis JW Jr, et al. Small-cell bronchogenic carcinoma: CT evaluation. AJR Am J Roentgenol 1988;150:265–8.
17. Patel AM, Davila DG, Peters SG. Paraneoplastic syndromes associated with lung cancer. Mayo Clin Proc 1993;68:278–87.
18. Utz JP, Patel AM, Edell ES. The role of transcarinal needle aspiration in the staging of bronchogenic carcinoma. Chest 1993;104:1012–6.
19. Schenk DA, Bower JH, Bryan CL, et al. Transbronchial needle aspiration staging of bronchogenic carcinoma. Am Rev Respir Dis 1986;134:146–8.
20. Schenk DA, Strollo PJ, Pickard JS, et al. Utility of the Wang 18-gauge transbronchial histology needle in the staging of bronchogenic carcinoma. Chest 1989;96:272–4.
21. Harrow EM, Abi-Saleh W, Blum J, et al. The utility of transbronchial needle aspiration in the staging of bronchogenic carcinoma. Am J Respir Crit Care Med 2000;161:601–7.
22. Davenport RD. Rapid on-site evaluation of transbronchial aspirates. Chest 1990;98:59–61.
23. Schenk DA, Chambers SL, Derdak S, et al. Comparison of the Wang 19-gauge and 22-gauge needles in the mediastinal staging of lung cancer. Am Rev Respir Dis 1993;147:1251–8.
24. Vansteenkiste J, Lacquet LM, Demedts M, et al. Transcarinal needle aspiration biopsy in the staging of lung cancer. Eur Respir J 1994;7:265–8.
25. Ratto GB, Mereu C, Motta G. The prognostic significance of preoperative assessment of mediastinal lymph nodes in patients with lung cancer. Chest 1988;93:807–13.
26. Garpestad E, Goldberg S, Herth F, et al. CT fluoroscopy guidance for transbronchial needle aspiration: an experience in 35 patients. Chest 2001;119:329–32.
27. Protopapas Z, Westcott JL. Transthoracic needle biopsy of mediastinal lymph nodes for staging lung and other cancers. Radiology 1996;199:489–96.
28. Mok TS, Wu YL, Thongprasert S, et al. Gefitinib or carboplatin-paclitaxel in pulmonary adenocarcinoma. N Engl J Med 2009;361:947–57.
29. Mitsudomi T, Morita S, Yatabe Y, et al. Gefitinib versus cisplatin plus docetaxel in patients with non-small-cell lung cancer harbouring mutations of the epidermal growth factor receptor (WJTOG3405): an open label, randomised phase 3 trial. Lancet Oncol 2010;11:121–8.
30. Maemondo M, Inoue A, Kobayashi K, et al. Gefitinib or chemotherapy for non-small-cell lung cancer with mutated EGFR. N Engl J Med 2010;362:2380–8.
31. Abstracts of the 35th European Society for Medical Oncology Conference. October 8–12, 2010. Milan, Italy. Ann Oncol 2010;21(Suppl 8):viii22–416.
32. Scagliotti GV, Park K, Patil S, et al. Survival without toxicity for cisplatin plus pemetrexed versus cisplatin plus gemcitabine in chemonaive patients with advanced non-small cell lung cancer: a risk-benefit analysis of a large phase III study. Eur J Cancer 2009;45:2298–303.

33. Scagliotti GV, Parikh P, von Pawel J, et al. Phase III study comparing cisplatin plus gemcitabine with cisplatin plus pemetrexed in chemotherapy-naive patients with advanced-stage non-small-cell lung cancer. J Clin Oncol 2008;26:3543–51.
34. Ciuleanu T, Brodowicz T, Zielinski C, et al. Maintenance pemetrexed plus best supportive care versus placebo plus best supportive care for non-small-cell lung cancer: a randomised, double-blind, phase 3 study. Lancet 2009;374: 1432–40.
35. Scagliotti G, Hanna N, Fossella F, et al. The differential efficacy of pemetrexed according to NSCLC histology: a review of two Phase III studies. Oncologist 2009; 14:253–63.
36. Johnson DH, Fehrenbacher L, Novotny WF, et al. Randomized phase II trial comparing bevacizumab plus carboplatin and paclitaxel with carboplatin and paclitaxel alone in previously untreated locally advanced or metastatic non-small-cell lung cancer. J Clin Oncol 2004;22:2184–91.
37. Cohen MH, Gootenberg J, Keegan P, et al. FDA drug approval summary: bevacizumab (Avastin) plus Carboplatin and Paclitaxel as first-line treatment of advanced/metastatic recurrent nonsquamous non-small cell lung cancer. Oncologist 2007;12:713–8.
38. Kodama K, Higashiyama M, Yokouchi H, et al. Prognostic value of ground-glass opacity found in small lung adenocarcinoma on high-resolution CT scanning. Lung Cancer 2001;33:17–25.
39. Suzuki K, Asamura H, Kusumoto M, et al. "Early" peripheral lung cancer: prognostic significance of ground glass opacity on thin-section computed tomographic scan. Ann Thorac Surg 2002;74:1635–9.
40. Takamochi K, Nagai K, Yoshida J, et al. Pathologic N0 status in pulmonary adenocarcinoma is predictable by combining serum carcinoembryonic antigen level and computed tomographic findings. J Thorac Cardiovasc Surg 2001;122: 325–30.
41. Sakurai H, Maeshima A, Watanabe S, et al. Grade of stromal invasion in small adenocarcinoma of the lung: histopathological minimal invasion and prognosis. Am J Surg Pathol 2004;28:198–206.
42. Adler B, Padley S, Miller RR, et al. High-resolution CT of bronchioloalveolar carcinoma. AJR Am J Roentgenol 1992;159:275–7.
43. El-Sherif A, Gooding WE, Santos R, et al. Outcomes of sublobar resection versus lobectomy for stage I non-small cell lung cancer: a 13-year analysis. Ann Thorac Surg 2006;82:408–15 [discussion: 415–6].
44. Nakamura H, Kawasaki N, Taguchi M, et al. Survival following lobectomy vs limited resection for stage I lung cancer: a meta-analysis. Br J Cancer 2005;92: 1033–7.
45. Okada M, Koike T, Higashiyama M, et al. Radical sublobar resection for small-sized non-small cell lung cancer: a multicenter study. J Thorac Cardiovasc Surg 2006;132:769–75.
46. Detterbeck FC, Boffa DJ, Tanoue LT, et al. Details and difficulties regarding the new lung cancer staging system. Chest 2010;137:1172–80.
47. Rusch VW, Crowley J, Giroux DJ, et al. The IASLC Lung Cancer Staging Project: proposals for the revision of the N descriptors in the forthcoming seventh edition of the TNM classification for lung cancer. J Thorac Oncol 2007;2:603–12.

A Review of Noninvasive Staging of the Mediastinum for Non–Small Cell Lung Carcinoma

Daaron McField, MD[a], Thomas Bauer, MD[b,c,d],*

KEYWORDS

• Non–small cell lung carcinoma • Mediastinum
• Noninvasive • Staging

Lung cancer causes significant morbidity and mortality. Annually lung cancer claims the life of 1.2 million people worldwide, and is the leading cause of cancer death in both men and women.[1] In the United States there were an estimated 222,000 new cases of lung cancer and 157,000 deaths in 2010.[2]

Over the last century both the absolute and relative frequency of lung cancer rose dramatically as smoking became more widespread. In the 1950s, lung cancer became the most common cause of cancer deaths in men, and in 1985 it became the leading cause of cancer deaths in women.[2] Although lung cancer deaths have begun to decline in men, the death rate in women continues to rise, and almost one-half of all lung cancer deaths now occur in women. Lung cancer is responsible for more cancer-related deaths than the next three most common cancers combined (breast, colon, and prostrate).[2]

Lung cancer and bronchogenic carcinoma are malignancies originating from the airways and pulmonary parenchyma. Most (approximately 90%) lung cancers are classified as non–small cell lung cancer (NSCLC). This distinction carries important

The authors have nothing to disclose.
[a] Department of Surgery, Christiana Care, MAP II, Suite 2121, 4735 Ogletown-Stanton Road, Newark, DE 19713, USA
[b] Department of Surgery, Thoracic Surgery, Helen F. Graham Cancer Center, Christiana Care, 4755 Ogletown-Stanton Road, JHA Education Center, Suite 2, East 70b, Newark, DE 19718, USA
[c] Department of Surgery, Jefferson Medical College, 1025 Walnut Street, Philadelphia, PA 19107, USA
[d] Department of Biological Sciences, University of Delaware, 118 Wolf Hall, Newark, DE 18716, USA
* Corresponding author. Helen F. Graham Cancer Center, S-2100, 4701 Ogletown-Stanton Road, Newark, DE 19713.
E-mail address: tbauer@christianacare.org

differences for staging, treatment, and prognosis. This article presents a review of mediastinal staging for patients with NSCLC.

For patients newly diagnosed with lung cancer, evaluation of the mediastinum is critical because it guides treatment and predicts survival. Local disease (stages I and II) is primarily treated with surgery, whereas locoregional, locally advanced, and advanced disease are primarily treated with nonoperative modalities. In patients without evidence of distant metastatic disease the evaluation for invasion into nonresectable structures and mediastinal lymph nodes metastasis becomes the key determinant for tumor stage, prognosis, and treatment. Historically, mediastinoscopy has been the gold standard for evaluating mediastinal nodes. However, with advances in current noninvasive imaging there has been increasing use of noninvasive imaging to evaluate the mediastinum.

CHEST RADIOGRAPHY

As a single imagine modality, chest radiography is rarely solely used for staging because it cannot accurately detect lymph node metastases, chest wall invasion, or invasion of mediastinal structures, although it can detect pleural effusions and multiple pulmonary masses. Despite its limited use, chest radiographs are readily available, inexpensive, and provide a lot of information with a minimal effective radiation dose.

COMPUTED TOMOGRAPHY

Chest computed tomography (CT) scans are performed in nearly everyone with a suspected NSCLC. Many of the older studies evaluating the use of CT scans are based on older technology limited to 5- to 10-mm cuts. Newer multislice scanners are able to obtain cuts with a slice thickness of 1.25 to 2.5 mm. The CT scan should include all of the thoracic structures starting from the neck, and continuing down through the abdomen to include the liver and adrenals. Intravenous contrast should be used to help distinguish vascular structures from mediastinal structures and lesions. Intravenous contrast also facilitates assessment of potential vascular involvement of the superior vena cava, pulmonary veins, pulmonary arteries, systemic mediastinal arterial structures, and cardiac structures.

CT scans are safe, quick, painless, and produce a great deal of information. It has become the initial imaging procedure for the staging of bronchiogenic carcinoma. Of particular importance is the presence or absence of mediastinal nodal (N2 and N3) disease. Lymph node enlargement (measured in the short axis) presumes lymph node metastasis in the context of a newly diagnosed or suspected NSCLC. The predictive accuracy depends on the size of the lymph nodes chosen as the upper limit of normal. CT images cannot distinguish malignant from inflammatory nodal tissue, so reactive lymph adenopathy may be mistaken for metastatic disease.

Normal mediastinal lymph nodes are usually less than 10 mm, although normal subcarinal lymph nodes can reach a diameter of 13 to 15 mm (**Box 1**). Any lymph nodes exceeding these sizes are significantly more likely to contain malignant disease. Normal lymph nodes are rarely seen in the retrocrural region, para-aortic region, or pericardial fat. Lymph nodes exceeding 8 mm in these regions should be considered suspicious.

In a meta-analysis of 35 studies, and 5111 patients by Silvestri and coworkers,[3] CT scans were used to evaluate for mediastinal nodal disease. In this population disease prevalence was found to be 28. CT predicted mediastinal lymph node metastasis with a sensitivity and specificity of 51 and 86, respectively.

Box 1
Mediastinal lymph node stations

1.	Highest mediastinal
2.	Upper paratracheal
3.	Prevascular and retrotracheal
4.	Lower paratracheal (including azygos nodes)
	N2 = single digit, ipsilateral
	N3 = single digit, contralateral or supraclavicular
5.	Subaortic (A-P window)
6.	Para-aortic (ascending aortic or phrenic)
7.	Subcarinal
8.	Paraesophageal (below carina)
9.	Pulmonary ligament
10.	Hilar
11.	Interlobar
12.	Interlobar
13.	Segmental
14.	Subsegmental

Data from Navani N, Spiro SG, Janes SM. Mediastinal staging of NSCLC with endoscopic and endobronchial ultrasound. Nat Rev Clin Oncol 2009;6:278–86.

Mediastinal lymph nodes are graded as N0, N1, N2, or N3 (**Fig. 1**). The assignment should be considered tentative, because the use of lymph node enlargement as a surrogate for malignant disease is imperfect. Metastatic disease can exist in normal size lymph nodes, whereas hyperplastic, benign lymph nodes can exceed 10 mm.

To address this issue, Arita and colleagues[4] specifically examined lung cancer metastases to normal-sized mediastinal lymph nodes in 90 patients. Using a cut off of 10 mm, 14 patients with negative CT scans were found to have occult N2 or N3 metastasis after thoracotomy resulting in a 16% false-negative rate.

Efforts have been made to identify low-risk tumors where a negative CT scan would eliminate the need for mediastinoscopy. Dillemans and colleagues[5] reported a selective mediastinoscopy strategy, proceeding straight to thoracotomy without mediastinoscopy for T1 peripheral tumors without enlarged mediastinal lymph nodes on preoperative CT. This strategy resulted in a 16% incidence of positive nodes discovered only at the time of thoracotomy. For identifying N2 disease, chest CT scans had a sensitivity and specificity of 69% and 71%, respectively. When both a CT scan and a subsequent mediastinoscopy were used the accuracy improved (89% vs 71%).

Thus, because of the low sensitivity and poor negative predictive value of CT scan tissue sampling is required to confirm the presence or absence of regional lymph node involvement in the mediastinum.

POSITRON EMISSION TOMOGRAPHY

Positron emission tomography (PET) is unique in that it detects tumor physiology, as opposed to anatomy. PET may be more sensitive than CT scans especially if reactive lymph adenopathy may be present. If postobstructive pneumonitis is present, there is little correlation between the size of the mediastinal lymph nodes and the tumor involvement.[6]

PET is accomplished by injecting a radioisotope bound to an analog of D-glucose (18-fluoro-2-deoxyglucose [FDG]) into the patient. All cells take up some of the FDG for glycolysis, but cells with increased metabolic activity accumulate more FDG

A

International Association for the Study of Lung Cancer

IASLC

TNM Stage Grouping Table

T and M		N0	N1	N2	N3
6th edition TNM	7th edition TNM	Stg	Stg	Stg	Stg
T1 (≤3 cm)	T1a (≤2 cm)	IA	IIA	IIIA	IIIB
	T1b (>2–3 cm)	IA	IIA	IIIA	IIIB
T2 (>3 cm)	T2a (>3–5 cm)	IB	IIA (IIB)	IIIA	IIIB
	T2b (>5–7 cm)	IIA (IB)	IIB	IIIA	IIIB
	T3 (>7 cm)	IIB (IB)	IIIA (IIB)	IIIA	IIIB
T3 invasion	T3	IIB	IIIA	IIIA	IIIB
T4 (same lobe nodules)	T3	IIB (IIIB)	IIIA (IIIB)	IIIA (IIIB)	IIIB
T4 (extension)	T4	IIIA (IIIB)	IIIA (IIIB)	IIIB	IIIB
M1 (ipsilateral lung)	T4	IIIA (IV)	IIIA (IV)	IIIB (IV)	IIIB (IV)
T4 (pleural effusion)	M1a	IV (IIIB)	IV (IIIB)	IV (IIIB)	IV (IIIB)
M1 (contralateral lung)	M1a	IV	IV	IV	IV
M1 (distant)	M1b	IV	IV	IV	IV

© International Association for the Study of Lung Cancer

☐ Change in classification with 7th edition of TNM from 6th edition in ( )

Proceedings leading up to and culminating in the 7th edition of TNM staging classifications were funded by a grant from Eli Lilly and Company to IASLC. Lilly had no input into the proceedings or the TNM staging classifications. This material is provided as an educational service of Lilly USA, LLC, with the permission of IASLC.

Fig. 1. (*A, B*) Mediastinal lymph node grading. (*Courtesy of* the International Association for the Study of Lung Cancer.)

because glycolysis is upregulated (the Warburg effect). Cells with increased metabolic activity (ie, inflammatory and some malignancies) appear brighter than the surrounding tissues. Ultimately, the FDG is extruded from the cell, filtered by the glomerulus, and excreted in the urine.

PET may be more sensitive than CT because it can detect metastatic disease in lymph nodes of normal size, thus overcoming one of the major limitations of CT scans.[7] Chin and colleagues[8] found that PET, when used to stage mediastinal lymph nodes, was 78% sensitive and 81% specific with a negative predictive value of 89%.

B

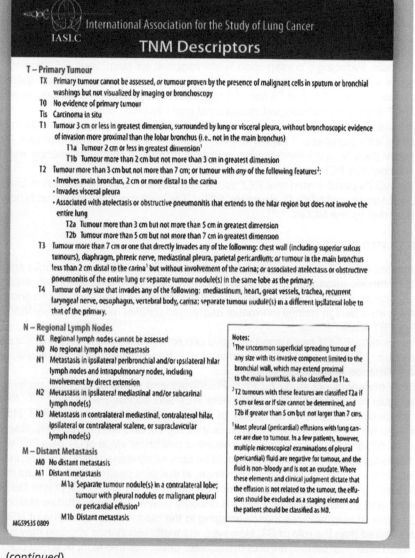

International Association for the Study of Lung Cancer
IASLC
TNM Descriptors

T – Primary Tumour

TX   Primary tumour cannot be assessed, or tumour proven by the presence of malignant cells in sputum or bronchial washings but not visualized by imaging or bronchoscopy

T0   No evidence of primary tumour

Tis   Carcinoma in situ

T1   Tumour 3 cm or less in greatest dimension, surrounded by lung or visceral pleura, without bronchoscopic evidence of invasion more proximal than the lobar bronchus (i.e., not in the main bronchus)

   T1a   Tumour 2 cm or less in greatest dimension[1]

   T1b   Tumour more than 2 cm but not more than 3 cm in greatest dimension

T2   Tumour more than 3 cm but not more than 7 cm; or tumour with any of the following features[2]:
   • Involves main bronchus, 2 cm or more distal to the carina
   • Invades visceral pleura
   • Associated with atelectasis or obstructive pneumonitis that extends to the hilar region but does not involve the entire lung

   T2a   Tumour more than 3 cm but not more than 5 cm in greatest dimension
   T2b   Tumour more than 5 cm but not more than 7 cm in greatest dimension

T3   Tumour more than 7 cm or one that directly invades any of the following: chest wall (including superior sulcus tumours), diaphragm, phrenic nerve, mediastinal pleura, parietal pericardium; or tumour in the main bronchus less than 2 cm distal to the carina[1] but without involvement of the carina; or associated atelectasis or obstructive pneumonitis of the entire lung or separate tumour nodule(s) in the same lobe as the primary.

T4   Tumour of any size that invades any of the following: mediastinum, heart, great vessels, trachea, recurrent laryngeal nerve, oesophagus, vertebral body, carina; separate tumour nodule(s) in a different ipsilateral lobe to that of the primary.

N – Regional Lymph Nodes

NX   Regional lymph nodes cannot be assessed

N0   No regional lymph node metastasis

N1   Metastasis in ipsilateral peribronchial and/or ipsilateral hilar lymph nodes and intrapulmonary nodes, including involvement by direct extension

N2   Metastasis in ipsilateral mediastinal and/or subcarinal lymph node(s)

N3   Metastasis in contralateral mediastinal, contralateral hilar, ipsilateral or contralateral scalene, or supraclavicular lymph node(s)

M – Distant Metastasis

M0   No distant metastasis

M1   Distant metastasis

   M1a   Separate tumour nodule(s) in a contralateral lobe; tumour with pleural nodules or malignant pleural or pericardial effusion[3]

   M1b   Distant metastasis

MG59535 0809

> **Notes:**
> [1] The uncommon superficial spreading tumour of any size with its invasive component limited to the bronchial wall, which may extend proximal to the main bronchus, is also classified as T1a.
>
> [2] T2 tumours with these features are classified T2a if 5 cm or less or if size cannot be determined, and T2b if greater than 5 cm but not larger than 7 cms.
>
> [3] Most pleural (pericardial) effusions with lung cancer are due to tumour. In a few patients, however, multiple microscopical examinations of pleural (pericardial) fluid are negative for tumour, and the fluid is non-bloody and is not an exudate. Where these elements and clinical judgment dictate that the effusion is not related to the tumour, the effusion should be excluded as a staging element and the patient should be classified as M0.

Fig. 1. (continued)

Kernstine and colleagues compared PET scan for identifying N2 and N3 disease in NSCLC.[9,10] The PET scan was found to be more sensitive than the CT scan for identifying mediastinal node disease (70% vs 65%).

PET has a good negative predictive value, but poor positive predictive value.[11] Some clinicians have suggested that patients with positive mediastinal PET scan results may be treated as stage III (with definitive chemoradiation or with induction therapy followed by surgery) without histologic confirmation of N2 disease or exclusion of N3 disease. There is no evidence in the literature to support this approach. False-positive results may be obtained when patients present with obstructive pneumonia and inflammatory disease. False-positive results are relatively common with

PET, which could lead to the assignment of an inappropriately high stage of disease, resulting in a missed opportunity for surgical cure.

This problem was addressed by Gonzalez-Stawinski,[12] who found that a strategy to equate a positive mediastinal PET scan result with stage III disease would result in inappropriate therapy in most (52%) patients.

Thus, a positive PET is not sufficient to make a diagnosis of mediastinal lymph node metastasis. Pathologic confirmation is still required for suspicious PET findings. For patients with primary tumors at high risk of mediastinal nodal disease (peripheral T2a, central T1ab, T2, and T3 lesions) mediastinoscopy is recommended even if the PET-CT scan does not suggest mediastinal node involvement.

In contrast, because of the low prior probability of lymph node involvement in patients with peripheral T1a, N0 lesions[13] current National Comprehensive Cancer Network (NCCN) guidelines permit omission of routine mediastinoscopy for those with a negative PET scan.

The NCCN panel stated that PET scans can play a role in the evaluation and more accurate staging of NSCLC. However, PET-CT is even more sensitive and is now recommended by the NCCN.[14–16]

INTEGRATED PET-CT

Integrated PET-CT is a modality that combines PET and CT providing both anatomic and metabolic information. Integrated PET-CT has the anatomic detail required to designate the primary tumor T stage. It also distinguishes malignant lesions (increased uptake) from benign lesions (normal or decreased uptake) more accurately than either CT or PET alone.[17,18]

Integrated PET-CT has a good negative predictive value, but a poor positive predictive value.[19–23] The use of PET alone may lead to frequent false-positive results, and an overestimation of the stage of disease.

In an observational study by Pozo-Rodriguez and coworkers,[20] 132 patients with potentially resectable NSCLC underwent PET and contrast-enhanced CT, followed by mediastinoscopy. The sensitivity of CT plus PET, CT alone, and PET alone for the detection of lymph node metastases was 98, 86, and 94, respectively. Specificity was 44, 67, and 59, respectively. The negative predictive value of CT plus PET was 98.

If patients with advanced disease could be accurately staged using PET-CT, inappropriate surgery could be avoided.[14] However, at this time positive PET-CT scan findings still need pathologic confirmation. Precisely how PET-CT scans will fit into the overall staging and surveillance of NSCLC will become clearer as newer studies mature.

The role of magnetic resonance imaging in the diagnosis and staging of NSCLC is more limited than the role of CT. However, magnetic resonance imaging may be helpful when brain metastasis, adrenal metastasis, chest wall invasion, or spinal cord invasion is suspected.

OTHER NONINVASIVE OR MINIMALLY INVASIVE TECHNIQUES
Endoscopic Ultrasound–guided Fine-needle Aspiration

Patients with suspicious mediastinal lymphadenopathy suggested by either size on CT or metabolically active lymph nodes by PET generally undergo lymph node sampling by mediastinoscopy. Endoscopic ultrasound–guided fine-needle aspiration (EUS–FNA) biopsy is a relatively new alternative to obtaining a tissue diagnosis for suspicious mediastinal findings. A minimally invasive modality is often preferred by patients because it is painless, it can be performed on outpatient basis, and it does not require general anesthesia.

Endoscopic ultrasound is performed with an echoendoscope and can obtain reliable images at a depth ranging from 3 mm to 8 cm from the transducer. The posterior mediastinum is visualized through the esophageal wall. The heart, pleura, spine, and vascular structures can be readily identified. EUS-FNA provides an effective method of sampling lymph nodes in the posterior mediastinum (levels 8 and 9) and subcarina (level 7) sites that are particularly susceptible to metastasis. In addition, it may on occasion be able to sample lymph nodes in the aortopulmonary window (level 5).

Metastases to mediastinal lymph nodes are identified by EUS-FNA with an accuracy of 83% to 97%, and a sensitivity of 84% to 92%.[24–28] Additionally, visualization of the primary tumor with EUS can identify tumors that invade mediastinal structures, such as the left atrium, aorta, centrally located pulmonary vessels, vertebra, and esophagus with a sensitivity and specificity of 87% and 98%, respectively.[9] This degree of tumor invasion defines T4 lesions and precludes curative surgery.

The value of EUS in staging patients who have NSCLC but no enlarged mediastinal lymph nodes according to CT, is uncertain because most clinical experience and data are from patients with mediastinal lymphadenopathy.

Endobronchial Ultrasound

Endobronchial ultrasound (EBUS) is a bronchoscopic technique that uses ultrasound to visualize structures within and adjacent to the airway wall.[29,30] Similar to EUS, EBUS can be used to obtain a tissue diagnosis for patients who have positive CT-PET findings.

EBUS-guided transbronchial needle aspiration (EBUS-TBNA) is best suited for sampling lymph nodes in the anterior or superior mediastinum (high mediastinal, paratracheal, subcarinal, and hilar lymph nodes).

In a prospective cohort study of 108 patients, EBUS-guided TBNA successfully sampled 163 mediastinal or hilar lymph nodes from 105 patients with known or suspected NSCLC.[31] Malignancy was detected with a sensitivity, specificity, positive predictive value, negative predictive value, and diagnostic accuracy of 95%, 100%, 100%, 90%, and 96%, respectively. As a result, 50 more invasive sampling (eg, mediastinoscopy and thoracoscopy) procedures were unnecessary.

EBUS-TBNA and EUS-FNA are often combined because EUS has better access to posterior and inferior mediastinal lymph nodes. The combination seems to improve the diagnostic yield, compared with either procedure alone.[32,33]

The wall of the airways can be visualized with EBUS,[30,34,35] which allows for accurate determination of the distance from the carina to the proximal portion of the tumor. This distance may determine whether the lesion is T2 or T3, which can impact the disease stage.

EBUS may permit discrimination of tumor invasion into the airway wall from external compression. In a prospective cohort study of 131 consecutive patients who had either invasion or external compression of an airway by an adjacent tumor, EBUS identified airway wall invasion with a sensitivity, specificity, and accuracy of 89%, 100%, and 94%, respectively.[36] In comparison, CT scan identified airway wall invasion with a sensitivity, specificity, and accuracy of only 75%, 28%, and 51%, respectively.

The positive predictive value of EUS-EBUS tissue diagnosis is excellent. However, in patients with negative findings conventional mediastinoscopy should be considered to confirm the findings of a positive CT or PET scan.[37,38]

SUMMARY

All patients with a new diagnosis of NSCLC should have a CT scan of the chest and mediastinum extending through the liver and adrenals. Scans should be done with intravenous contrast with 5-mm cuts or smaller. PET or PET-CT should be preformed for all patients diagnosed with NSCLC. Patients with T1a peripheral tumors and negative lymph adenopathy by PET may omit further mediastinal staging. At this time there is not enough evidence to omit pathologic staging of the mediastinum for central T1a, T2, T3, and T4 tumors with PET-negative lymph nodes. Patients with PET-positive mediastinal lymphadenopathy still require pathologic conformation of lymph node metastasis. Mediastinoscopy remains the gold standard for lymph node evaluation; however, in centers with skilled clinicians EBUS and EUS may be used to confirm CT or PET findings. At this time negative findings on EBUS and EUS should be confirmed with conventional mediastinoscopy when initiated by a positive CT or PET scan.

REFERENCES

1. Parvin DM, Bray F, Ferlay J, et al. Global cancer statistics, 2002. CA Cancer J Clin 2005;55:74.
2. Jemal A, Siegel R, Xu J, et al. Cancer statistics, 2010. CA Cancer J Clin 2010;60:277.
3. Silvestri GA, Gould MK, Margolis ML, et al. Noninvasive staging of non-small cell lung cancer: ACCP evidence-based clinical practice guidelines (2nd edition). Chest 2007;132:178S.
4. Arita T, Kuramitsu T, Kawamura M, et al. Bronchogenic carcinoma: incidence of metastases to normal sized lymph nodes. Thorax 1995;50:1267–9.
5. Dillemans B, Deneffe G, Verschakelen J, et al. Value of computed tomography and mediastinoscopy in preoperative evaluation of mediastinal nodes in non-small cell lung cancer. Eur J Cardiothorac Surg 1994;8:37–42.
6. Kerr K, Lamb D, Wathen C, et al. Pathologic assessment of mediastinal lymph nodes in lung cancer: implications for non-invasive mediastinal staging. Thorax 1992;47:337–41.
7. Patz EF Jr, Lowe VJ, Goodman PC, et al. Thoracic nodal staging with PET imaging with 18FDG in patients with bronchogenic carcinoma. Chest 1995;108:1617.
8. Chin R Jr, Ward R, Keyes JW, et al. Mediastinal staging of non-small-cell lung cancer with positron emission tomography. Am J Respir Crit Care Med 1995;152(6 Pt 1):2090–6.
9. Kernstine KH, Stanford W, Mullan BF, et al. PET, CT, and MRI with Combidex for mediastinal staging in non-small cell lung carcinoma. Ann Thorac Surg 1999;68(3):1022–8.
10. Kernstine KH, Trapp JF, Croft DR. Comparison of positron emission tomography (PET) and computed tomography (CT) to identify N2 and N3 disease in non small cell lung cancer (NSCLC). J Clin Oncol (Meeting Abstracts) 1998;17:459.
11. Vansteenkiste JF, Stroobants SS. PET scan in lung cancer: current recommendations and innovation. J Thorac Oncol 2006;1:71.
12. Gonzalez-Stawinski GV. A comparative analysis of positron emission tomography and mediastinoscopy in staging non–small cell lung cancer. J Thorac Cardiovasc Surg 2003;126(6):1900–5.
13. Meyers BF, Haddad F, Siegel BA, et al. Cost-effectiveness of routine mediastinoscopy in computed tomography- and positron emission tomography-screened patients with stage I lung cancer. J Thorac Cardiovasc Surg 2006;131(4):822–9 [discussion: 822–9].
14. Maziak DE, Darling GE, Inculet RI, et al. Positron emission tomography in staging early lung cancer: a randomized trial. Ann Intern Med 2009;151(4):221–8.

15. Fischer B, Lassen U, Mortensen J, et al. Preoperative staging of lung cancer with combined PET-CT. N Engl J Med 2009;361(1):32–9.
16. De Wever W, Stroobants S, Coolen J, et al. Integrated PET/CT in the staging of nonsmall cell lung cancer: technical aspects and clinical integration. Eur Respir J 2009;33(1):201–12.
17. Yi CA, Lee KS, Kim BT, et al. Tissue characterization of solitary pulmonary nodule: comparative study between helical dynamic CT and integrated PET/CT. J Nucl Med 2006;47:443.
18. Kim SK, Allen-Auerbach M, Goldin J, et al. Accuracy of PET/CT in characterization of solitary pulmonary lesions. J Nucl Med 2007;48:214.
19. Gámez C, Rosell R, Fernández A, et al. PET/CT fusion scan in lung cancer: current recommendations and innovations. J Thorac Oncol 2006;1:74.
20. Pozo-Rodríguez F, Martín de Nicolás JL, Sánchez-Nistal MA, et al. Accuracy of helical computed tomography and [18F] fluorodeoxyglucose positron emission tomography for identifying lymph node mediastinal metastases in potentially resectable non-small-cell lung cancer. J Clin Oncol 2005;23:8348.
21. Antoch G, Stattaus J, Nemat AT, et al. Non-small cell lung cancer: dual-modality PET/CT in preoperative staging. Radiology 2003;229:526.
22. Lardinois D, Weder W, Hany TF, et al. Staging of non-small-cell lung cancer with integrated positron-emission tomography and computed tomography. N Engl J Med 2003;348:2500.
23. Cerfolio RJ, Ojha B, Bryant AS, et al. The accuracy of integrated PET-CT compared with dedicated PET alone for the staging of patients with nonsmall cell lung cancer. Ann Thorac Surg 2004;78:1017.
24. Devereaux BM, Leblanc JK, Yousif E, et al. Clinical utility of EUS-guided fine-needle aspiration of mediastinal masses in the absence of known pulmonary malignancy. Gastrointest Endosc 2002;56:397.
25. Gress FG, Savides TJ, Sandler A, et al. Endoscopic ultrasonography, fine-needle aspiration biopsy guided by endoscopic ultrasonography, and computed tomography in the preoperative staging of non-small-cell lung cancer: a comparison study. Ann Intern Med 1997;127:604.
26. Fritscher-Ravens A, Bohuslavizki KH, Brandt L, et al. Mediastinal lymph node involvement in potentially resectable lung cancer: comparison of CT, positron emission tomography, and endoscopic ultrasonography with and without fine-needle aspiration. Chest 2003;123:442.
27. Eloubeidi MA, Cerfolio RJ, Chen VK, et al. Endoscopic ultrasound-guided fine needle aspiration of mediastinal lymph node in patients with suspected lung cancer after positron emission tomography and computed tomography scans. Ann Thorac Surg 2005;79:263.
28. Varadarajulu S, Schmulewitz N, Wildi SM, et al. Accuracy of EUS in staging of T4 lung cancer. Gastrointest Endosc 2004;59:345.
29. Hürter T, Hanrath P. Endobronchial sonography: feasibility and preliminary results. Thorax 1992;47:565.
30. Kurimoto N, Murayama M, Yoshioka S, et al. Assessment of usefulness of endobronchial ultrasonography in determination of depth of tracheobronchial tumor invasion. Chest 1999;115:1500.
31. Yasufuku K, Chiyo M, Koh E, et al. Endobronchial ultrasound guided transbronchial needle aspiration for staging of lung cancer. Lung Cancer 2005;50:347.
32. Wallace MB, Pascual JM, Raimondo M, et al. Minimally invasive endoscopic staging of suspected lung cancer. JAMA 2008;299:540.

33. Vilmann P, Krasnik M, Larsen SS, et al. Transesophageal endoscopic ultrasound-guided fine-needle aspiration (EUS-FNA) and endobronchial ultrasound-guided transbronchial needle aspiration (EBUS-TBNA) biopsy: a combined approach in the evaluation of mediastinal lesions. Endoscopy 2005;37:833.

34. Baba M, Sekine Y, Suzuki M, et al. Correlation between endobronchial ultrasonography (EBUS) images and histologic findings in normal and tumor-invaded bronchial wall. Lung Cancer 2002;35:65.

35. Tanaka F, Muro K, Yamasaki S, et al. Evaluation of tracheo-bronchial wall invasion using transbronchial ultrasonography (TBUS). Eur J Cardiothorac Surg 2000;17: 570.

36. Herth F, Ernst A, Schulz M, et al. Endobronchial ultrasound reliably differentiates between airway infiltration and compression by tumor. Chest 2003;123:458.

37. Rintoul RC, Tournoy KG, El Daly H, et al. EBUS-TBNA for the clarification of PET positive intra-thoracic lymph nodes-an international multi-centre experience. J Thorac Oncol 2009;4(1):44–8.

38. Medford AR, Bennett JA, Free CM, et al. Mediastinal staging procedures in lung cancer: EBUS, TBNA and mediastinoscopy. Curr Opin Pulm Med 2009;15: 334–42.

Surgical Staging for Non–Small Cell Lung Cancer

Ziv Gamliel, MD

KEYWORDS

• Surgical • Staging • Lung cancer

In non–small cell lung cancer, as with many other malignancies, prognosis is dependent on disease stage.[1] It has been proposed that recent improvements in stage-specific survival are attributable to increased accuracy of pretreatment staging of non–small cell lung cancer.[2] As the treatment of non–small cell lung cancer has become increasingly stage specific, accurate pretreatment staging has become increasingly important.[3]

Modern pretreatment staging of non–small cell lung cancer utilizes a variety of methods to evaluate patients for possible spread of tumor to distant sites, or to local and regional lymph nodes. Staging methods include imaging with computed tomography (CT), magnetic resonance imaging (MRI), and positron emission tomography (PET) scans. Lesions suspicious for nodal involvement or distant metastatic spread that are identified on imaging are then biopsied for confirmation. Often a needle biopsy of such suspicious lesions can be achieved percutaneously under ultrasound or CT guidance, or endoscopically with the help of transesophageal endoscopic ultrasonography (EUS) or endobronchial ultrasonography (EBUS). Although it is possible to demonstrate the presence of metastatic disease with a positive needle biopsy, the absence of metastatic disease must be proven more rigorously, usually with a surgical biopsy.

SCALENE NODE BIOPSY

Non–small cell lung cancer may involve supraclavicular or scalene lymph nodes.[4] Under such circumstances, cure cannot be achieved by surgical resection.[5] Involvement of supraclavicular lymph nodes with metastatic cancer may be suspected if the lymph nodes appear enlarged on CT scan or hypermetabolic on PET scan. Percutaneous needle biopsy of involved supraclavicular lymph nodes, with or without ultrasound guidance, is often diagnostic of metastatic disease. In some instances, however, a hypermetabolic supraclavicular node may not be large enough to allow

The author has nothing to disclose.
Division of Thoracic Surgery, St Joseph Medical Center, 7501 Osler Drive, Towson, MD 21204, USA
E-mail address: zivgamliel@catholichealth.net

Surg Oncol Clin N Am 20 (2011) 691–700
doi:10.1016/j.soc.2011.07.010
1055-3207/11/$ – see front matter © 2011 Elsevier Inc. All rights reserved.

surgonc.theclinics.com

successful percutaneous needle biopsy. Under such circumstances, a formal scalene node biopsy may be helpful.

Technique

With the patient in the supine position under general endotracheal anesthesia, the neck is hyperextended by placing a roll under the shoulders. The arms are tucked at the patient's sides, the head is turned to the contralateral side, and the neck and upper chest are prepared and draped. A 3-cm horizontal supraclavicular incision is made over the lateral border of the sternocleidomastoid muscle. The muscle is retracted medially; to enhance exposure, its lateral fibers may be divided.

The scalene fat pad is bordered by the subclavian vein inferiorly, the internal jugular vein medially, and the omohyoid muscle laterally. Its deep border is formed by the scalenus anticus muscle, with the phrenic nerve lying in its sheath. The fat pad is excised using blunt dissection aided by judicious use of electrocautery. The transverse cervical and inferior thyroid vessels typically course through the scalene fat pad, and may be ligated and divided. Care should be taken to avoid injury to the phrenic nerve. On the left side, special care should be taken to avoid injury to the thoracic duct.

After the fat pad has been completely excised and hemostasis has been secured, the incision is closed in layers. Placement of a drain is not required. The platysma muscle and subcutaneous fat are reconstituted using a running absorbable suture. The skin is closed using a running subcuticular absorbable suture. Steristrips may be used, and a light adhesive bandage is applied.

MEDIASTINOSCOPY

In the presence of mediastinal lymph node involvement, it is unlikely that non–small cell lung cancer can be cured by surgical resection alone.[6] In such circumstances, neoadjuvant therapy is generally recommended before surgical resection is undertaken. The usefulness of PET scans for pretreatment staging of the mediastinum is limited by a high rate of false positives.[7,8] Moreover, the absence of abnormal hypermetabolism in mediastinal lymph nodes does not exclude the possibility of microscopic lymph node involvement. In recent years, transbronchial needle aspiration (TBNA) under EBUS guidance (EBUS-TBNA) of mediastinal lymph nodes has been utilized with increasing frequency. The positive predictive value of this method is practically 100%, but the negative predictive value is variable.[7,9–11] To date, mediastinoscopy remains the most reliable method for excluding mediastinal lymph node involvement with metastatic tumor. With the advent of the videomediastinoscope, this procedure can now be done under video guidance. Although some believe that this is superior to standard mediastinoscopy, the most important contribution of this technique is the opportunity to teach a very dangerous and complex procedure without the surgeon "having to take their eye off" the field.

Technique

With the patient in the supine position under general endotracheal anesthesia, the endotracheal tube is carefully secured with adhesive tape at the left side of the mouth. The patient is positioned at the extreme head of the operating table, and the neck is hyperextended by placing a roll under the shoulders. A pillow is placed under the knees, and safety straps are securely fastened above and below the patellae. The operating table is turned so that the anesthesiologist is at the patient's left side while the surgeon stands at the head. The anterior cervical and pectoral regions are prepared and draped.

A 2-cm horizontal incision is made in the suprasternal notch, below the thyroid isthmus and above the innominate artery, at a level where the trachea is most readily palpable. Ideally the incision can be hidden in a prominent skin crease. The incision is deepened through the platysma muscle. Anterior jugular veins may be ligated and divided. The strap muscles are separated in the midline with electrocautery. The pretracheal fascia is incised transversely with scissors. Blunt digital dissection is used to develop a pretracheal plane inferiorly.

The mediastinoscope is introduced into the pretracheal space, and additional blunt dissection is carried out with the insulated suction cautery to expose the anterior walls of the mainstem bronchi and the anterior aspect of the subcarinal space. A bronchial artery is usually seen coursing anterior to the proximal left mainstem bronchus into the subcarinal space. Before dividing this vessel with electrocautery, consideration should be given to ligating it using a short 5-mm endoscopic clip applier.

The subcarinal lymph node "packet" is dissected bluntly from the medial wall of the left mainstem bronchus and is reflected off of the anterior esophageal wall. Next, the subcarinal lymph node packet is dissected bluntly from the medial wall of the right mainstem bronchus. Electrocautery may be used to control the many bronchial vessels typically found in the subcarinal space. Care should be taken to avoid injury to the anterior esophageal wall and the posterior pericardium. Finally, the subcarinal lymph node packet is completely removed using biopsy forceps. Hemostasis is completed using electrocautery, and may be facilitated by epinephrine-soaked gauze packing.

Attention is turned to the paratracheal lymph nodes on the side contralateral to the primary lung tumor. Paratracheal lymph nodes are bluntly dissected, commencing inferiorly and proceeding cephalad. After the paratracheal nodes are completely dissected and excised from the contralateral side, attention is turned to the side ipsilateral to the primary tumor. Dissection of the right paratracheal nodes should include a careful search for lower pretracheal (station 3A) nodes. These nodes are typically found anteriorly, just medial to the right lower paratracheal (station 4R) nodes, and are dissected bluntly off the posterior pericardium.

On the right side, special care should be taken to avoid injury to the azygos vein and superior vena cava. The left recurrent laryngeal nerve courses especially close to the left lower paratracheal nodes. More distal dissection in the paratracheal space leads to the superior branches of the pulmonary artery. Using patient and gentle blunt dissection while minimizing the use of electrocautery, it is usually possible to mobilize intact lymph nodes almost completely before they are biopsied. In this manner, bleeding and recurrent laryngeal nerve injury can usually be avoided.

Hemostasis is completed with judicious use of electrocautery, aided by epinephrine-soaked gauze packing. A careful account is made of all packing as it is removed. With good hemostasis in effect, the mediastinoscope is removed and the incision is closed in layers. The strap muscles may be approximated using a single interrupted absorbable suture. The platysma muscle is reconstituted using a running absorbable suture. The skin is closed using a running subcuticular absorbable suture. Steristrips may be used and a Band-Aid is applied.

REDO MEDIASTINOSCOPY

When the spread of non–small cell lung cancer is limited to the mediastinal lymph nodes, neoadjuvant chemotherapy or concurrent chemoradiotherapy has been used successfully to downstage the disease, making it amenable to cure with surgical resection.[12] The persistence of mediastinal lymph node involvement following neoadjuvant therapy is predictive of a low likelihood of cure with surgical resection.[13,14] Typically the presence of mediastinal lymph node involvement is initially determined by pretreatment mediastinoscopy.

Following neoadjuvant therapy, restaging the mediastinum can be challenging. It is often unclear whether residual hypermetabolism in mediastinal lymph nodes is caused by inflammation resulting from neoadjuvant therapy, or is due to persistent mediastinal lymph node involvement with tumor.[15] Even in cases where previously involved mediastinal lymph nodes are no longer hypermetabolic, the presence of residual microscopic involvement must be suspected. To avoid futile high-risk lung resection, reliable exclusion of persistent mediastinal lymph node involvement is essential.

In some cases, EBUS-TBNA of enlarged, hypermetabolic mediastinal lymph nodes can successfully identify persistent involvement with metastatic tumor. However, when posttreatment EBUS-TBNA is negative or equivocal in the face of enlarged or hypermetabolic lymph nodes, larger mediastinal lymph node biopsies might be desirable. In certain cases, redo mediastinoscopy might be the preferred approach to obtain these biopsies.[16,17]

Due to the presence of dense fibrosis resulting from the initial mediastinoscopy and from neoadjuvant radiotherapy, performing a redo mediastinoscopy can be daunting. Concerns have been raised about the increased risk of recurrent laryngeal nerve injury[18] and major venous or pulmonary arterial injury, as well as the inability to successfully reach all of the relevant mediastinal lymph node stations.[19] Refuting such concerns, several investigators have published case series suggesting that redo mediastinoscopy can be performed safely and can effectively predict the presence or absence of persistent mediastinal lymph node involvement.[20–22] The need for redo mediastinoscopy can be avoided if pretreatment mediastinal lymph node involvement is demonstrated by EBUS-TBNA; mediastinoscopy can then be reserved for posttreatment restaging.[23,24]

Technique

Although the technique of redo mediastinoscopy is similar in most respects to the technique of initial mediastinoscopy, there are several special considerations that must be taken into account. The presence of dense fibrosis can make it difficult to gain access to the pretracheal space from the neck after prior mediastinoscopy. It may be more likely that anterior jugular veins will have to be divided. Strap muscles themselves might have to be divided. Dissection should be conducted directly on the anterior tracheal wall so as to avoid major vascular injury. Electrocautery should be used with great caution. Ultimately, it is usually possible to gain access to the pretracheal space and the subcarinal space below.

After reaching the subcarinal space, great care should be taken in dissecting the paratracheal spaces on either side. On the right side, injury to the azygos arch or superior vena cava is to be avoided. On the left side, recurrent laryngeal nerve injury is to be avoided. Lymph nodes are often more adherent than at initial mediastinoscopy; it is often wiser to biopsy only portions of lymph nodes rather than to attempt excisional biopsy of entire nodes. In any case, the key to making safe progress is patience and persistence.

ANTERIOR MEDIASTINOTOMY (CHAMBERLAIN PROCEDURE)

Standard transcervical mediastinoscopy does not reach the aortopulmonary window (station 5) or prevascular (station 6) lymph nodes. Particularly in the case of left lung cancers, it is essential to evaluate these nodal stations for possible tumor involvement before final treatment decisions are made. Before the widespread use of diagnostic thoracoscopy, anterior mediastinotomy was the preferred approach for sampling these lymph node stations.[25] This technique does not require inpatient admission and can be combined with transcervical mediastinoscopy. It does not allow access to paraesophageal (station 8) or inferior pulmonary ligament (station 9) lymph nodes. Nowadays it is a useful approach when thoracoscopic staging of left-sided lung cancers is not feasible.

Technique

With the patient in the supine position under general double-lumen tube endotracheal anesthesia, the arms are tucked securely at the patient's sides. The anterior chest is prepared and draped in the usual fashion. A 4-cm incision is made directly overlying the left second costal cartilage. The incision is deepened through the subcutaneous tissue with electrocautery. A muscle-splitting incision is made through the fibers of the pectoralis major muscle, exposing the costal cartilage. Long-acting local anesthetic can be infiltrated along the second neurovascular bundle. The perichondrium is opened with a scalpel and is dissected bluntly off the cartilage. After the costal cartilage is completely encircled, it is disarticulated from the sternum medially and from the rib laterally. The cartilage is removed in its entirety.

Ventilation is withheld from the left lung, and the posterior or deep side of the perichondrium is opened sharply, avoiding injury to the left lung as the left pleural cavity is entered. A mediastinoscope is introduced through the incision into the left pleural cavity and is used to inspect the aortopulmonary window. Using an insulated suction cautery, any visualized prevascular (station 6) and/or aortopulmonary window (station 5) nodes are dissected bluntly, taking care to avoid injury to the left phrenic nerve and the left recurrent laryngeal nerve. Biopsies are obtained with cup biopsy forceps. Hemostasis is completed with judicious use of electrocautery.

After the desired biopsies have been obtained, ventilation of the left lung is resumed. The posterior or deep aspect of the perichondrium is closed around a 20F chest tube, using a running absorbable suture. A Valsalva maneuver is performed, expelling as much free intrapleural air as possible. While maintaining the Valsalva maneuver, the chest tube is rapidly removed and the running suture is tied. The subcutaneous layer of the incision is closed with a running absorbable suture. The skin is reapproximated with a running subcuticular absorbable suture. Steristrips and a Band-Aid dressing are applied.

STAGING THORACOSCOPY

Standard mediastinoscopy cannot provide access to aortopulmonary window (station 5), prevascular (station 6), posterior subcarinal (station 7p), paraesophageal (station 8), or inferior pulmonary ligament (station 9) nodes. While some of these lymph node stations (stations 7p, 8, and 9) are accessible to EUS, others are not (stations 5 and 6). Before undertaking surgical resection for lung cancer with curative intent, it is essential to ascertain that these lymph node stations are free from involvement with metastatic disease.

Staging thoracoscopy provides an ideal approach to the aforementioned lymph node stations.[26,27] Because the preparation for staging thoracoscopy is virtually identical to that for lung resection, it is often performed at the same sitting as the initial step in lung resection. Once thoracoscopic mediastinal lymph node sampling has been completed, the patient is kept under anesthesia while frozen-section histology is used to determine whether lung resection is to be performed forthwith, or whether neoadjuvant therapy will be required. In addition, this technique can be used when a redo mediastinoscopy is not feasible after neoadjuvant therapy.

Technique

Under general double-lumen tube endotracheal anesthesia, placement of a contralateral radial arterial line and/or ipsilateral jugular venous line should be considered. The patient is placed in the lateral decubitus as for lateral thoracotomy, and the chest wall is prepared and draped. Ventilation is confined to the contralateral lung. A 12-mm thoracoscopy port is established in the seventh intercostal space in the posterior axillary line. A 10-mm operating thoracoscope with a 5-mm working channel is introduced, and the visceral and parietal pleural surfaces are carefully inspected. Any suspicious parietal pleural nodules are biopsied using a 5-mm cup forceps passed through the working channel of the scope.

In the absence of any evidence of parietal pleural metastases, a second 12-mm thoracoscopy port is established in the fifth intercostal space in the anterolateral line. The surface of the lung is carefully inspected, in search of subpleural lung metastases. A curved (Landreneau) lung grasper is introduced through the second port site. The thoracoscope and lung grasper may be introduced via either thoracoscopy port site to facilitate visualization and retraction. Any suspicious subpleural lung nodule is biopsied via wedge resection. The nodule is grasped using a long 5-mm (Davis & Geck, Danbury, CT) grasper passed through the working channel of the thoracoscope. An endostapler is introduced through the other thoracoscopy port. A plastic endobag is used to retrieve any wedge resection specimens.

In the absence of any pleural or lung metastases, attention is turned to mediastinal lymph node sampling. The thoracoscope is introduced through the inferior port site and the lung grasper is introduced through the anterolateral port site. The inferolateral edge of the lower lobe is grasped and retracted cephalad, placing the inferior pulmonary ligament on tension. Endoscopic scissors are introduced through the working channel of the thoracoscope and are used to divide the inferior pulmonary ligament from its inferior edge cephalad. Electrocautery may be used judiciously. As dissection proceeds cephalad, paraesophageal (station 8) lymph nodes may be identified. As dissection of the inferior pulmonary ligament approaches the inferior pulmonary vein, its lymph node (station 9) usually comes into view.

Using blunt dissection, the lymph node to be biopsied is completely mobilized. The working channel of the thoracoscope is used to pass endoscopic scissors, a long 5-mm suction irrigation device, long 5-mm Kittner cotton-tipped dissectors, or a long 5-mm cup forceps. Small vessels coursing into the lymph node are divided using electrocautery. The completely dissected lymph node is grasped using long 5-mm cup forceps, passed through the working channel of the thoracoscope. The thoracoscope is removed from the chest, retrieving the intact lymph node behind it in the grip of the long 5-mm cup forceps.

At this point, attention is turned to the subcarinal space. The thoracoscope is reintroduced through the lower thoracoscopy port. The lung grasper is used via the anterolateral thoracoscopy port to grasp the superior segment of the lower lobe and retract it anteriorly. The table is tilted slightly toward the patient's front. Using endoscopic scissors passed through the working channel of the thoracoscope, the mediastinal pleura overlying the posterior subcarinal space is opened. Blunt dissection and retrieval of the subcarinal (station 7) lymph node "packet" is carried out as for the inferior pulmonary ligament node.

On the right side, the right paratracheal (stations 2R and 4R) lymph node packet may be dissected and retrieved using similar technique. Here, the lung grasper is used to grasp the posterior segment of the upper lobe and retract it anteroinferiorly. The paratracheal lymph node "packet" is dissected from the superior border of the azygos arch, from the posterior border of the superior vena cava, from the anterolateral border of the trachea, and from the lateral border of the ascending aorta.

On the left side, the aortopulmonary window (station 5) and prevascular (station 6) nodes can be dissected and retrieved. This time, the thoracoscope is passed via the anterolateral thoracoscopy port. The lung grasper is passed via the inferolateral port and is used to grasp the anteromedial edge of the left upper lobe and retract it posteroinferiorly, taking care not to avulse or overcompress the pulmonary artery. Dissection and retrieval of the aortopulmonary and prevascular nodes is carried out as already described, taking special care to avoid injury to the phrenic nerve and to the recurrent laryngeal nerve below the aortic arch.

When all reachable lymph node stations have been sampled and with good hemostasis in effect, intercostal nerve blocks are infiltrated along the neurovascular bundles above and below each thoracoscopy port site incision. This maneuver is best accomplished percutaneously under thoracoscopic visualization. The thoracoscope is then passed via the anterolateral thoracoscopy port site as a straight 32F chest tube is passed via the inferolateral thoracoscopy port site incision. The tube is guided posterosuperiorly toward the apex. The thoracoscope is removed and the lung is expanded. The chest tube is secured to the skin. The anterolateral port site incision is closed in layers, using a figure-of-8 absorbable suture to close the subcutaneous fat, and a running subcuticular absorbable suture to reapproximate the skin. Steristrips may be used, and a Band-Aid is applied.

APPLICATION OF SURGICAL STAGING TECHNIQUES

The first step in staging non–small cell lung cancer is to rule out distant metastatic disease. In general, this can be accomplished through various imaging techniques including CT, PET/CT, and MRI. Suspected sites of metastatic disease can be further evaluated with percutaneous needle biopsy under CT or ultrasound guidance. Occasionally a small peripheral lung nodule suspicious for metastasis might be too small to biopsy percutaneously with a needle. In such cases, thoracoscopic lung wedge resection can be used to obtain a definite tissue diagnosis.

In the absence of distant metastatic disease, the presence of palpable cervical lymphadenopathy in suspected non–small cell lung cancer warrants ultrasound-guided percutaneous needle biopsy. In the event that needle biopsy is negative, or when hypermetabolic cervical nodes are inaccessible to needle biopsy, excisional scalene node biopsy may be considered.

When extrathoracic spread has been ruled out, pretreatment staging of non–small cell lung cancer should always include a thorough evaluation of the mediastinum. Although the use of PET/CT scans for mediastinal lymph node staging has become routine in the staging of non–small cell lung cancer, it is widely accepted that the false-positive rate is unacceptably high. Most investigators reporting on the use of PET/CT in non–small cell lung cancer recommend tissue biopsy of abnormally hypermetabolic mediastinal lymph nodes. The use of EBUS-TBNA for this purpose has been increasing. While a positive result is confirmatory, a negative result still leaves room for doubt. Mediastinoscopy remains the most trusted method of staging mediastinal lymph nodes.

Although most clinicians use mediastinoscopy selectively, some do so routinely. There is no widespread agreement about when mediastinoscopy is unnecessary. When no abnormal hypermetabolism is found in mediastinal lymph nodes, some investigators suggest that mediastinoscopy is unnecessary because of the low likelihood of finding metastatic disease.[28,29] Others argue that mediastinoscopy should be performed in patients with large, central, or upper lobe tumors or in the face of intrapulmonary (N_1) nodal involvement.[15,30,31] Still others use mediastinoscopy routinely, citing a low complication rate and a significant benefit if metastatic disease is found unexpectedly.

When no evidence of mediastinal lymph node involvement is found at mediastinoscopy, it is still necessary to rule out involvement of mediastinal lymph nodes in stations that are not accessible to mediastinoscopy. This assessment is accomplished most conveniently at the time of planned lung resection. Typically only 2 to 4 lymph node stations remain to be sampled. The results of frozen-section histology should be awaited before committing to undertake lung resection. If thoracoscopic mediastinal lymph node biopsies are positive, the planned lung resection may be aborted and deferred until after completion of neoadjuvant therapy.

With the use of adjuvant chemotherapy for stage II (and some stage I) non–small cell lung cancers, and the use of neoadjuvant therapy in stage III non–small cell lung cancer, survival rates are likely to improve. The consequence of missed lymph node involvement is understaging and undertreatment, with a potentially reduced likelihood of cure. Microscopic (rather than macroscopic) lymph node involvement is generally below the threshold of detection by radiologic imaging modalities. In such patients, the likelihood of a false-negative result using needle biopsy techniques (eg, EBUS-TBNA) is unknown. Surgical biopsy seems to be a preferable method of ruling out microscopic mediastinal lymph node involvement.

By virtue of their relatively more limited disease, non–small cell lung cancer patients who are found to have microscopic lymph node involvement are ostensibly more likely to be cured by multimodality therapy than their counterparts with macroscopic lymph node involvement. With this in mind, it seems logical that these patients in particular stand to benefit from aggressive pretreatment staging methods that are potentially more likely to identify their microscopic lymph node involvement. As long as surgical staging methods can be applied with low rates of complications and morbidity, it would seem appropriate to use them routinely in every patient who presents with nonmetastatic disease.

SUMMARY

The treatment and prognosis of non–small cell lung cancer are determined by pretreatment staging. Stage migration, resulting from the use of aggressive staging methods, has been associated with improved stage-specific survival. Although needle biopsy techniques (eg, EBUS-TBNA) are able to identify lymph node involvement, surgical staging methods such as mediastinoscopy or thoracoscopic lymph node biopsy may be more reliable in excluding lymph node involvement. Identifying even microscopic lymph node involvement before treatment begins is associated with significant ramifications on treatment and prognosis. Surgical staging methods such as mediastinoscopy and thoracoscopy can be applied with low rates of complications and morbidity. These methods should be used routinely before undertaking surgical resection of non–small cell lung cancer with curative intent.

REFERENCES

1. Mountain CF. The new international staging system for lung cancer. Surg Clin North Am 1987;67:925–35.
2. Feinstein AR, Sosin DM, Wells CK. The Will Rogers phenomenon—stage migration and new diagnostic techniques as a source of misleading statistics for survival in lung cancer. N Engl J Med 1985;312:1604–8.

3. Tsim S, O'Dowd CA, Milroy R, et al. Staging of non-small cell lung cancer (NSCLC): a review. Respir Med 2010;104:1767–74.
4. Daniels AC. A method of biopsy useful in diagnosing certain intrathoracic diseases. Dis Chest 1949;16:360–7.
5. Harken DE, Black H, Clauss R, et al. A simple cervicomediastinal exploration for tissue diagnosis of intrathoracic disease. N Engl J Med 1954;251:1041–4.
6. Carlens E. Mediastinoscopy: a method for inspection and tissue biopsy in the superior mediastinum. Dis Chest 1959;36:343–52.
7. Annema JT, van Meerbeeck JP, Rintoul RC, et al. Mediastinoscopy vs endosonography for mediastinal nodal staging of lung cancer: a randomized trial. JAMA 2010;304:2245–52.
8. Darling GE, Maziak DE, Inculet RI, et al. Positron emission tomography-computed tomography compared with invasive mediastinal staging in non-small cell lung cancer: results of mediastinal staging in the early lung positron emission tomography trial. J Thorac Oncol 2011. [Epub ahead of print].
9. Cerfolio RJ, Bryant AS, Eloubeidi MA, et al. The true false negative rates of esophageal and endobronchial ultrasound in the staging of mediastinal lymph nodes in patients with non-small cell lung cancer. Ann Thorac Surg 2010;90:427–34.
10. Defranchi SA, Edell ES, Daniels CE, et al. Mediastinoscopy in patients with lung cancer and negative endobronchial ultrasound guided needle aspiration. Ann Thorac Surg 2010;90:1753–7.
11. De Leyn P, Lardinois D, Van Schil PE, et al. ESTS guidelines for preoperative lymph node staging for non-small cell lung cancer. Eur J Cardiothorac Surg 2007;32:1–8.
12. Albain KS, Swann RS, Rusch VW, et al. Radiotherapy plus chemotherapy with or without surgical resection for stage III non-small-cell lung cancer: a phase III randomised controlled trial. Lancet 2009;374:379–86.
13. De Waele M, Hendriks J, Lauwers P, et al. Nodal status at repeat mediastinoscopy determines survival in non-small cell lung cancer with mediastinal nodal involvement, treated by induction therapy. Eur J Cardiothorac Surg 2006;29:240–3.
14. Stamatis G, Fechner S, Hillejan L, et al. Repeat mediastinoscopy as a restaging procedure. Pneumologie 2005;59:862–6.
15. Cerfolio RJ, Bryant AS, Ojha B. Restaging patient with N2 (stage IIIa) non-small cell lung cancer after neoadjuvant chemoradiotherapy: a prospective study. J Thorac Cardiovasc Surg 2006;131:1229–35.
16. De Waele M, Serra-Mitjans M, Hendriks J, et al. Accuracy and survival of repeat mediastinoscopy after induction therapy for non-small cell lung cancer in a combined series of 104 patients. Eur J Cardiothorac Surg 2008;33:824–8.
17. Louie BE, Kapur S, Farivar AS, et al. Safety and utility of mediastinoscopy in non-small cell lung cancer in a complex mediastinum. Ann Thorac Surg 2011;92:278–83.
18. Roberts JR, Wadsworth J. Recurrent laryngeal nerve monitoring during mediastinoscopy: predictors of injury. Ann Thorac Surg 2007;83:388–91.
19. de Cabanyes Candela S, Detterbeck FC. A systematic review of restaging after induction therapy for stage IIIa lung cancer: prediction of pathologic stage. J Thorac Oncol 2010;5:389–98.
20. Call S, Rami-Porta R, Obiols C, et al. Repeat mediastinoscopy in all its indications: experience with 96 patients and 101 procedures. Eur J Cardiothorac Surg 2011;39:1022–7.
21. De Waele M, Hendriks J, Lauwers P, et al. Different indications for repeat mediastinoscopy: single institution experience of 79 cases. Minerva Chir 2009;64:415–8.
22. Marra A, Hillejan L, Fechner S, et al. Remediastinoscopy in restaging of lung cancer after induction therapy. J Thorac Cardiovasc Surg 2008;135:843–9.

23. Van Schil P, De Waele M, Hendriks J, et al. Remediastinoscopy. J Thorac Oncol 2007;2:365–6.

24. Van Schil PE, De Waele M. A second mediastinoscopy: how to decide and how to do it? Eur J Cardiothorac Surg 2008;33:703–6.

25. McNeill TM, Chamberlain JM. Diagnostic anterior mediastinotomy. Ann Thorac Surg 1966;2:532–9.

26. Cerfolio RJ, Bryant AS, Eloubeidi MA. Accessing the aortopulmonary window (#5) and the paraaortic (#6) lymph nodes in patients with non-small cell lung cancer. Ann Thorac Surg 2007;84:940–5.

27. Howington JA. The role of VATS for staging and diagnosis in patients with non-small cell lung cancer. Semin Thorac Cardiovasc Surg 2007;19:212–6.

28. Defranchi SA, Cassivi SD, Nichols FC, et al. N2 disease in T1 non-small cell lung cancer. Ann Thorac Surg 2009;88:924–8.

29. Detterbeck FC, Jantz MA, Wallace M, et al. Invasive mediastinal staging of lung cancer: ACCP evidence-based clinical practice guidelines (2nd edition). Chest 2007;132:202S–20S.

30. Al-Sarraf N, Aziz R, Gately K, et al. Pattern and predictors of occult mediastinal lymph node involvement in non-small cell lung cancer patients with negative mediastinal uptake on positron emission tomography. Eur J Cardiothorac Surg 2008;33:104–9.

31. Lee PC, Port JL, Korst RJ, et al. Risk factors for occult mediastinal metastases in clinical stage I non-small cell lung cancer. Ann Thorac Surg 2007;84:177–81.

The Surgical Management of Stage I and Stage II Lung Cancer

Lyall A. Gorenstein, MD, Joshua R. Sonett, MD*

KEYWORDS

- Stage I lung cancer • Stage II lung cancer
- Surgical management • Non–small cell lung cancer

In 2010, there were 225,000 new cases of lung cancer, of which approximately 25% to 30% were early stage (American Joint Committee on Cancer stages I and II) and potentially curable with surgical resection. Stages I and II lung cancer include many different subsets, ranging from very small tumors (T1aN0) (<2 cm), to more advanced cancers (ie, T4N0) (multiple nodules within the same lobe). Yet despite there being many subsets within these 2 stages (**Table 1**), they are defined by the fact that a complete resection can always be achieved by an anatomic resection, either lobectomy or pneumonectomy. In the case of T3 tumors that invade adjacent structures (chest wall, pericardium, or diaphragm) complete resection can be achieved with en bloc resection. Therefore, surgical resection, to include the tumor with complete intra-operative hilar and mediastinal nodal staging, is the preferred treatment of patients with early-stage lung cancer. Although chemotherapy and radiation have roles in treating patients with lung cancer, there has never been a randomized trial comparing these modalities with surgery for early-stage lung cancer. Based on the expected 5-year survival after resection of 60% to 80% for stage I non–small cell lung cancer (NSCLC), and 40% to 60% for stage II NSCLC, complete surgical resection of early-stage lung cancer affords patients the best chance for long-term survival.[1]

When large central tumors invade vascular structures or the proximal bronchus either directly or through nodal extension (N1), and complete resection cannot be achieved by a lobectomy, then a bilobectomy or pneumonectomy is necessary. There is no benefit to the patient when an incomplete resection is performed.[2] In keeping with the basic tenet of achieving a complete resection, and preserving lung function,

Division of Thoracic Surgery, Columbia Presbyterian Medical Center, New York Presbyterian Hospital, 161 Fort Washington Avenue #301, New York, NY 10032, USA
* Corresponding author. Columbia University, 622 West 168th Street, PH-14 East Room 104, New York, NY 10032.
E-mail address: js2106@columbia.edu

Surg Oncol Clin N Am 20 (2011) 701–720
doi:10.1016/j.soc.2011.07.009
1055-3207/11/$ – see front matter © 2011 Elsevier Inc. All rights reserved.

Table 1
Stages I and II lung cancer subsets

T		N0	N1
Sixth Edition TNM	Seventh Edition TNM	Stage	Stage
T1 (≤3 cm)	T1a (≤2 cm)	IA	IIA
	T1b (>2–3 cm)	IA	IIA
T2 (>3 cm)	T2a (>3–5 cm)	IB	IIA (IIB)
• Involves main bronchus	T2b (>5–7 cm)	IIA (IB)	IIB (IIB)
• >2 cm from carina	T3 (>7 cm)	IIB (IB)	IIIA
• Invades visceral pleura			
• Atelectasis to hilum but not entire lung			
T3 Invasion	T3	IIB	IIIA
• <2 cm from carina			
• Invasion of chest wall, diaphragm, pericardium, mediastinal pleura			
T4	T3	IIB (IIIB)	IIIA (IIIB)
• Multiple malignant nodules same lobe			

Based on the seventh edition of TNM lung cancer staging from the International Association for the Study of Lung Cancer.
The stage given in parentheses is based on the sixth edition of TNM lung cancer.

occasionally in patients with central tumors, a sleeve resection of the bronchus, the pulmonary artery, and rarely both structures, can be performed to avoid performing a pneumonectomy.[3] (See article by Rendina elsewhere in this issue.)

The quest to preserve pulmonary function after surgical resection raises the question of performing lesser resections than lobectomy, especially in patients with very small peripheral tumors (ie, clinical stage T1aN0 tumors and particularly with noninvasive or microinvasive carcinoma [formerly defined as bronchioloalveolar carcinoma (BAC)]). In patients with compromised lung function, sublobar resection, either wedge resections or segmental resections, are well-established acceptable treatment alternatives to nonsurgical therapy, and are routinely performed in higher-risk surgical patients.[4,5] There is mounting evidence to support consideration of sublobar resections in certain subsets of patients with small (<2 cm) NSCLC tumors.[6]

Although the incidence of stage II NSCLC is less frequent than the other stages, metastases to regional lymph nodes greatly influence both treatment and survival in NCSLC. Nodal involvement with direct extension into hilar structures affects the extent of resection, thereby requiring a larger resection than lobectomy, with greater inherent surgical morbidity and mortality.[7,8] Yano and colleagues[9] reported that hilar nodal involvement affected 5-year survival greater than presence of lobar nodes (64.5% vs 39.7%). Over the past decade, the roles of both adjuvant and neoadjuvant therapies have been defined. Several randomized studies have independently identified patients with stages I and II lung cancer who will likely benefit from adjuvant chemotherapy.[10–12]

Preoperative imaging and staging, as discussed in the staging article, is paramount in selecting patients with locally advanced tumors who should receive neoadjuvant therapy.

LOBECTOMY

After the report by Graham and colleagues[13] of a successful pneumonectomy for lung cancer in 1932, pneumonectomy became the standard of care in the surgical management of patients with bronchogenic carcinoma. Over the next several decades reports of lesser resections, namely lobectomy, for patients with peripheral tumors were reported, using surgical techniques incorporating individual lobar vascular and bronchial division. After the report by Churchill and colleagues[14] in 1950 of long-term survival in patients with early-stage lung cancer after lobectomy, lobectomy began to replace pneumonectomy as the preferred surgical treatment of small peripheral lung tumors. This report coincided with the increasing incidence of bronchogenic cancers in North America and Western Europe from tobacco exposure, subsequently resulting in widespread acceptance and performance of anatomic lobectomy for lung cancer. The oncologic principle involves removal of the primary tumor within the lobe, and thereby the lymphatic drainage associated with the tumor. Intraoperative staging, which is critical in the surgical management of lung cancer, includes removal of lymph nodes based on their anatomic location as outlined by the American Thoracic Society (ATS) guidelines.[15]

The major surgical developments in the management of patients with operable lung cancers between 1960 and 1990 included improving postthoracotomy pain management,[16] developing surgical selection criteria based on exercise tolerance[17] and pulmonary function testing,[18] and the evolution of surgical staplers. These devices combined with better postoperative pain management allowed surgeons to perform pulmonary resections through smaller incisions, even in patients with chronic obstructive pulmonary disease (COPD) and elderly patients, who frequently have multiple medical comorbidities.

The most recently published data on morbidity and mortality associated with open lobectomy come from the Society of Thoracic Surgeons (STS) database of 5957 patients, thereby establishing the current guidelines with which to compare all treatments for lung cancer. Morbidity after open lobectomy was 32% and the 30-day mortality was 2%.[19]

VIDEO-ASSISTED THORACIC SURGERY LOBECTOMY

Video-assisted thoracic surgery (VATS) lobectomy represents the further evolution in the surgical management of early-stage lung cancer. Initial reports of VATS lobectomy from the early 1990s were highly criticized because it was believed that both oncologic principles and patient safety might be compromised during lung resections without a thoracotomy.[20] In the first single-institution randomized trial of VATS lobectomy, Kirby and colleagues[21] randomized 61 patients to either VATS lobectomy (n = 31) or muscle-sparing thoracotomy (n = 30). The complication rate was lower in the VATS group (6% vs 16%), indicating that VATS lobectomy could be performed safely. Sugi and colleagues[22] randomized 100 patients with clinical stage I lung cancer to either VATS lobectomy or a standard thoracotomy and lobectomy. There was no significant difference in 5-year survival between VATS lobectomy and open lobectomy (90% vs 85%), indicating that VATS lobectomy did not compromise oncologic principles.

McKenna and colleagues[23] reported the largest single-institution study of VATS lobectomy. In their series of 1100 patients with various stages of lung cancer, mortality was 0.8%, and morbidity 15.3%, with a conversion rate to open thoracotomy of 2.5%. As a result of this and other large series,[24-27] there has been a gradual acceptance within the surgical community of VATS lobectomy, for patients with early-stage NSCLC. CALGB 39,802, a prospective multi-institution study of the feasibility of total video-assisted resection reported that VATS lobectomy is safe and associated with low morbidity.[28] Comparative studies between VATS lobectomy and open lobectomy are primarily single-institution retrospective reviews (Table 2). VATS lobectomy

Table 2
Morbidity and mortality of VATS and open lobectomy

Study	Conversion Rate (%)	n VATS	n Open	Blood Loss VATS	Blood Loss Open	Complication Rate (%) VATS	Complication Rate (%) Open	Chest Tube (d) VATS	Chest Tube (d) Open	Length of Stay (d) VATS	Length of Stay (d) Open	Mortality (%) VATS	Mortality (%) Open
Kirby et al,[21] 1995 prospective	10	25	30	<250	<250	24	53	6.5	4.6	7.1	8.3	0	0
Petersen et al,[29] 2007 retrospective	5	43	57	NR	NR	9	11	3.1	4.7	4.2	4.3	0	0
Whitson et al,[30] 2007 retrospective	15.7	59	88	251	255	NR	NR	5.0	6.1	6.4	7.7	0	0
Villamizar et al,[31] 2009 retrospective	4.6	284	284	NR	NR	31	51	3	4	4	5	3	5
Flores et al,[32] 2009 retrospective	17.5	398	343	NR	NR	23	33	NR	NR	5	7	0.3	0.3
Whitson et al,[33] 2008 Systematic review	NR	3114	3256	251	255	16.4	32	5	6.1	6.4	7.7	NR	NR
Yan et al,[34] 2009 Systematic review	8.1	1391	1250	146	235	NR	NR	4.6	5.3	12	12.2	0.4	0.7
Scott et al,[35] 2010 retrospective	6.7	74	62	NR	NR	34	39	3	5	4	7	1.6	1.4

Abbreviation: NA, not reported.

compares favorably in regards to surgical morbidity, mortality, and the incidence of serious complications. As surgeons became more experienced with performance of VATS lobectomy and recognized its benefits compared with open lobectomy, establishing a large intergroup randomized trial to compare the 2 operations became difficult because of difficulty in enrolling patients. A multi-institution registry designed to collect data prospectively comparing open and VATS lobectomy (CALGB 140,501) failed to proceed as well. The review by Whitson and colleagues[33] of publications between 1992 and 2007 yielded 39 articles comparing open with VATS lobectomy. Although the reduction in surgical morbidity was not statistically significant, the reductions in both length of stay (absolute reduction 5 days) and duration of chest tube drainage (absolute difference 1.5 days) were both statistically significant. VATS lobectomy can be performed safely and does not increase the surgical risk of anatomic lobectomy. However, the most important outcome when comparing cancer treatments is survival. Although there are no large randomized trials comparing the 2 operations, the published data indicate that long-term survival and locoregional recurrence are not compromised by VATS lobectomy (**Table 3**). In the meta-analysis by Yan and colleagues,[34] 21 comparative studies were reviewed. VATS lobectomy had no significant impact on locoregional recurrence. There was a statistically significant decrease in systemic recurrence and improved 5-year survival with VATS lobectomy compared with open lobectomy. Data suggest that the improved 5-year survival in early-stage NSCLC may result from modulation of the inflammatory and cellular immune responses after VATS lobectomy,[39,40] similar to that seen in other minimally invasive surgical procedures.[41] In a randomized controlled trial by Craig and colleagues,[42] VATS lobectomy was associated with decreased acute phase inflammatory response. More data are necessary before any conclusions regarding the relationship between immune response and survival after VATS lobectomy can be made.

VATS lobectomy results in decreased postoperative pain[43] and earlier ambulation, which is likely responsible for the reduction in pulmonary complications.[44] There is decreased pulmonary morbidity with improved pulmonary function and performance status with VATS,[45] allowing anatomic resections to be offered to patients who would otherwise be considered high risk for thoracotomy and lobectomy such as elderly patients,[46] patients with poor performance status,[44] or those with reduced pulmonary function.[45] Many octogenarians diagnosed with clinical stage I lung cancer are denied anatomic lobectomy despite its oncologic advantages over nonanatomic resections, or other alternative strategies such as stereotactic radiation, merely because of their

Table 3
Long-term survival after VATS lobectomy

Author, Year	Clinical Stage	Technique	n	Results 5-Year Survival (%)
Sugi et al,[22] 2000	I	VATS	48	90
		Open	52	85
Walker et al,[17] 2003	I and II	VATS	159	Stage I = 78
				Stage II = 51
Thomas et al,[36] 2002	I	VATS	110	62.9
		Open	404	62.8
Rovario et al,[37] 2004	I	VATS	257	63.6
Shiraishi et al,[38] 2006	I	VATS	81	89
		Open	79	77
Flores et al,[31] 2009	I	VATS	398	79
		Open	343	75

age, and the presumed morbidity and mortality associated with a thoracotomy.[47] The data on VATS lobectomy in elderly patients are encouraging, with a mortality of 1.8% and morbidity of 18% having been reported in a single-institution series.[26] Similarly, patients with compromised pulmonary function who would be expected to have significant pulmonary morbidity from a thoracotomy can safely undergo a VATS lobectomy.[45] No large multi-institutional randomized trial of open lobectomy versus VATS lobectomy has been performed that conclusively confirms its perceived advantages. However, considering all the available clinical evidence, VATS lobectomy is recommended as the procedure of choice and should now be considered the gold standard for patients with early-stage NSCLC.

TECHNIQUE OF VATS LOBECTOMY

The fundamental approach to VATS lobectomy is no different from an open lobectomy. Each anatomic structure, namely the pulmonary artery, pulmonary vein, and bronchus, is isolated and individually ligated and divided. In the course of the dissection, the lymph nodes that lie on the artery (the interlobar lymph nodes, ATS level 11), and the hilar lymph nodes (ATS level 10) are removed, which is critical to complete staging. The order in which each structure is isolated and stapled varies by the lobe being removed and surgeon preference. Generally, the structures are approached from anterior to posterior, without dissection within the fissure, until the vascular structures are divided.

Patient positioning is critical to successful VATS lobectomy. Rather than placing the patient in a full lateral position as when performing a standard posterolateral thoracotomy, the hips are rotated posteriorly, thereby exposing the anterior chest, and the table is maximally flexed to allow the anterior hip to drop away, and give full range of motion to the camera (**Fig. 1**). Most surgeons prefer to stand on the

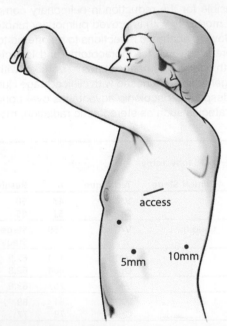

Fig. 1. Positioning of patient for left VATS lobectomy. The access incision is placed in the fourth interspace for upper lobectomy and fifth interspace for a lower lobectomy.

contralateral side of the patient (ie, the patient's left when performing a right VATS lobectomy).

The camera is placed in the eighth or ninth intercostal space at the level of the posterior axillary line. The currently available high-definition cameras and monitors provide excellent resolution with a 5-mm 30° telescope. The utility incision is placed either in the fourth or fifth intercostal space, depending on the lobe being removed. The posterior extent of the incision begins at the anterior border of the trapezius. We prefer to place a wound protector in the utility incision, to facilitate easy introduction of instruments. Depending on surgeon preference and experience 1 or 2 other incisions are made for retraction and instrumentation (see **Fig. 1**).

When performing a right upper lobectomy, the anterior hilum of the lung is exposed and the upper lobe vein isolated. After the vein is stapled and divided, the arterial branches are isolated and stapled (**Fig. 2**). The first arterial branch (truncus anterior) supplies the anterior and apical segments. The second arterial branch supplies the posterior segment to the upper lobe; its size and location are extremely variable. After dividing the arterial branches to the upper lobe, the bronchus is isolated and divided (**Fig. 3**), then allowing completion of the minor fissure and the posterior aspect of the major fissure. This technique minimizes dissection in the fissure, which reduces postoperative air leak, allowing more rapid chest tube removal, and patient discharge from hospital.

PNEUMONECTOMY
Incidence and Surgical Mortality

Pneumonectomy may be required to obtain a complete resection in either stage I or II lung cancer because of central invasion of hilar structures by either the tumor (T status), or N1 lymph nodes. The most current data regarding the incidence of pneumonectomy in clinical stage I or II lung cancer come from ACOS Z0030, a randomized study designed to analyze the impact of lymph node dissection on survival.[8] In this multicenter randomized study, in which the participating centers were high-volume thoracic surgical centers, the incidence of pneumonectomy was 4%. The detection

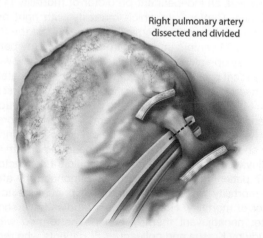

Right pulmonary artery
dissected and divided

Fig. 2. Commonly performed right upper lobectomy. After exposing and stapling the upper lobe vein, the truncus anterior is stapled.

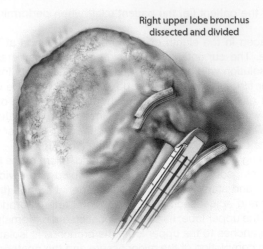

Right upper lobe bronchus
dissected and divided

Fig. 3. After stapling the arterial braches to the upper lobe, the bronchus is cleared of lymph nodes and stapled. The fissure is than completed, thus reducing the incidence of air leaks.

of early lung cancer is increasing,[48] and the incidence of pneumonectomy has been decreasing. In a study by Watanabe and colleagues,[49] which compared the surgical treatment of lung cancer over a 15-year interval, the incidence of pneumonectomy declined from 16.2% to 5.6% in the later period.

Significant morbidity and mortality are associated with pneumonectomy, and therefore all attempts at avoiding pneumonectomy should be used, including bronchoplasty or vascular reconstruction of the pulmonary artery. Many single-institution retrospective analyses have reported mortality and morbidity of pneumonectomy, and have identified risk factors that predict major morbidity.[49–57] Surgical mortality with pneumonectomy for NSCLC generally ranges from 2% to 12%; however, if pulmonary complications occur postoperatively mortality increases significantly.[49] Right pneumonectomy was an independent predictor of mortality in the series from the MD Anderson Cancer Center,[50] in which mortality with right pneumonectomy was 12% versus 1% for left pneumonectomy. In an analysis of the STS database in which 1267 patients from 80 centers underwent pneumonectomy between the years 2002 and 2007, the 30-day operative mortality was 5.6%.[55] The following criteria were identified to be independent predictors of major morbidity: age greater than 65 years, male sex, congestive heart failure, forced expiratory volume in the first second of expiration (FEV_1) less than 60% predicted, benign lung disease, and extrapleural pneumonectomy. In this analysis right pneumonectomy did not increase mortality. Neoadjuvant therapy has also been identified to be a risk factor for increased surgical mortality.[58–60] Martin and colleagues[58] identified the need to perform a right pneumonectomy after neoadjuvant chemotherapy to be a significant risk factor. In their retrospective review of 97 patients undergoing right pneumonectomy after neoadjuvant therapy, the 30-day mortality was 20%, whereas left pneumonectomy was not an independent predictor of mortality. However, other studies have shown that a right pneumonectomy after neoadjuvant therapy can be performed without increased mortality.[58] In the study by Krasna and colleagues,[61] patients who received neoadjuvant chemotherapy and radiation to an average dose of 6100 cGy, right pneumonectomy, had no impact on surgical mortality or morbidity.

Preoperative Assessment for Pneumonectomy

Many of the complications associated with pneumonectomy, including arrhythmias, increased A-a gradient, hypoxia, and myocardial ischemia, arise from the significant hemodynamic changes that occur from acute reduction of pulmonary capillary compliance, resulting in increased pulmonary arterial pressure. It is essential to thoroughly evaluate preoperatively patients who may require pneumonectomy. There is a significant body of data dealing with patient selection criteria for pneumonectomy.[62–65] If the FEV_1 is greater than 2 L, then pneumonectomy should be tolerated. If the FEV_1 is less than 2 L, a quantitative V/Q lung scan should be obtained to predict the postoperative FEV_1.[62] A predicted postoperative FEV_1 greater than 1 L is generally believed to be adequate after pneumonectomy. The studies using only FEV_1 to predict postoperative morbidity after pneumonectomy often do not take age, size of patient, or the presence of interstitial lung disease into consideration. A predicted postoperative FEV_1 of 800 mL, which is 60% or 70% of the patient's total FEV_1, indicates an acceptable risk for resection. On the other hand, a patient with a predicted postresection FEV_1 of 800 mL, corresponding to a FEV_1 of 35%, is at higher risk for pulmonary complications.[65] The predicted postoperative DLCO (carbon monoxide diffusion in the lung) is also important in stratifying the risk of pneumonectomy. A predicted postoperative DLCO greater than 40% is considered adequate. In patients in whom the predicted FEV_1 and DLCO are borderline to safely consider resection, exercise stress can be tested. Most of the data dealing with mV_{O2} and pulmonary resection aimed to assess risk of pneumonectomy rather than lobectomy. Patients with $mV_{O2}max$ greater than 15 mL/kg/min or greater than 75% of predicted are considered operable. Those with mV_{O2} max less than 10 mL/kg/min or 60% of predicted are at high risk for pulmonary complications after pneumonectomy.[65]

Complications Associated with Pneumonectomy

Aside from the significant hemodynamic and pulmonary consequences of a pneumonectomy, nonhealing of the bronchial stump, resulting in bronchopleural fistula (BPF), is a major predictor of mortality after pneumonectomy.[51,57,58] To prevent this complication the following technical steps should be followed. Avoid stripping the bronchial stump of all its adventitial tissue, especially on the right. Extensive lymphadenectomy of both the subcarinal and paratracheal tissues is believed to contribute to the higher incidence of BPF after right pneumonectomy.[66] Using a mechanical stapler to close the bronchial stump, and dividing the bronchus as close as possible to its origin, thereby minimizing the length of the residual bronchus, reduces the risk of BPF.[67] Covering the bronchial stump with healthy tissue, especially on the right side with pleura, pericardium, or intercostal muscle, reduces the risk of BPF. After left pneumonectomy, the incidence of BPF is lower, because the bronchial stump retracts into the mediastinal between the aorta and esophagus, and coverage is less important.[68]

SUBLOBAR RESECTION

Anatomic lobectomy with regional lymphadenectomy is the preferred treatment of patients with resectable early-stage NSCLC. However, in patients with significant medical comorbidities or insufficient pulmonary function, believed to be at high surgical risk for an anatomic lobectomy, sublobar resection by either wedge resection or segmental resection have long been practiced.[69,70] However, a major concern is the impact of sublobar resection on both local recurrence and long-term survival. Segmental resection was believed to be superior to nonanatomic wedge resection because it required division of the segmental bronchovascular structures, thereby encompassing the lymphatic drainage. However, because tumors often cross segmental boundaries, and increased morbidity resulted from prolonged air leak, enthusiasm for segmental resection remained limited.[71]

The surgical experience gained from performing lung volume reduction surgery (LVRS) in patients with advanced COPD has allowed patients who otherwise would be considered inoperable to undergo surgical resection. Ideally, the cancer is situated within the severely emphysematous lung, and resection of the tumor simultaneously achieves a lung volume reduction procedure with improvement in pulmonary function testing. DeRose and colleagues[72] reported 14 patients who underwent combined LVRS and resection of a pulmonary nodule. The mean preoperative FEV_1 was 680 mL (24% predicted), and 10 patients were oxygen dependent. In 9 of 14 patients, the nodule resected was NSCLC. At 6-month follow-up all patients showed improvement in dyspnea index and FEV_1. Choong and colleagues[73] reported on 21 patients with advanced COPD undergoing simultaneous LVRS and resection of an NSCLC. The mean preoperative FEV_1 was 29% of predicted. In only 9 of the 21 patients was the cancer located in the emphysematous lung. Eighteen patients in this group underwent anatomic lobectomy. The postoperative FEV_1 at 1 year was 43% of predicted.

The Lung Cancer Study Group performed a multi-institutional randomized trial, in which patients with clinical stage I lung cancer with adequate pulmonary reserve, and peripheral tumors amenable to sublobar resection, were randomized to either lobectomy or sublobar resection.[74] The sublobar resection could be either wedge resection or segmentectomy depending on location of the tumor and surgeon preference. The results confirmed the superiority of lobectomy over the sublobar resection in patients with resectable stage I NSCLC. There was a 75% increased risk of local recurrence, yet in those patients who underwent pulmonary function testing 1 year postoperatively, there was no significant difference between the 2 groups. Sublobar resection did not result in a meaningful benefit in regards to preservation of lung function, but placed patients at significant increased risk for both local recurrence and increased mortality. Based on this study, lobectomy remained the operation of choice in patients with resectable early-stage NSCLC. Proponents of sublobar resection argue that this study was flawed in that patients with tumors up to 3 cm were included. In a retrospective analysis by Okada and colleagues,[75] 1272 consecutive patients who underwent complete resection of pathologic stage I cancer, tumor size had a significant impact on survival. Patients were stratified into 4 groups according to tumor size: (1) 10 mm or less; (2) 11 to 20 mm; (3) 21 to 30 mm; (4) 30 mm or greater. The cancer-specific 5-year survival rates were 100%, 83.5%, 76.5%, and 57.9%, respectively. In a retrospective series of 784 patients from a single-institution undergoing surgery for stage I lung cancer, there was no difference in 5-year survival between patients with pathologic stage IA tumors who underwent lobectomy or sublobar resection. However, in patients with pathologic stage IB tumors who underwent sublobar resection, both overall 5-year survival (40% vs 54%) and disease-free survival (58% vs 50%) were inferior compared with patients who underwent lobectomy.[76] Ohta and colleagues[77] reported a correlation between tumor size and the incidence of occult regional lymph node metastases, which translated into decreased 5-year survival with increasing tumor size. This finding could explain the impact of tumor size on survival and locoregional recurrence in patients undergoing sublobar resection.

Over the past decade, there has been renewed interest in sublobar resection for patients with early-stage NSCLC.[78] This enthusiasm for sublobar resection has arisen predominantly because of the changing demographics of NSCLC. There seems to be an increasing incidence of smaller peripheral early-stage tumors with a declining incidence of large central tumors.[79] The frequent use of computed tomography (CT) scans identifies subclinical lung tumors in elderly patients with associated comorbidities, who may not otherwise be considered operable. The ELCAP (Early Lung Cancer Action Program) data[48] identified an increased proportion of small stage I lung cancers in high-risk patients who underwent CT lung cancer screening. In Japan, CT screening to detect early-stage lung cancer has been in practice for decades. Japanese surgeons have developed significant experience treating patients with these small asymptomatic incidental tumors with sublobar resection.[77,79–81]

PATIENT SELECTION FOR SUBLOBAR RESECTION OF NSCLC

There is a growing body of literature indicating that in patients with peripheral clinical stage I tumors less than 2 cm, segmental resection compares favorably with lobectomy in regards to both local recurrence and survival. In 2001, Okada and colleagues[81] performed a prospective study of extended segmentectomy compared with lobectomy in patients with clinical stage IA (tumors ≤ 2 cm). The 5-year survival compared favorably with lobectomy (87%). Other factors aside from tumor size also may affect patient selection for sublobar resection. Tumors (≤ 2 cm) with a predominant ground-glass appearance on CT scan and bronchoalveolar (BAC) histology, have an excellent prognosis after sublobar resection.[78] Borczuk and colleagues[82] performed a retrospective analysis of patients with adenocarcinoma. Multivariate analysis identified invasive component greater than 6 mm to be an independent predictor of prognosis in 121 patients with pathologic stage I adenocarcinoma. When there was no invasive component (BAC), or less than 6 mm of invasion, nodal micrometastases were absent (0/32 patients). When the invasive component was greater than 6 mm, the incidence of nodal metastases was 23%. Patient age should also be considered. Several reviews identified advanced age as an independent predictor of increased surgical morbidity and mortality after anatomic lobectomy for NSCLC. In a retrospective review of lobectomy in elderly patients, Naunheim and colleagues[83] reported a mortality of 16% in patients older than 75 years of age. Several studies have shown that lobectomy has no survival advantage compared with sublobar resection in elderly patients. Ikeda and colleagues[84] compared lobectomy with sublobar resection in patients more than 80 years of age. In patients with stage I NSCLC, there was no difference in 5-year survival (59%) after lobectomy compared with sublobar resection. In a study comparing lobectomy with segmentectomy in patients more than 75 years of age, Kilic and colleagues[85] reported no difference in either survival (45% vs 50%) or locoregional recurrence (4% vs 6%). In general, unless the patient has poor pulmonary function, a decision to perform a sublobar resection should not be based on age alone.

WEDGE RESECTION VERSUS SEGMENTECTOMY

The current literature suggests that segmentectomy, or rather extended segmentectomy in which additional lung from the adjacent segment to ensure an adequate surgical margin is included in the resection, is preferable to wedge resection.[78,81] The risk of local recurrence seems to be reduced with segmental resection, although there has never been a randomized trial evaluating these 2 procedures, or the impact of surgical margin on local recurrence. There is no consensus as to what constitutes an adequate margin after wedge resection. A surgical margin of at least 1 cm is recommended, with higher rates of recurrence being identified in several retrospective studies, when smaller margins are present (**Fig. 4**). Sawabata and colleagues[86] have recommended a surgical margin equal in size to the diameter of the tumor to decrease the risk of local recurrence.

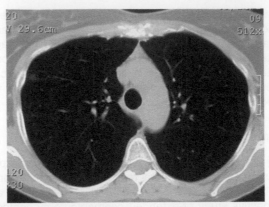

Fig. 4. A peripheral lung nodule, with a ground-glass quality in a patient with COPD. It lies along the border between the anterior and posterior segments. Wedge resection can achieve an adequate resection margin.

Surgical Approach to Sublobar Resection

Thoracoscopy is the preferred approach to sublobar resection, because it is associated with decreased postoperative pain, morbidity, and mortality, compared with thoracotomy in patients undergoing lobectomy. In most instances, peripheral tumors can be palpated and a simple wedge resection performed. For those tumors that are difficult to palpate because of their location or histology, a variety of techniques can help to identify the tumor. The most promising may be electromagnetic navigational bronchoscopy.

Although each anatomic segment can be resected, practically, some segments are more conducive to localized resection than others. Tumors arising in the superior segment of the lower lobes, the lingula segment, or (**Figs. 5** and **6**) upper lobe segments are most amenable to VATS segmentectomy. Schuchert and colleagues[87] reported the results of open versus VATS segmentectomy in patients with NSCLC. VATS segmentectomy compared favorably with open segmentectomy in regards to mortality, morbidity, recurrence, and survival.

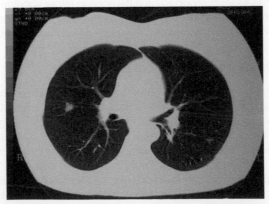

Fig. 5. 2-cm nodule with both ground-glass and solid components within the posterior segment of the right upper lobe. An extended segmental resection of the posterior segment can achieve adequate margins.

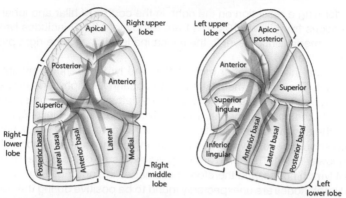

Fig. 6. Segmental anatomy of the right and left lungs.

Lobectomy with hilar lymph node dissection is recommended as the surgical treatment of stage I NSCLC. In selected patients sublobar resection can be considered (**Box 1**). Sublobar resection may also be considered for patients with adequate pulmonary function provided the tumor is less than 2 cm and within a segment that is amenable to an extended segmental resection. Otherwise anatomic lobectomy is the preferred treatment of stage I NSCLC.

LYMPH NODE DISSECTION

Hilar and mediastinal lymph node dissection, in combination with lobectomy, pneumonectomy, or sublobar resection are well-established components in the surgical therapy for NSCLC. The role of lymph node dissection is multifactorial; it affords accurate staging, which is essential in predicting prognosis as well as determining the need for adjuvant therapy, and removal of microscopic nodal disease may affect local recurrence.

What constitutes a thorough lymphadenectomy remains controversial. The Eastern Cooperative Oncology Group in the ECOG 3590 study defined lymphadenectomy as the removal of 10 or more lymph nodes from at least 2 or more mediastinal lymph node stations.[88] The advantage of a complete mediastinal lymphadenectomy (MLND) compared with mediastinal lymph node sampling (MLNS) is more accurate staging. Keller and colleagues[89] found a higher incidence of multistation N2 disease (30% vs 12%) in patients in whom MLND was performed. In the American College of Surgery Oncology Group Z0030, patients were randomized to either MLNS or MLND. In 4% of patients in whom the MLNS was negative, complete MLND revealed occult-positive mediastinal lymph nodes.[8]

Box 1
Indications for sublobar resection in NSCLC

1. Peripheral tumor 2 cm or less

2. Predominant ground-glass appearance on CT scan

3. Patient age 75 years or older

4. FEV_1 less than 60% of predicted

5. Presence of synchronous tumors

When performing a resection on the right, in the course of hilar and lobar mobilization, lymph nodes from levels 10 and 11 are removed. MLND includes lymph nodes from the lower mediastinum level 9, the subcarina level 7, and the right paratracheal nodes levels 2, 3, and 4.

On the left side, hilar and lobar mobilization and lymphadenectomy are similar to that on the right. The inferior mediastinal and subcarinal lymph node dissections are also performed in a similar fashion. Unique to the left side are the presence of lymph node stations 5, the aorta pulmonary window lymph nodes, and level 6, representing nodes along the ascending aorta between the phrenic nerve and vagus nerve. These lymph nodes should be removed when performing pulmonary resections of either the left upper or lower lobes. The aortic arch impairs exposure of the left paratracheal level 2 and level 4 lymph nodes, and therefore these nodes are not routinely removed. If the level 5 or 6 lymph nodes are unexpectedly found to be positive during the course of the pulmonary resection, the aortic arch can be mobilized to allow the paratracheal lymph nodes to be removed. If the preoperative staging indicates a high level of suspicion of the level 2 or 4 lymph nodes, then either endobronchial ultrasonography or mediastinoscopy is performed before resection.

There are potential risks and morbidity associated with complete MLND. These risks include bleeding, injury to the thoracic duct resulting in chylothorax, recurrent laryngeal nerve or phrenic nerve injury, devascularization of the bronchial stump, and prolonged chest tube drainage. There have been several randomized trials aimed at evaluating the role of MLND. The study by Keller and colleagues,[89] a prospective multicenter nonrandomized study of MLND in 373 patients, showed no increase in operative time or bleeding compared with MLNS. In the ACOSOG Z0030 study, the largest prospective multicenter trial comparing MLND versus MLNS, there was no difference in morbidity or length of stay, although median operating time was increased by 15 minutes in patients undergoing MLND.[8]

Several studies have looked at the impact of MLND on survival. Gajra and colleagues[90] retrospectively reviewed patients with clinical stage I lung cancer and found a correlation between the number of lymph nodes removed and 5-year survival. Lardinois and colleagues[91] found a higher incidence of local recurrence in patients with stage I lung cancer who underwent MLNS. The controversy regarding the impact of MLND on survival seems to have been resolved. ACOSOG Z0030, which was designed to evaluate the role of MLND on survival, showed that there is no survival advantage with MLND compared with thorough MLNS in patients with either clinical stage I or II NSCLC. Our personal bias is to perform MLND rather than MLNS, because of its greater accuracy in diagnosing occult N2 mediastinal lymph node disease, which identifies patients who would benefit from adjuvant systemic therapy. However, individual patient factors should be taken into consideration, such as age, comorbidities, and size and histology of the primary tumor when deciding on whether to perform MLND.

VATS can perform a complete mediastinal lymph node dissection as thoroughly as performed by thoracotomy. Several Japanese reports comparing lymphadenectomy[92–94] have shown that both the number of lymph nodes and the lymph node stations sampled are similar, when lymphadenectomy is performed by either thoracotomy or VATS. In the course of exposing the hilar structures to the lobe being resected, the level 10 and 11 nodes are removed. When performing a VATS lobectomy, many surgeons prefer to perform the MLND after the pulmonary resection, because this affords better exposure and visualization of the mediastinum. We prefer to perform the subcarinal lymph node dissection initially, especially in conjunction with a lower lobectomy. Removing the subcarinal lymph nodes and exposing the bronchus intermedius and level 11 lymph nodes posteriorly simplifies later mobilization of the interlobar pulmonary artery and exposure of the bronchus. When performing an upper lobectomy, we generally complete the MLND, after the lobe has been removed.

SUMMARY

Over the past several decades there have been major advances in all aspects of the treatment of NSCLC, including early detection, patient selection, pain management, surgical techniques, and the role of both neoadjuvant and adjuvant chemotherapy. Surgical resection remains the cornerstone in the treatment of patients with stages I and II NSCLC. Anatomic lobectomy combined with hilar and MLND, constitutes the oncologic basis of surgical resection. Pneumonectomy, commonly performed in the past, is less frequently required because of the changing demographics of NSCLC, and the development of a variety of bronchial and vascular reconstructive techniques that allow preservation of pulmonary function, without compromising oncologic principles when tumors invade hilar structures. VATS lobectomy is a significant development in the surgical management of lung cancer. The surgical data overwhelmingly favor VATS lobectomy over open lobectomy and have established VATS lobectomy as a gold standard in the surgical resection of early-stage NSCLC. As the application of CT screening and other early detection techniques evolves, more patients with small lung cancers will present for surgical resection. Current standards still favor VATS lobectomy; however, in these patients the role of sublobar pulmonary resection, either anatomic segmentectomy or nonanatomic wedge resection, in patients with subcentimeter nodules will be clarified in the future.

REFERENCES

1. Scott WJ, Howington J, Feigenberg S, et al. Treatment of non-small cell lung cancer stage I and stage II ACCP evidence-based clinical practice guidelines (2nd edition). Chest 2007;132(Supp 3):234S–42S.
2. Deslauriers J. Current surgical treatment of nonsmall cell lung cancer 2001. Eur Respir J Suppl 2002;35:61s–70s.
3. Delauriers J, Gregoire J, Jacques LF, et al. Sleeve lobectomy versus pneumonectomy for lung cancer: a comparative analysis of survival and sites of recurrences. Ann Thorac Surg 2004;77:1152–6.
4. Haasbeek CJ, Senan S, Smit EF, et al. Critical review of non surgical treatment options for stage I non-small cell lung cancer. Oncologist 2008;13(3):309–19.
5. Miller JI, Hatcher CR. Limited resection of bronchogenic carcinoma in the patient with marked impairment of pulmonary function. Ann Thorac Surg 1987;44:340–3.
6. Tsubota N, Ayabe K, Doi O, et al. Ongoing prospective study of segmentectomy for small lung tumors. Ann Thorac Surg 1998;66:1781–90.
7. Ginsburg RJ, Hill LD, Eagan RT, et al. Modern thirty-day operative mortality for surgical resections in lung cancer. J Thorac Cardiovasc Surg 1983;86:654–8.
8. Allen MS, Darling GE, Peche TT, et al. Morbidity and mortality of major pulmonary resections in patients with early stage lung cancer: initial results of the randomized, prospective ACOSOG Z0030 trial. Ann Thorac Surg 2006;81:1013–20.
9. Yano T, Yokohama H, Inoue T, et al. Surgical results and prognostic factors of pathologic N1 disease in non-small-cell carcinoma of the lung. Significance of N1 level: lobar or hilar nodes. J Thorac Cardiovasc Surg 1994;107:1398–402.
10. The International Adjuvant Lung Cancer Trial Collaborative Group. Cisplatin-based adjuvant chemotherapy in patients with completely resected NSCLC. N Engl J Med 2004;350:351–60.

11. Winton TL, Livingston R, Johnson D, et al. Vinorelbine plus cisplatinim vs. observation in resected NSCLC. N Engl J Med 2005;352:2589–97.
12. Strauss GM, Herndon J, Maddaus MA, et al. Adjuvant paclitaxel plus carboplatin compared with observation in stage IB non–small-cell lung cancer: CALGB 9633 with the cancer and Leukemia Group B, Radiation Therapy Oncology Group, and North Central Cancer Treatment Group Study Groups. J Clin Oncol 2008;26(31): 5043–51.
13. Graham EA, Singer JJ. Successful removal of an entire lung for carcinoma of the bronchus. JAMA 1933;101:1371.
14. Churchill ED, Sweet RH, Sutter L, et al. The surgical management of carcinoma of the lung. A study of cases treated at the Massachusetts General Hospital from 1930-50. J Thorac Surg 1950;20:349–65.
15. Mountain CF, Dresler CM. Regional lymph node classification for lung cancer staging. Chest 1997;111:1718–23.
16. Ballantyne JC, Carr DB, deFerranti S, et al. The comparative effects of postoperative analgesic therapies on pulmonary outcome: cumulative meta-analysis of randomized controlled trials. Anesth Analg 1998;86:598–612.
17. Reilly DF, McNeely MJ, Doerner D, et al. Self-reported exercise tolerance and the risk of serious perioperative complications. Arch Intern Med 1999;159(8): 2185–92.
18. Beckles MA, Spiro SG, Colice GL, et al. The physiologic evaluation of patients with lung cancer being considered for resectional surgery. Chest 2003; 123(Suppl 1):105S–14S.
19. Boffa DJ, Allen MS, Grab JD, et al. Data from the Society of Thoracic Surgeons General Thoracic Surgery database: the surgical management of primary lung tumors. J Thorac Cardiovasc Surg 2008;135:247–54.
20. Lewis RJ. The role of video assisted thoracic surgery for carcinoma of the lung: wedge resection to lobectomy by simultaneous individual stapling. Ann Thorac Surg 1993;56:762–8.
21. Kirby T, Mack M, Landreneau J, et al. Lobectomy: video-assisted thoracic surgery versus muscle sparing thoracotomy–a randomized trial. J Thorac Cardiovasc Surg 1995;109:997–1001.
22. Sugi K, Kaneda Y, Esato K, et al. Video-assisted thoracoscopic lobectomy achieves a satisfactory long-term prognosis in patients with clinical stage IA lung cancer. World J Surg 2000;24:27–30.
23. McKenna RJ Jr, Houck W, Fuller CB. Video assisted thoracic surgery lobectomy: experience with 1,100 cases. Ann Thorac Surg 2006;81:421–5.
24. Onaitis MW, Peterson RP, Bladerson SS, et al. Thoracoscopic lobectomy is a safe and versatile procedure. Experience with 500 consecutive patients. Ann Thorac Surg 2006;244:420–5.
25. Walker WS, Codispoti M, Soon SY, et al. Long term outcomes of VATS lobectomy for non small cell bronchogenic carcinoma. Eur J Cardiothorac Surg 2003;23: 397–402.
26. McVay CL, Pickens A, Fuller C, et al. VATS anatomic pulmonary resection in octogenarians. Am Surg 2005;71:791–3.
27. Kim K, Kim HK, Park JS, et al. Video-assisted thoracic surgery: single institution experience with 704 cases. Ann Thorac Surg 2010;89(6):S2118–22.
28. Swanson SJ, Herndon JE, D'Amico TA, et al. Video-assisted thoracic surgery lobectomy. Report of CALGB 39802–a prospective, multiinstitutional feasibility study. J Clin Oncol 2007;25:4993–7.

29. Petersen RP, Pham D, Burfeind WR, et al. Thoracoscopic lobectomy facilitates the delivery of chemotherapy after resection for lung cancer. Ann Thorac Surg 2007; 83(4):1245–9.
30. Whitson BA, Andrade RS, Bardales R, et al. Video-assisted thoracoscopic surgery is more favorable than thoracotomy for resection of clinical stage I non-small cell lung cancer. Ann Thorac Surg 2007;83:1965–70.
31. Villamazar NR, Darrabie MD, Buirfiend WR, et al. Thoracoscopic lobectomy is associated with lower morbidity compared with thoracotomy. J Thorac Cardiovasc Surg 2009;138:419–25.
32. Flores RM, Park BJ, Dycoco J, et al. Lobectomy by video-assisted thoracic surgery (VATS) versus thoracotomy for lung cancer. J Thorac Cardiovasc Surg 2009;138:11–8.
33. Whitson BA, Groth SS, Duval SJ, et al. Surgery for early stage non small cell lung cancer: a systemic review of video assisted thoracic surgery versus thoracotomy approaches to lobectomy. Ann Thorac Surg 2008;86:2008–18.
34. Yan TD, Black D, Bannon PG, et al. Systematic review and meta-analysis of randomized and non randomized trials on safety and efficacy of video- assisted thoracic surgery lobectomy for early stage non- small-cell lung cancer. J Clin Oncol 2009;27(15):2553–62.
35. Scott WJ, Matteotti RS, Egelston BL, et al. A comparison of perioperative outcomes of video-assisted thoracic surgical (VATS) lobectomy with open thoracotomy and lobectomy: results of an analysis using propensity score based weighting. Ann Surg Innov Res 2010;4(1):1.
36. Thomas P, Doddoli C, Thirion X, et al. VATS is an adequate oncological operation for stage I non-small cell lung cancer. Eur J Cardiothorac Surg 2002;21:1094–9.
37. Roviaro G, Varoli F, Vergani, et al. Long term survival after videothoracoscopic lobectomy for stage I lung cancer. Chest 2004;126:725–32.
38. Shiraishi T, Shirakusa T, Hiratsuka M. Video-assisted thoracoscopic surgery lobectomy for c-T1N0M0 primary lung cancer: its impact on locoregional control. Ann Thorac Surg 2006;82(3):1021–6.
39. Walker WS, Leaver HA. Immunologic and stress responses following video-assisted thoracic surgery and open pulmonary lobectomy in early stage lung cancer. Thorac Surg Clin 2007;17(2):241–9.
40. Whitson BA, D'Cunha J, Andrade RS, et al. Thoracoscopic versus thoracotomy approaches to lobectomy: differential impairment of cellular immunity. Ann Thorac Surg 2008;86(6):1735–44.
41. Kuntz C, Wunsch A, Bay F, et al. Prospective randomized study of stress and immune response after laparoscopic vs. conventional colonic resection. Surg Endosc 1998;12(7):963–7.
42. Craig SR, Leaver HA, Yap PL, et al. Acute phase responses following minimal access and conventional thoracic surgery. Eur J Cardiothorac Surg 2001;20: 455–63.
43. Handy JR Jr, Asaph JW, Douville EC, et al. Does video-assisted thoracoscopic lobectomy for lung cancer provide improved functional outcomes compared with open lobectomy? Eur J Cardiothorac Surg 2010;37:451–5.
44. Demmy TL, Curtis JJ. Minimally invasive lobectomy directed toward frail and high risk patients: a case-control study. Ann Thorac Surg 1999;68:194–200.
45. Kachare S, Dexter EU, Nwogu C, et al. Perioperative outcomes of thoracoscopic anatomic resections in patients with limited pulmonary reserve. J Thorac Cardiovasc Surg 2011;141(2):459–62.

46. Cattaneo SM, Park BJ, Wilton AS, et al. Use of video-assisted thoracic surgery for lobectomy in the elderly results in fewer complications. Ann Thorac Surg 2008;85: 231–6.

47. Rivera C, Dahan M, Bernard A, et al. Surgical treatment of lung cancer in the octogenarians: results of a nationwide audit. Eur J Cardiothorac Surg 2011; 39(6):981–6.

48. Henschke CI, Shaham D, Yankelvitz DF, et al. CT screening for lung cancer: past and ongoing studies. Semin Thorac Cardiovasc Surg 2005;17:99–106.

49. Watanabe S, Asamura H, Suzuki K, et al. Recent results of postoperative mortality for surgical resections in lung cancer. Ann Thorac Surg 2004;78:999–1002.

50. Wahi R, McMurtrey MJ, Decaro LF, et al. Determinants of perioperative morbidity and mortality after pneumonectomy. Ann Thorac Surg 1989;48:33–7.

51. Darling GE, Abdurahman A, Yi QL, et al. Risk of a right pneumonectomy: role of bronchopleural fistula. Ann Thorac Surg 2005;79(2):433–7.

52. Licker MJ, Widikker I, Robert J, et al. Operative mortality and respiratory complications after lung resection for cancer: impact of chronic obstructive pulmonary disease and time trends. Ann Thorac Surg 2006;81(5):1837–8.

53. Licker M, Spiliopoulos A, Frey JG, et al. Risk factors for early mortality and major complications following pneumonectomy for non small call carcinoma of the lung. Chest 2002;121(6):1890–7.

54. Joo JB, DeBord JR, Montgomery CE, et al. Perioperative factors as predictors of operative mortality and morbidity in pneumonectomy. Am Surg 2001;67(4): 318–21.

55. Shapiro M, Swanson SJ, Wright CD, et al. Predictors of major morbidity and mortality after pneumonectomy utilizing the Society for Thoracic Surgeons General Thoracic Surgery Database. Ann Thorac Surg 2010;90(3):927–34.

56. Algar FJ, Alvarez A, Salvatierra A, et al. Predicting pulmonary complications after pneumonectomy for lung cancer. Eur J Cardiothorac Surg 2003;23(2):201–8.

57. Vaporciyan AA, Merriman KW, Ece F, et al. Incidence of major pulmonary morbidity after pneumonectomy: association with timing of smoking cessation. Ann Thorac Surg 2002;73(2):425–6.

58. Martin J, Ginsberg R, Abolhoda A, et al. Morbidity and mortality after neoadjuvant therapy for lung cancer; the risk of right pneumonectomy. Ann Thorac Surg 2001; 72:1149–54.

59. Alifano M, Boudaya MS, Salvi M, et al. Pneumonectomy after chemotherapy: morbidity, mortality, and long term outcome. Ann Thorac Surg 2008;85(6): 1866–72.

60. Mansour Z, Kochetkova EA, Ducrocq X, et al. Induction chemotherapy does not increase the operative risk of pneumonectomy. Eur J Cardiothorac Surg 2007;31: 181–5.

61. Krasna MJ, Gamliel Z, Burrows WM, et al. Pneumonectomy for lung cancer after preoperative concurrent chemotherapy and high-dose radiation. Ann Thorac Surg 2010;89(1):200–6.

62. Kristersson S, Lindell SE, Svanberg L, et al. Prediction of pulmonary function loss due to pneumonectomy using 133 Xe-radiospirometry. Chest 1972;62:694.

63. Gass GD, Olsen GN. Preoperative pulmonary function testing to predict postoperative morbidity and mortality. Chest 1986;89:127–35.

64. Ferguson MK. Assessment of operative risk for pneumonectomy. Chest Surg Clin N Am 1999;9(2):339–51.

65. Benzo R, Kelley GA, Recchi L, et al. Complications of lung resection and exercise capacity: a meta-analysis. Respir Med 2007;101(8):1790–7.

66. Haraguchi S, Koizumi K, Hirata T, et al. Analysis of risk factors for postpneumonectomy bronchopleural fistulas in patients with lung cancer. J Nippon Med Sch 2006;73(6):314–9.
67. Javadpour H, Sidhu P, Luke DA. Bronchopleural fistula after pneumonectomy. Ir J Med Sci 2003;172(1):13–5.
68. Lindner M, Hapfelmeier A, Morressi-Hauf A, et al. Bronchial stump coverage and postpneumonectomy bronchopleural fistula. Asian Cardiovasc Thorac Ann 2010; 18(5):443–9.
69. Jacobson MJ, Zand L, Fox RT, et al. Comparison of the wedge and segmental resection of the lung. Thorax 1976;31(4):365–8.
70. Jensik RJ, Faber LP, Kittle CF. Segmental resection for bronchogenic carcinoma. Ann Thorac Surg 1979;28(5):475–83.
71. Warren WH, Faber LP. Segmentectomy versus lobectomy in patients with stage I pulmonary carcinoma. J Thorac Cardiovasc Surg 1994;107:1087–94.
72. DeRose JJ, Argenziano M, El-Amir N, et al. Lung reduction operation and resection of pulmonary nodules in patients with severe emphysema. Ann Thorac Surg 1998;65(2):314–8.
73. Choong CK, Meyers BF, Battafarano RJ, et al. Lung cancer resection combined with lung volume reduction in patients with severe emphysema. J Thorac Cardiovasc Surg 2004;127:1323–31.
74. Ginsberg RJ, Rubinstein LV, Lung Cancer Study Group. Randomized trial of lobectomy versus limited resection for T1 N0 non-small cell lung cancer. Ann Thorac Surg 1995;60:615–23.
75. Okada M, Nishio W, Sakamoto T, et al. Effect of tumor size on prognosis in patients with non-small cell lung cancer: the role of segmentectomy as type of lesser resection. J Thorac Cardiovasc Surg 2005;129:87–93.
76. El-Sherif A, Gooding WE, Santos R, et al. Outcomes of sublobar resection versus lobectomy for stage I non-small cell lung cancer: a 13 year analysis. Ann Thorac Surg 2006;82:408–16.
77. Ohta Y, Oda M, Wu J, et al. Can tumor size be a guide for limited surgical intervention in patients with peripheral non-small cell lung cancer? Assessment from the point of view of nodal micrometastases. J Thorac Cardiovasc Surg 2001; 122(5):900–6.
78. Narsule CK, Ebright MI, Fernando HC. Sublobar versus lobar resection: current status. Cancer J 2011;17(1):23–7.
79. Okada M, Nishio W, Sakamoto T, et al. Evolution of surgical outcomes for non-small cell lung cancer: time trends in 1,465 consecutive patients undergoing complete resection. Ann Thorac Surg 2004;77:1926–30.
80. Sobue T, Suzuki T, Naruke T. A control study for evaluating lung cancer screening in Japan. Japanese Lung-Cancer-Screening Research Group. Int J Cancer 1992; 50:230–7.
81. Okada M, Yoshikawa K, Hatta T, et al. Is segmentectomy with lymph node assessment an alternative to lobectomy for non-small cell lung cancer of 2 cm or smaller? Ann Thorac Surg 2001;71:956–60.
82. Borczuk AC, Qian F, Kazeros A, et al. Invasive size is an independent predictor of survival in pulmonary adenocarcinoma. Am J Surg Pathol 2009; 33(3):462–9.
83. Naunheim KS, Kesler KA, D'Orazio SA, et al. Lung cancer surgery in the octogenarian. Eur J Cardiothorac Surg 1994;8:453–6.
84. Ikeda N, Hayashi A, Iwasaki K, et al. Surgical strategy for non small cell lung cancer in octagenarians. Respirology 2007;12:712–8.

85. Kilic A, Schuchert MJ, Pettiford BL, et al. Anatomic segmentectomy for stage I non-small cell lung cancer (NSCLC) in the elderly. Ann Thorac Surg 2009;87: 1662–6.

86. Sawabata N, Ohta M, Matsumura A, et al. Optimal distance of malignant negative margin in excision of non-small cell lung cancer: a multicenter prospective study. Ann Thorac Surg 2004;77:415–20.

87. Schuchert MJ, Pettiford BL, Pennathur A, et al. Anatomic segmentectomy for stage I non-small cell lung cancer. Comparison of video-assisted thoracic surgery versus open approach. J Thorac Cardiovasc Surg 2009;138:1318–25.

88. Keller SM, Adak S, Wagner H, et al, The Eastern Cooperative Oncology Group. Mediastinal lymphadenectomy in non-small cell lung cancer: effectiveness in patients with or without nodal micrometastases-results of a preliminary study. Eur J Cardiothorac Surg 2002;21:520–6.

89. Keller SM, Adak S, Wagner H, et al. Mediastinal lymph node dissection improves survival in patients with stages II and IIIA non-small cell lung cancer. Ann Thorac Surg 2000;70:358–66.

90. Gajra A, Newman N, Gamble P, et al. Effects of number of lymph nodes sampled on outcome in patients with stage I non-small cell lung cancer. J Clin Oncol 2003; 21:1029–33.

91. Lardinois D, Suter H, Hakki H, et al. Morbidity survival and site recurrence after mediastinal lymph node dissection versus systematic sampling after complete resection for non-small cell lung cancer. Ann Thorac Surg 2005;27:680–5.

92. Naruke T, Tsuchiya R, Kondo H, et al. Lymph node sampling in lung cancer: how should it be done? Eur J Cardiothorac Surg 1999;(16):S17–24.

93. Shigemura N, Akashi A, Funaki S, et al. Long term outcomes after a variety of video-assisted thoracoscopic lobectomy approaches for clinical stage IA lung cancer: a multi-institutional study. J Thorac Cardiovasc Surg 2006;132:507–12.

94. Sagawa M, Sato M, Sakurda A, et al. A prospective trial of systematic nodal dissection for lung cancer by video-assisted thoracic surgery: can be perfect? Ann Thorac Surg 2002;73:900–4.

Role of Surgery Following Induction Therapy for Stage III Non–Small Cell Lung Cancer

Benedict D.T. Daly, MD[a,b],*, Robert J. Cerfolio, MD[c,d],
Mark J. Krasna, MD[e]

KEYWORDS

- Non–small cell lung cancer • Neoadjuvant induction therapy
- Tumor resection • Radiotherapy

EVOLUTION OF NEOADJUVANT THERAPY

The treatment of stage IIIA non–small cell lung cancer and subsequently resectable stage IIIB disease has evolved over the last 30 years. Before the advent of the cisplatin era that began in the early 1980s, the overall survival of patients with stage IIIA-N2 disease was dismal, and a major focus of management was surgical staging.[1] In their classic article in 1982 Pearson and colleagues[2] reported a 9% 5-year survival in 62 patients with a positive mediastinoscopy who underwent a complete surgical resection, compared with a 24% 5-year survival in 79 patients who had a negative mediastinoscopy and who after a complete resection were found to have unsuspected mediastinal nodal disease. Postoperative adjuvant chemotherapy and radiotherapy had little impact on the survival of these patients.[3]

Early phase 2 trials of neoadjuvant chemotherapy using mitomycin, vinblastine, and cisplatin performed at the Memorial Sloan-Kettering Cancer Center and the University of Toronto demonstrated improved survivals of 20% in patients with preoperatively

[a] Cardiothoracic Surgery Boston Medical Center, 88 East Newton Street Robinson B402, Boston, MA 02118, USA
[b] Cardiothoracic Surgery Boston University School of Medicine, Boston, MA, USA
[c] Thoracic Surgery, JH Estes Endowed, Birmingham, AL, USA
[d] University of Alabama, Birmingham, 703 19th Street, S ZRB 739, Birmingham, AL 35294-0016, USA
[e] Meridian Health System, Neptune, NJ, USA
* Corresponding author.
E-mail address: benedict.daly@bmc.org

Surg Oncol Clin N Am 20 (2011) 721–732
doi:10.1016/j.soc.2011.07.006
1055-3207/11/$ – see front matter © 2011 Elsevier Inc. All rights reserved.

surgonc.theclinics.com

identified N2 disease.[4,5] Similar results were seen in early phase 2 studies performed combining radiation (3000–4500 cGy) with platinum-containing chemotherapy.[6] In 1994 small phase 3 trials demonstrated improved survival with induction chemotherapy followed by surgery compared with surgery alone. In the trial by Roth and colleagues[7] at M.D. Anderson, patients underwent induction therapy with a combination of cyclophosphamide, etoposide, and cisplatin, followed by surgery and then 3 additional cycles postoperatively. Thirty-five percent of the patients had a major clinical response, and their 2-year and 3-year survivals were 60% and 50% compared with the surgery-alone group (25% and 15%). In the trial from Barcelona[8] patients were treated with induction mitomycin, ifosfamide, and cisplatin followed by surgery and postoperative radiation in comparison with surgery and radiation. The 2-year and 5-year survivals were 29% and 17% in the chemotherapy/surgery/radiation arm, and 5% and 0% in the surgery/radiation arm.

In 1989 the Cancer and Leukemia Group B (CALGB) designed a multi-institutional phase 2 trial of high-intensity trimodality therapy for patients with surgically staged IIIA-N2 non–small cell lung cancer, and published these results in 1995 (CALGB 8935A).[9] The trial combined 2 cycles of neoadjuvant cisplatin and vinblastine with surgical resection and radical lymphadenectomy, followed by 2 additional cycles of adjuvant chemotherapy followed by radiation therapy (5400–6000 cGy). This study was performed by 30 separate teams. Their definition for a complete resection was defined as all margins negative as well as the highest lymph node resected. Seventy-four patients were entered into the study. Eighty-six percent of all patients were explored and 62% of all eligible patients underwent resection. The operative mortality was 3.2% and the morbidity 30%. However, only 31% of the patients had an R0 resection by their criteria. Nonetheless, the study was important because it demonstrated that an aggressive approach that included induction therapy could be delivered with a then relatively low treatment-related mortality of 5.4%, which compared favorably with an earlier study by CALGB that included an induction regimen of cisplatin, vinblastine, and fluorouracil and concomitant radiation to 3000 cGy whereby the treatment-related mortality was 15%. The study also demonstrated the importance of an R0 resection. These patients had a 3-year survival of 46% compared with 21% for those having an incomplete resection and 0% for unresectable patients.

In 1995 the mature results of Southwest Oncology Group (SWOG) 8805 were published.[10] This phase 2 trial evaluated the impact of induction chemotherapy and concomitant radiotherapy on survival in 126 patients with stage IIIA/B non–small cell lung cancer. All patients had biopsy-proven N2 or N3 disease or T4 lesions. The induction regimen consisted of 2 cycles of cisplatin and etoposide with concurrent radiation to 4500 cGy. Seventy-five patients had stage IIIA-N2 and 51 patients had stage IIIB disease. Twenty-seven of the patients with stage IIIB disease were N3. Operation consisted of resection and lymph node sampling. Unresectable patients or patients with positive nodes received additional chemotherapy and radiation postoperatively. In this study 85% of patients with stage IIIA-N2 and 80% of patients with stage IIIB were resected. There were 10% treatment-related deaths. With this aggressive induction approach, 21% of patients had a complete pathologic response and 37% had only residual microscopic disease. There was no difference in the survival of patients with stage IIIA and stage IIIB disease. The 2-year survivals were 37% and 39% and the 3-year survivals 27% and 24%, respectively. However, this study demonstrated the importance of downstaging on survival, and the strongest predictor of survival was an absence of tumor in the mediastinal lymph nodes. The median and 5-year survivals for these patients were 30 months and 44% versus 10 months and 18% for patients with residual nodal disease.

In 2001 Rusch and colleagues[11] published the initial results of SWOG 9416, which adopted the protocol of 8805 and applied it to superior sulcus tumors. Eighty T3 and 31 T4 patients were enrolled. The resection rate was 91% for T3 tumors and 87% for T4 tumors. Once again the impact of the induction regimen on downstaging was impressive, with 28 patients having a complete pathologic response and only 26 patients having microscopic residual disease. The long-term results of this study, published in 2007, demonstrated a 54% survival for patients undergoing a complete resection.[12]

In 2005 Albain and colleagues[13] reported the initial results of a randomized trial of definitive chemoradiotherapy (194 patients) versus induction chemoradiotherapy followed by surgical resection (202 patients) for patients with stage III-N2 non–small cell lung cancer (RTOG 9309, Intergroup Trial 0139). All patients received 2 cycles of chemotherapy with cisplatin and etoposide. Both groups received concomitant radiation. However, the radiation doses were significantly different between the two groups. The patients randomized to go onto surgical resection received a total dose of 4500 cGy and the patients randomized to definitive radiation received a total dose of 6100 cGy. The mature results of this trial were reported in 2009.[14] Although all patients were to receive 2 additional cycles of chemotherapy, this was only accomplished in 55% of the surgical group and 74% of the nonsurgical group. While there was a difference in the progression-free survival between the two groups (12.8 months in the surgical group vs 10.5 months in the nonsurgical group; $P = .017$), there was no difference in the overall survival (23.6 months vs 22.2 months; $P = .24$). However, the operative mortality for patients undergoing pneumonectomy was 26%. In the lobectomy group there was a difference in survival (33.6 months vs 21.7 months in a matched chemotherapy-radiation group; $P = .002$). However, despite these results many centers have considered patients with N2 disease inoperable. Surgery, however, was not the only variable in this study, as there is a significant difference in the biological effectiveness between 4500 and 6000 cGy of radiation.

The authors of this article have reported their single-institution experiences using neoadjuvant concurrent chemoradiotherapy using platinum-based chemotherapy protocols and high-dose radiation (ca 6000 cGy) followed by surgical resection for patients with stage III A/B non–small cell lung cancer and for locally advanced T3N0 or T4N0 tumors or tumors of the superior sulcus (**Table 1**). The major difference between other studies and these ones has been the radiation dose, which approximates the dose of radiation in the Intergroup 0139 Trial. The authors' collective experience highlights the importance of surgical resection for local control even after relatively high doses of radiation. As **Table 1** shows, approximately 50% of patients will have residual tumor at the time of resection. In addition, in patients with stage IIIA/B lung cancers and involved lymph nodes these regimens have relatively high success in effecting nodal downstaging. There is no question that operating after higher doses of radiation can be technically challenging, and that pneumonectomy carries significant risk that has to be weighed against potential benefit. Each of the authors has used different slightly different strategies in the management of these patients, but these operations can be performed safely and these regimens are now being used by more surgeons.

GOALS OF NEOADJUVANT THERAPY

The major goal of neoadjuvant therapy is to increase the survival of patients with advanced M0 lung cancer. In patients with locally invasive cancers or bulky adenopathy a complete resection may not be possible and, unfortunately, most patients with

Table 1
Reports of neoadjuvant platinum based chemotherapy and concurrent high-dose radiation

Authors	Year	No. of Patients	Clinical Stage	Study Focus	% CPR	% Nodal Downstaging	No. of Pneumonectomies	% Pneumonectomy Mortality
Sonett et al[15]	1999	19	IB, IIB, IIIA/B	—	42	83	6	0.0
Vora et al[16]	2000	33	IIIA/B	—	27	64	9	0.0
Sonett et al[17]	2004	40	IIB, IIIA/B, IV	—	45	85	11	0.0
Cerfolio et al[18]	2005	54	IIIA-N2	—	28	83	9	16.7
Kwong et al[19]	2005	36	IIB, IIIA/B, IV	All Pancoast tumors	41	—	3	—
Daly et al[20]	2006	30	IIA/B, IIIA/B	All pneumonectomy	29	47	30	13.3
Edelman et al[21,a]	2008	40	IIIA/B	hfXRT to 6960 cGy	17	73	4	0.0
Krasna et al[22]	2010	29	IIB, IIIA/B	All pneumonectomy	55	91	29	0.0
Daly et al[23]	2011	47	IIB, IIIB	All N0	45	—	12	8.3

Abbreviations: CPR, complete pathologic response; hfXRT, hyperfractionated radiotherapy.
[a] This study also evaluated chemotherapy dose escalation. Twenty-nine node-negative patients went to surgery and 28 were resected.

mediastinal nodal disease recur distally. Furthermore, most patients with less than an R0 resection are not cured. Neoadjuvant therapy, therefore, has a fourfold purpose: to increase the resectability of locally advanced disease, permit an R0 resection, downstage the mediastinal lymph nodes, and eliminate the presence of micrometastatic disease. In some patients this may make a lobectomy rather than a pneumonectomy possible, and thereby reduce the operative risk. Although postoperative radiotherapy may improve local control and postoperative chemotherapy may reduce the risk of systemic metastases, particularly in patients with unsuspected nodal disease, these regimens are less likely to be effective in patients with gross disease, and these patients may not tolerate or complete postoperative therapy.

Several reports from both multi-institutional and single-institution studies using neoadjuvant chemotherapy or chemoradiotherapy are shown in **Table 2**. The resectability rate for patients with stage III non–small cell lung cancer entered into these studies is variable, ranging from 50% to 80% on average. It is also clear that the percentage of patients undergoing an R0 resection is approximately 10% to 20% lower than the percentage of patients resected. These regimens, therefore, are only partially successful in fulfilling the goals of neoadjuvant therapy. Many of these trials include adjuvant therapy in their protocols, but in virtually all of these studies patients undergoing an incomplete resection do significantly poorer. It is also unclear whether radiation added to the induction regimen improves the resectability rate. The study by Thomas and colleagues,[38] reporting the results of a randomized trial of the German Lung Cancer Cooperative Group in 481 patients, demonstrated only a 5% difference in resectability between patients receiving induction chemotherapy and those receiving induction chemotherapy followed by concurrent chemotherapy and radiation, favoring the group that did not receive the radiation. Although the resectability rates of patients receiving high-dose radiation and chemotherapy. (Daly, Unpublished data, 2011) In the authors' experience it has been approximately 75% to 80%. It is possible, therefore, that the resectability in this group of patients may be higher, but this awaits further study.

Achieving a complete pathologic response with induction therapy is variable, but overall appears to be higher in those patients receiving neoadjuvant chemotherapy and concurrent high-dose radiation as opposed to chemotherapy alone or chemotherapy and lower doses of radiation. The significance of this ultimately remains to be determined, although it has been suggested that patients who achieve a complete pathologic response have a survival advantage.[25,42] A more important determinant of survival has been the downstaging of involved mediastinal lymph nodes from N3 or N2 to N0 or N1, and this finding has been consistently demonstrated in multiple studies (**Table 3**). Whereas the definition of absence of tumor in the mediastinal lymph nodes may be variously classified as no viable tumor or no tumor seen, and there may be interobserver variability from institution to institution, there is no disagreement that nodal downstaging is an important determinant of survival in patients with stage III disease. The only study using high-dose radiation in the neoadjuvant protocol and limited to patients with N2 disease was published by Cerfolio and colleagues.[18] This retrospective study demonstrated higher mediastinal nodal downstaging in patients receiving high-dose radiation (83%) than in those receiving low-dose radiation (median 4500 cGy; 74%). Consistent with other studies, there was an increase in the disease-free survival in the high-dose radiation group compared with the low-dose radiation group (estimated 3-year survival 65% vs 30%; $P = .047$). Overall, patients receiving high-dose radiation have a higher rate of nodal downstaging than those in studies using either chemotherapy alone or chemotherapy and lower doses of radiation in the induction protocol, as well as significant survival (see **Table 1**). In

Table 2
Reports of neoadjuvant chemotherapy with or without radiotherapy

Authors	Year	Stage	Induction Regimen[a]	No. of Patients	No. Resected[b]	% Resected	No. of CPR	N2 to N1/0
Weiden and Piantadosi[24]	1991	IIIA/B	P, FL with 3000 cGy	85	43 (29R0)	51 (34)	8 (17%)	—
Yashar et al[25]	1992	III-N2	P with 5500 cGy	36	31	86	10 (28%)	17 (47%)
Strauss et al[26]	1992	III	P, VB, F with 3000 cGy	41	25	56	4 (16%)	—
Burkes et al[5]	1992	III-N2	P, VD, MM	39	22 (18 R0)	56	1 (5%)	8 (36%)
Sugarbaker et al[9]	1995	IIIA-N2	P, VB × 2 cycles	74	46 (23 R0)[a]	62 (31)	—	10 (22%)
Albain et al[10]	1995	IIIA-N2	P, ET with 4500 cGy	75	57	76	19 (21%)	51% estimated
Albain et al[10]	1995	IIIB	P, ET with 4500 cGy	51	32	63	—	—
Mathisen et al[26]	1996	IIIA-N2	P, VB, F with 2100 cGy-hf	40	35	88	2 (6%)	14 (40%)
Eberhardt et al[27]	1998	IIIA/B	P, ET × 2 then P, ET × 1 with 4500 cGy	94	62 (50 R0)	66 (53)	24 (39%)	—
Rice et al[28]	1998	III	P, PT with 3000 cGy (150 cGy twice a day)	45	32 (R0)	71	14 (31%)	—
Stamatis et al[29]	1999	IIIB	P, ET × 3; P, ET × 1 with 4500 cGy-hf	56	27 (R0)	48	—	—
Junker et al[30]	2001	III	C, ET, IF × 2; CB, VD with 4500 cGy	54	40	74	—	—
Grunenwald et al[31]	2001	IIIB	P, VD, FL with 4200 cGy (2100 cGy × 2)	40	29 (23 R0)	73 (56)	4 (14%)	10 (30%)
Rusch et al[11]	2001	Pancoast	P, ET with 4500 cGy	111	83 (76 R0)	75 (68)	28 (34%)	—
Cyjon et al[32]	2002	III	P, ET; P, 4500 cGy	57	30	53	5 (17%)	—
Granetzny et al[33]	2003	IIIA/B	CB, ET, IF × 2; CB, VD with 4500 cGy	33	26 (24 R0)	79 (73)	6 (23%)	10 (38%)
Betticher et al[34]	2003	IIIA-N2	P, DT × 3	90	75 (39 R0)	83 (43)	45 (60%)	—
Galetta et al[35]	2003	IIIB	P, FL with 5040 cGy	39	21	54	9 (43%)	—
Ichinose et al[36]	2003	IIIB	P, UT with 4000 cGy	27	22	81	5 (23%)	—
DeCamp et al[37]	2003	IIIA/B	P, PT with 3000 cGy-hf	105	83 (R0)	79	12 (16%)	35% N2, 30% N3
Thomas et al[38]	2004	III	P, ET × 3; CB, VD × 2 with 4500 cGy-hf	245	111 (R0)	45	—	—
Thomas et al[38]	2004	III	P, ET × 3	236	118 (R0)	50	—	—
Machtay et al[39]	2004	III	P, ET or CB, PT with 4500–5400 cGy	53	45 (38 R0)	85 (72)	7 (16%)	—
Steger et al[40]	2009	III-N2/3	CB, PT × 4 with 4500 cGy-hf	55	55	100	19 (35%)	38 (69%)
Caglar et al[41]	2009	IIIA/B	CB, PT × 2; CB, PT with 54 cGy (average dose)	44	—	—	—	32 (73%)

Abbreviations: C, cisplatin; CP, carboplatinum; CPR, complete pathologic response; DC, docetaxel; FL, fluorouracil; hf, hyperfractionated radiation 150 cGy twice a day; IF, ifosfamide; MM, mitomycin; PT, paclitaxel; R0, R0 resection; UT, uracil plus tegafur; VB, vinblastine; VD, vindesine.

[a] Abbreviations

[b] Total number resected.

Number in parentheses indicates number having an R0 resection when both the total number and number of complete resections are reported.

Table 3
Reports demonstrating survival with and without nodal downstaging

Authors	Year	No. of Resected Patients	Nodal Downstaging (%)	Survival of Node-Positive Patients	Survival of Node-Negative Patients	P Value
Albain et al[10]	1995	57	51	10 mo median	30 mo median	0
Mathisen et al[26]	1996	35	40	26 mo median	Not reached (11/16 alive)	0.04
Bueno et al[43]	2000	103	52	15.9 mo median (N1/2)	21.3 mo median (N0)	0.02
Grunenwald et al[31]	2001	29	30	12% estimated 5 y	40% estimated 5 y	0
Rice et al[28]	1998	40	31	33% estimated 2 y	83% estimated 2 y	0.01
Granetzny et al[33]	2003	26	38	11.4 mo median	34.7 mo median	0.01
Betticher et al[34]	2003	75	45	8.4 mo overall	Not reached	0
Steger et al[40]	2009	55	69	27 mo mean	54 mo mean	0
Stefani et al[44]	2010	175	39	22% estimated 5 y	45% estimated 5 y	0
Paul et al[45]	2011	136	52	20% estimated 5 y	45% estimated 5 y	0

Daly's experience, of the 32 patients with N2 disease treated with concurrent platinum-based chemotherapy and high-dose radiation, the median and estimated 5-year survivals for the 14 patients who had mediastinal nodal downstaging were 58 months and 49%, compared with the 18 patients with residual mediastinal nodal disease who had a median survival of 38 months and an estimated 5-year survival of 41%. At present, a study (RTOG 0839) is evaluating patients with potentially operable N2 disease treated with induction chemotherapy and high-dose radiation, with or without panitumumab. This study will provide further insight into the impact of nodal staging on survival.

When one reflects on the prognosis of patients with stage III lung cancer and particularly those with involved lymph nodes, all of the neoadjuvant studies reported here demonstrate significantly improved survival over their historical controls. This improvement has occurred as a result of increased resectability and better control of both local and distant disease. Nonetheless, significant controversies continue to exist.

CONTROVERSIES

The first controversy is whether patients with N2 disease should be operated on at all. The authors strongly disagree with those who support this position, based on their own results and those they have referenced. This controversy is primarily based on the early results of the Intergroup 0139 study that showed no difference in the overall survival of patients undergoing neoadjuvant chemoradiotherapy followed by surgery versus definitive chemoradiotherapy.[13] The more mature results of this study, however, do show a difference for patients undergoing lobectomy.[14] The poor results in the pneumonectomy group are largely due to the high operative mortality of 26% in these patients. When one looks at the number of patients with residual disease in the primary tumor who have been resected after high-dose radiation and concurrent chemotherapy (see **Table 1**), it is likely that 50% of patients will ultimately fail locally if they do not succumb to metastases. Thus, the rationale for surgery in non–small cell lung cancer after treatment with concurrent chemotherapy and high-dose radiation is local control.

The second controversy is whether patients with gross mediastinal nodal disease, multistation mediastinal nodal disease, or even residual nodal disease after induction therapy should be offered resection. While it is intuitive that patients with gross or multistation N2 disease are more likely to do poorly with any treatment algorithm, this is not universally accepted.[46,47] It is clear from **Table 3**, however, that in most studies of patients with stage III-N2 disease, survival is significantly compromised when residual nodal disease is present after induction therapy, and that they might do as well overall without surgery. However, the authors have seen a median survival of 41 months in patients with residual nodal disease with an induction regimen that includes high-dose radiation, and continue to offer these patients resection.

The most significant controversy is whether pneumonectomy should be offered to patients undergoing resection after induction therapy particularly when radiation is included in the induction regimen, and some surgeons omit radiation when pneumonectomy is contemplated. Unfortunately, many of these patients have advanced disease and the incidence of pneumonectomy in these patients is relatively high.[29] The operative mortality rate in several recent series is significant, and in several recent large series has varied from 6% to 12% with 90-day mortalities significantly higher.[48,49] In fact it has been suggested that for these patients 90-day mortality should be the gold standard for reporting. On the other hand, the higher mortality is not a universal experience.[50] In the recent study by Weder and colleagues,[51] 176 patients (21% of the resections) underwent pneumonectomy (49% right) for stage III disease following neoadjuvant treatment, and 141 of these received chemoradiotherapy. The 90-day mortality rate was only 3%. Krasna and coleagues[22] encountered no mortality in their group of pneumonectomy patients even though they received high-dose radiation. Although the operative risk is higher with pneumonectomy, the overall survival of this group of patients is probably higher than if they did not undergo resection. Even so, these patients tend to have a shorter survival than a comparable group of patients undergoing lobectomy, likely due to both their more advanced disease and the physiologic consequences of the resection. Some investigators express additional caution when considering right pneumonectomy, although this has not been an issue in the authors' series.[19,20,52]

Although the optimal dose of preoperative radiation as well as fractionation and sequence remain controversial, more groups are using higher effective doses of radiation (6000 cGy and higher) because this provides definitive treatment for those patients who do not go on to surgery for a variety of reasons. In most series this approximates to 20% or more of patients (see **Table 3**). Based on experience there is the additional advantage of better nodal downstaging and potential survival advantage. In addition, the number of cycles of chemotherapy given preoperatively, the number of drug combinations in the protocol, and whether chemotherapy postoperatively affords an additional benefit are other issues that have not been definitively determined. These issues will change as other drug and drug combinations become available, genetic profiling or in vitro testing for drug sensitivity becomes more widely used, and immunotherapy advances.

Based on the results of the experience with neoadjuvant treatment of stage III disease, several groups extended these aggressive regimens to the treatment of patients with superior sulcus tumors. The SWOG (9416, Intergroup Trial 0160) has shown the superiority of neoadjuvant chemoradiotherapy in treating these patients, with a complete resection rate of 94% and 5-year survival of 54% for patients undergoing a complete resection.[12] Kwong and colleagues[19] demonstrated similar results in their study in which high-dose radiation was used in the induction protocol. Their median survival was 2.6 years, and for the 40.5% of patients who had a complete pathologic response it was 7.8 years. Daly and colleagues[23] further extended their aggressive approach to include patients with T3N0 lung cancers, and demonstrated a median survival of 120 months. The efficacy of these approaches, however, requires confirmation in randomized trials.

SUMMARY

Neoadjuvant treatment followed by surgical resection has significantly improved the overall results of treatment for patients with stage III disease as well as for patients with locally invasive tumors. Significant controversies still exist regarding treatment. Different chemotherapy regimens have been used, although in the majority of studies some combination of drugs that include cisplatin are the standard. Radiation when given as part of the induction protocol appears to offer a higher rate of resection and complete resection, and higher doses of radiation (6000 cGy or higher) are associated with better nodal downstaging. Pneumonectomy should be undertaken with caution, and in patients with residual nodal disease risk assessment is important. In the final analysis every patient is different, and the overall risks and benefits of surgical resection have to be evaluated individually. Randomized and multi-institutional trials will clarify the issues regarding treatment, and new drugs or drug combinations, especially targeted therapy, will improve results further. Whether postoperative adjuvant chemotherapy adds to the benefit of neoadjuvant therapy followed by surgery remains to be determined.

REFERENCES

1. Martini N, Flehinger BJ. The role of surgery in N2 lung cancer. Surg Clin North Am 1987;67:1037–49.
2. Pearson FG, DeLarue NC, Ilves R, et al. Significance of positive superior mediastinal nodes identified at mediastinoscopy in patients with resectable lung cancer. J Thorac Cardiovasc Surg 1982;83:1–11.
3. Jaklitsch MT, Strauss GM, Sugarbaker DJ. Neoadjuvant and adjuvant therapy in the management of locally advanced non-small cell lung cancer. World J Surg 1993;17:729–34.
4. Martini N, Kris M, Flehinger BJ, et al. Preoperative chemotherapy for stage IIIa (N2) lung cancer: the Sloan-Kettering experience with 136 patients. Ann Thorac Surg 1993;55:1365–73.
5. Burkes RL, Ginsberg RJ, Sheperd FA, et al. Induction chemotherapy with mitomycin, vindesine, and cisplatin for Stage III unresectable non-small cell lung cancer; results of the Toronto phase II trial. J Clin Oncol 1992;10:580–6.
6. Ginsberg RJ. Neoadjuvant (induction) treatment for non-small cell lung cancer. Lung Cancer 1995;12:S33–40.
7. Roth JA, Fosella F, Komaki R, et al. A randomized trial comparing perioperative chemotherapy and surgery with surgery alone in resectable Stage IIIA non-small cell lung cancer. J Natl Cancer Inst 1994;86:673–80.

8. Rosell R, Gomez-Codina J, Camps C, et al. A randomized trial comparing preoperative chemotherapy plus surgery with surgery alone in patients with non-small cell lung cancer. N Engl J Med 1994;330:153–8.

9. Sugarbaker DJ, Herndon J, Kohman LJ, et al. Cancer and Leukemia Group B Thoracic Surgery Group. Results of cancer and leukemia group B protocol 8935A mutiinstitutional phase II trimodality trial for Stage IIIa (N2) non-small-cell lung cancer. J Thorac Cardiovasc Surg 1995;109:473–85.

10. Albain KS, Rusch VW, Crowley JJ, et al. Concurrent cisplatin/etoposide plus chest radiotherapy followed by surgery for Stages IIIA (N2) and IIIB non-small-cell lung cancer: mature results of Southwest Oncology Group phase II study 8805. J Clin Oncol 1995;13:1880–92.

11. Rusch VW, Giroux DJ, Kraut MJ, et al. Induction chemoradiation and surgical resection for non-small cell lung carcinomas of the superior sulcus: initial results of Southwest Oncology Group Trial 9416 (Intergroup trial 0160). J Thorac Cardiovasc Surg 2001;121:472–83.

12. Rusch VW, Giroux DJ, Kraut MJ, et al. Induction chemoradiation and surgical resection for superior sulcus non-small cell lung carcinomas: long-term results of Southwest Oncology Group Trial 9416 (Intergroup trial 0160). J Clin Oncol 2007;25:313–8.

13. Albain KS, Scott CB, Rusch VR, et al. Phase III study of concurrent chemotherapy plus radiotherapy (CT/RT) and CT/RT followed by surgical resection for stage IIIA(pN2) non-small cell lung cancer: initial results from intergroup trial 0139 (RTOG 93-09) [abstract]. Proc Am Soc Clin Oncol 2003;22:621.

14. Albain KS, Swann RS, Rusch VW, et al. Radiotherapy plus chemotherapy with or without surgical resection for stage III non-small-cell lung cancer: a phase III randomized controlled trial. Lancet 2009;374:379–86.

15. Sonett JR, Krasna MJ, Suntharalingam M, et al. Safe pulmonary resection after chemotherapy and high-dose thoracic radiation. Ann Thorac Surg 1999;68:316–20.

16. Vora SA, Daly BD, Blaszkowsky L, et al. High dose radiation therapy and chemotherapy as induction treatment for stage III nonsmall cell lung carcinoma. Cancer 2000;89:1946–52.

17. Sonett JR, Suntharalingam M, Edelman MJ, et al. Pulmonary resection after curative intent radiotherapy (>59 Gy) and concurrent chemotherapy in non-small-cell lung cancer. Ann Thorac Surg 2004;78:1200–6.

18. Cerfolio RJ, Bryant AS, Spencer SA, et al. Pulmonary resection after high-dose and low-dose chest irradiation. Ann Thorac Surg 2005;80:1224–30.

19. Kwong KF, Edelman MJ, Suntharalingam M, et al. High-dose radiotherapy in trimodality treatment of Pancoast tumors results in high pathologic complete response rates and excellent long-term survival. J Thorac Cardiovasc Surg 2005;129:1250–5.

20. Daly BD, Fernando HC, Ketchedjian A, et al. Pneumonectomy after high-dose radiation and concurrent chemotherapy for nonsmall cell lung cancer. Ann Thorac Surg 2006;82:227–31.

21. Edelman MJ, Suntharalingam M, Burrows W, et al. Phase I/II trial of hyperfractionated radiation and chemotherapy followed by surgery in stage III lung cancer. Ann Thorac Surg 2008;86:903–11.

22. Krasna MJ, Gamliel Z, Burrows WM, et al. Pneumonectomy for lung cancer after preoperative concurrent chemotherapy and high-dose radiation. Ann Thorac Surg 2010;89:200–6.

23. Daly BD, Ebright MI, Walkey AJ, et al. Impact of neoadjuvant chemoradiotherapy followed by surgical resection on node-negative T3 and T4 non-small cell lung cancer. J Thorac Cardiovasc Surg 2011;141(6):1392–7.

24. Weiden PL, Piantadosi S. Preoperative chemotherapy (cisplatin and fluorouracil) and radiation therapy in stage III non-small-cell lung cancer: a phase II study of the Lung Cancer Study Group. J Natl Cancer Inst 1991;83:266–73.
25. Yashar J, Weitberg AB, Glicksman AS, et al. Preoperative chemotherapy and radiation therapy for stage IIIa carcinoma of the lung. Ann Thorac Surg 1992; 53:445–8.
26. Mathisen DJ, Wain JC, Wright C, et al. Assessment of preoperative accelerated radiotherapy and chemotherapy in stage IIIA (N2) non-small-cell lung cancer. J Thorac Cardiovasc Surg 1996;111:123–33.
27. Eberhardt W, Wilke H, Stamatis G, et al. Preoperative chemotherapy followed by concurrent chemoradiation therapy based on hyperfractionated accelerated radiotherapy and definitive surgery in locally advanced non-small-cell lung cancer: mature results of a phase II trial. J Clin Oncol 1998;16:622–34.
28. Rice TW, Adelstein DJ, Ciezki JP, et al. Short-course induction chemoradiotherapy with paclitaxel for stage III non-small-cell lung cancer. Ann Thorac Surg 1998;66:1909–14.
29. Stamatis G, Eberhardt W, Stuben G, et al. Preoperative chemoradiotherapy and surgery for selected non-small cell lung cancer IIIB subgroups: long-term results. Ann Thorac Surg 1999;68:1144–9.
30. Junker K, Langner K, Klinke F, et al. Grading of tumor regression in non-small cell lung cancer: morphology and prognosis. Chest 2001;120:1584–91.
31. Grunenwald DH, Andre F, Le Pechoux C, et al. Benefit of surgery after chemoradiotherapy in stage IIIB (T4 and/or N3) non-small cell lung cancer. J Thorac Cardiovasc Surg 2001;122:796–802.
32. Cyjon A, Nili M, Fink G, et al. Advanced non-small cell lung cancer: induction chemotherapy and chemoradiation before operation. Ann Thorac Surg 2002; 74:342–7.
33. Granetzny A, Striehn E, Bosse U, et al. A phase II single-institution study of neoadjuvant stage IIIA/B chemotherapy and radiochemotherapy in non-small cell lung cancer. Ann Thorac Surg 2003;75:1107–12.
34. Betticher DC, Schmitz SH, Totsch M, et al. Mediastinal lymph node clearance after docetaxel-cisplatin neoadjuvant chemotherapy is prognostic of survival in patients with stage IIIA pN2 non-small-cell lung cancer: a multicenter phase II trial. J Clin Oncol 2003;21(9):1752–9.
35. Galetta D, Cesario A, Margaritora S, et al. Enduring challenge in the treatment of nonsmall cell lung cancer with clinical stage IIIB: results of a trimodality approach. Ann Thorac Surg 2003;76:1802–9.
36. Ichinose Y, Fukuyama Y, Asoh H, et al. Induction chemoradiotherapy and surgical resection for selected stage IIIB non-small-cell lung cancer. Ann Thorac Surg 2003;76:1810–5.
37. DeCamp MM, Rice TW, Adelstein DJ, et al. Value of accelerated multimodality therapy in stage IIIA and IIIB non-small cell lung cancer. J Thorac Cardiovasc Surg 2003;126:17–27.
38. Thomas M, Macha HN, Ukena D, et al. Cisplatin/etoposide (PE) followed by twice-daily chemoradiation (hfRT/CT) versus PE alone before surgery in stage III non-small cell lung cancer (NSCLC): a randomized phase III trial of the German Lung Cancer Cooperative Group (GLCCG). J Clin Oncol 2004;22:14S.
39. Machtay M, Lee JH, Stevenson JP, et al. Two commonly used neoadjuvant chemotherapy regimens for locally advanced stage III non-small cell lung carcinoma: long-term results and associations with pathologic response. J Thorac Cardiovasc Surg 2004;127:108–13.

40. Steger V, Walles T, Kosan B, et al. Trimodal therapy for histologically proven N2/3 non-small cell lung cancer: mid-term results and indicators for survival. Ann Thorac Surg 2009;87:1676–83.

41. Caglar HB, Baldini EH, Othus M, et al. Outcomes of patients with stage III non-small cell lung cancer treated with chemotherapy and radiation with and without surgery. Cancer 2009;115:4156–66.

42. Strauss GM, Herndon JE, Sherman DD, et al. Neoadjuvant chemotherapy and radiotherapy followed by surgery in stage IIIA non-small-cell carcinoma of the lung: report of a Cancer and Leukemia Group B phase II study. J Clin Oncol 1992;10:1237–44.

43. Bueno R, Richards WC, Swanson SJ, et al. Nodal stage after induction therapy for stage IIIA lung cancer determines patient survival. Ann Thorac Surg 2000;70: 1826–31.

44. Stefani A, Alifano M, Bobbio A, et al. Which patients should be operated on after induction chemotherapy for non-small cell lung cancer? Analysis of a 7-year experience in 175 patients. J Thorac Cardiovasc Surg 2010;140:356–63.

45. Paul S, Mirza F, Port JL, et al. Survival of patients with clinical stage IIIA non-small cell lung cancer after induction therapy: age, mediastinal downstaging, and extent of resection as independent predictors. J Thorac Cardiovasc Surg 2011; 141:48–55.

46. Adelstein DJ, Rice TW, Rybicki LA, et al. Long-term follow-up after chemoradiotherapy (CRT) in patients (pts) with stage III non-small cell lung cancer (NSCLC): is bulky mediastinal nodal disease of prognostic importance? [abstract]. J Clin Oncol 2004;22:14S.

47. Okada M, Tsubota N, Yoshimura M, et al. Induction therapy for non-small cell lung cancer with involved mediastinal nodes in multiple stations. Chest 2000;118: 123–8.

48. Doddoli CD, Barlesi F, Trousse D, et al. One hundred consecutive pneumonectomies after induction therapy for non-small cell lung cancer; an uncertain balance between risks and benefits. J Thorac Cardiovasc Surg 2005;130:416–25.

49. Allen AM, Mentzer SJ, Yeap BY, et al. Pneumonectomy after chemoradiation: the Dana-Farber cancer Institute/Brigham and Women's Hospital Experience. Cancer 2008;112:1106–13.

50. Gudbjartsson T, Gyllstedt E, Pikwer A, et al. Early surgical results after pneumonectomy for non-small cell lung cancer are not affected by preoperative radiotherapy and chemotherapy. Ann Thorac Surg 2008;86:376–82.

51. Weder W, Colland S, Eberhardt WE, et al. Pneumonectomy is a valuable treatment option after neoadjuvant therapy for stage III non-small-cell lung cancer. J Thorac Cardiovasc Surg 2010;139:1424–30.

52. Martin J, Ginsberg RJ, Abolhoda A, et al. Morbidity and mortality after neoadjuvant therapy for lung cancer: the risks of right pneumonectomy. Ann Thorac Surg 2001;72:1149–54.

Extensive Resections: Pancoast Tumors, Chest Wall Resections, En Bloc Vascular Resections

Antonio D'Andrilli, MD[a],*, Federico Venuta, MD[b],
Cecilia Menna, MD[a], Erino A. Rendina, MD[a]

KEYWORDS
- Lung cancer • Pancoast tumor • Chest wall
- Superior vena cava • Aorta

Infiltration by lung tumor of adjacent anatomic structures including major vessels (pulmonary artery [PA], superior vena cava [SVC], aorta, and supra-aortic vessels), main bronchi, and chest wall not only influences the oncologic severity of the disease but also increases the technical complexity of surgery, requiring extended resections and demanding reconstructive procedures. Completeness of resection represents in every case one of the main factors influencing the long-term outcome of patients.

Although increasing experience in the last years has contributed toward improving the results of such complex operations, the diffusion of some of these interventions to multiple institutions still remains limited, due to the concern for higher perioperative complication and mortality rates.

Technical and oncologic aspects of extended operations, including resection of Pancoast tumors and the chest wall, bronchovascular sleeve resections, and en bloc resections of major thoracic vessels, are reported in this article.

PANCOAST TUMORS

Pancoast tumor was first described in 1924[1,2] as a tumor of the apex of the lung with chest wall infiltration above the second rib and clinical signs of nerve injury such as

The authors have nothing to disclose.
[a] Department of Thoracic Surgery, Sant'Andrea Hospital, University LaSapienza, Via di Grottarossa 1035, 00189 Rome, Italy
[b] Department of Thoracic Surgery, Policlinico Umberto I, Sant'Andrea Hospital, University LaSapienza, Viale del Policlinico 155, 00161 Rome, Italy
* Corresponding author.
E-mail address: adandrilli@hotmail.com

pain, Horner syndrome, and muscle atrophy of the hand. Due to the involvement of the apex of the lung, invasion of the lower part of the brachial plexus, first ribs and vertebrae, subclavian vessels, and stellate ganglion may be present at the time of diagnosis, justifying the associated symptoms. More recently, to simplify the inclusion criteria of patients in multimodality treatment protocols a renewed definition of Pancoast tumor[3] has been proposed, including all tumors that invade the parietal pleura or the chest wall at the level of the second rib or above, regardless the presence of neurologic symptoms (**Fig. 1**).

These tumors may present at variable clinical stages ranging from IIB to IV, but patients amenable to surgical resection are usually limited to the T3–T4, N0–1 subgroup. Due to the particular location of the tumor and the complex anatomy of the area involved, Pancoast tumor represents a major surgical challenge, as suggested by the increased rates of incomplete resections, local recurrences, and perioperative morbidity reported in many experiences, especially in the early era of surgical treatment.

Historical Notes

The first successful surgical treatment of a superior sulcus tumor followed by postoperative radiation was reported by Chardack and MacCallum in 1956.[4] Until that time, Pancoast tumors had been unvaryingly considered as an unresectable and incurable type of lung cancer, and definitive radiotherapy with palliative intent represented the best standard of care, although no long-term success had been reported with this therapeutic approach.

In the same year, Shaw and colleagues[5] successfully performed a radical resection of a superior sulcus tumor in a patient previously undergoing radiotherapy with palliative intent, who presented postirradiation resolution of pain and reduction of tumor size. Based on this encouraging result, Shaw[6] standardized this treatment strategy for the following period, observing improved local control and longer survival when compared with historical controls.

The surgical approach used consisted in an extended posterolateral thoracotomy, allowing good exposure of the posterior chest wall. As a result of the Shaw experience,

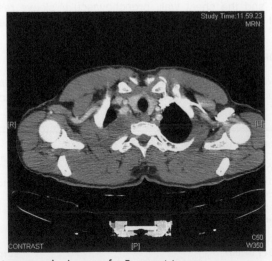

Fig. 1. Computed tomography image of a Pancoast tumor.

the administration of induction radiotherapy followed by en bloc resection became the treatment strategy of choice for this type of tumor until the 1980s. In particular the advantages of preoperative administration of radiotherapy have been emphasized, based on the possibility to verify the marked tumor regression on the surgical specimen. The posterior incision proposed by Shaw represented the sole surgical approach used for Pancoast tumors until the early 1990s, when innovative anterior approaches[7] were introduced that allowed for safer control of the subclavian vessels.

Although no randomized study comparing radiotherapy alone with radiotherapy plus surgical resection has been conducted, a large number of reports appeared between the 1970s and 1990s showing improved survival with the radiosurgical approach. A recent review[8] considering 23 studies that analyze the results of radiotherapy plus surgery for Pancoast tumors has reported a mean 5-year survival rate of 36.5%. This rate was clearly higher than that (6.2%) reported in the 18 studies analyzing the results of radiotherapy alone.

Modern Multimodality Treatment Strategy

The treatment strategy for superior sulcus tumors has further changed since the late 1990s, when the introduction of trimodality regimens based on the preoperative association of chemotherapy to irradiation appeared able to produce a clear improvement of results in terms of local control and long-term prognosis. Several studies published in the last decade, reporting the use of induction chemoradiotherapy followed by surgery with radical intent, have confirmed a significant increase in complete resection rates, pathologic response rates, and long term survival.

The largest study reporting the results of multimodality treatment for Pancoast tumors was published by the Southwestern Oncology Group (SWOG) in 2007.[9] This trial included 110 patients with N0–1 disease undergoing an induction regimen of concurrent chemotherapy (cisplatin and etoposide) and radiotherapy (45 Gy) followed by surgery and postoperative boost of chemotherapy with the same scheme. The treatment was well tolerated, with low morbidity and mortality rates. In 88 operated patients, the complete or near complete pathologic response rate was 61% and the complete resection rate was 94%. Overall actuarial 5-year survival was 44%, and was 54% in patients showing complete response. The main limitation of this study was the heterogeneity in the surgical treatment, due to the large number of participating institutions.

In another North American study by Kwong and colleagues,[10] the administration of a higher dose of radiotherapy in the trimodality treatment allowed favorable results even with less restrictive criteria in the selection of patients. This series included 36 patients, 14% of whom presented with N3 disease or single brain metastasis, undergoing a preoperative platinum-based chemotherapy concurrent with 45-Gy large-field radiotherapy followed by 14.2-Gy small-field boost radiotherapy. A complete pathologic response was observed in 40% of these patients, and the complete resection rate was 97%. Despite the more advanced stage of the patients, 5-year survival was 50% and was not influenced by the occurrence of brain relapses.

In a German experience published by Marra and colleagues[11] including 31 operated patients, an aggressive multimodality treatment was used for patients with advanced stage (N2–3 disease in 29% of cases, T4 in 19% of cases). Induction regimen consisted of 3 cycles of chemotherapy with cisplatin and etoposide followed by concurrent chemoradiotherapy (one course of cisplatin/etoposide plus 45 Gy hyperfractionated accelerated irradiation). This unique multimodality approach resulted in a high complete or near complete response rate (69%) with radical (R0) resection achieved in all patients. Overall 5-year survival was 46%, with significantly better results in patients showing response to induction therapy and with N0–1 disease. A 6.4% postoperative mortality was reported.

A high pathologic response rate has been also reported in a recent large series (72 patients) published by Pourel and colleagues,[12] with a less aggressive induction chemoradiotherapy regimen (cisplatin and etoposide plus 45 Gy radiotherapy). In this study the tumoral tissue was found to be completely replaced by necrosis and desmoplastic fibrosis induced by the preoperative treatment in 39.5% of patients. The reported 5-year survival reached 51% with a 98% complete resection rate.

Similar pathologic response rate was achieved in a study of the Japanese Clinical Oncology Group,[13] with a 5-year survival rate of 56% despite the inclusion of N2 patients. Results of the main trimodality treatment series are reported in **Table 1**.[9–13] Improvements in survival obtained with trimodality treatment are principally explained by the decrease of local recurrences. The incidence of recurrent disease at thoracic level has been observed as less than 30% after trimodality regimens, in comparison with 70% and more after radiotherapy and chemotherapy alone, and 40% with concurrent chemoradiotherapy alone.[13–17]

Analyzing literature data, the most significant negative factors influencing long-term survival include the presence of mediastinal nodal metastases, spine and/or subclavian vessel involvement (T4 disease), and incomplete resection.[15,18,19] The presence of metastatic mediastinal nodes has been considered an exclusion criterion in some studies. Among trials including N2 patients,[10–13] this prognostic variable, especially with persistent positive lymph node disease after chemoradiation, negatively affects long-term survival in all studies except one.[10]

Some investigators[15,20] have reported Horner syndrome and invasion of brachial plexus to be additional negative factors influencing prognosis.

The prognostic significance of the ipsilateral supraclavicular nodes in superior sulcus tumors is still the object of debate. According to the actual International Union Against Cancer classification, metastases to these nodes are classified as N3 disease. Because these nodes are adjacent to the primary tumor, such particular anatomic location could justify a clinical behavior more similar to that of N1 than that of N3 disease.[8,15]

The presence of T4 disease has been also reported as an adverse variable influencing the probability of complete resection in most surgical experiences. In a study by Rusch and colleagues,[9] the complete resection rate achieved in T3N0 patients was 25% higher than that achieved in T4N0 patients.

Distant metastases, mainly to the brain, represent the most frequent cause of death in patients with Pancoast tumor undergoing trimodality treatment in principal studies.[12,21] The incidence of brain metastases as first site of recurrence is reported as between 15% and 30% in the largest series. For this reason, prophylactic cranial irradiation has been proposed by some investigators to minimize the risk for distant recurrence.[11]

Surgical Approaches and Technical Aspects

Although an original incision for the treatment of Pancoast tumor was first reported by Chardack and MacCallum in the early 1950s,[4] the most popular surgical approach was the so-called high posterior thoracotomy described by Shaw and colleagues[5] some years later.

This technique is an extension of the conventional posterolateral thoracotomy, with posterior enlargement of the incision that curves around the tip of the scapula and continues upward between the posterior edge of the scapula and the spinous processes of the vertebrae up to C7 (**Fig. 2**). It allows good exposure of the posterior

Table 1
Multimodality treatment of Pancoast tumors: results of series with more than 30 patients

Authors, Year	No. of Operated Patients	Stage	Inclusion/ Exclusion Criteria	Treatment	Complete Resection (%)	Pathologic Complete Response (%)	5-Year Survival (%)	Median Survival (mo)
Kwong et al,[10] 2005	36	IIB–IV	N2, M1 incl.	CT/RT (59.2 Gy) + S	97	40	50	31
Marra et al,[11] 2007	31	IIB–IIIB	N2–3 incl.	CT+ CT/RT (45 Gy) + S	100	69	46	54
Rusch et al,[9] 2007	88	IIB–IIIB	N0–1 only	CT/RT (45 Gy) + S + CT	94	61	44	NR
Kunitoh et al,[13] 2008	57	IIB–IIIB	N2 incl.	CT/RT (45 Gy) + S	68	21	56	NR
Pourel et al,[12] 2008	72	IIB–IIIB	N2 incl.	CT/RT (45 Gy) + S	98	NR	51 (3 y)	36.5

Abbreviations: CT, chemotherapy; NR, not reported; RT, radiotherapy; S, surgery.

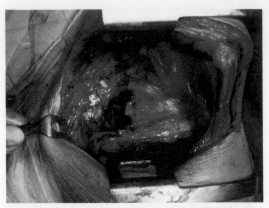

Fig. 2. Chest wall resection for Pancoast tumor through a high posterior thoracotomy (Shaw-Paulson approach).

chest wall, including the vertebrae and the roots of the thoracic nerves and brachial plexus. The main advantage of this access is represented by the association of improved exposure of the upper thoracic district with optimal vision of the pulmonary hilum and the entire pleural cavity, facilitating the accomplishment of major lung resection. However, the exposure of vascular structures, especially of subclavian vessels, may be not adequate. This restricted access to the anterior structures can be responsible for the higher rates of incomplete resections[20] and the higher surgical morbidity and mortality[21] reported by some investigators. To improve the exposure of subclavian vessels, a modification of this approach has been proposed more recently[22,23] with a hook-formed extension that runs anteriorly toward the sternoclavicular joints.

The search for improved exposure of the anterior structures of the thoracic inlet produced between the late 1980s and early 1990s some innovative techniques that approach the tumor by anterior incisions.

An anterior cervicothoracic transclavicular approach was first described and popularized by Dartevelle and colleagues.[7] Through a large L-shaped incision running along the anterior border of the sternocleidomastoid muscle and continuing laterally above the clavicle, the medial clavicular portion is removed. This action allows dissection or resection of the subclavian vein, sectioning of the scalenus anterior muscle, and isolation or resection of the cervical part of the phrenic nerve if involved. Moreover, exposure of the subclavian artery is gained and dissection of the brachial plexus up to the spinal foramen can be done. The removal of the medial part of the clavicle proves particularly useful in the case of tumors involving the subclavian vessels at their confluences with the cervical trunks (innominate vein and brachiocephalic artery), allowing their safer dissection. In the experience of Dartevelle and colleagues, this approach has allowed them to treat most patients with superior sulcus tumors without the need for large posterolateral thoracotomy. However, the transection of the clavicle may cause postoperative alterations in shoulder mobility and cervical posture,[14,24] and this aspect has limited the diffusion of this incision. This problem led therefore to further modifications of this technique.

A variation of this approach has been reported by Grunenwald and Spaggiari,[25] which they term the transmanubrial osteomuscular sparing approach. This technique consists of an L-shaped skin incision along the sternocleidomastoid muscle and 2 cm below the clavicle. This incision allows sparing of the insertions of the sternocleidomastoid and the pectoralis muscle on the clavicle. An L-shaped section of the manubrium with the resection of the first rib cartilage and the costoclavicular ligament is then performed. The modified technique preserves shoulder mobility and avoids deformities due to the clavicle resection, ensuring equal surgical exposure to the Dartevelle incision.

An interesting alternative to these anterior approaches has been described by Masaoka and colleagues[26]: this is an anterior transsternal approach consisting of a median sternotomy with an extension into the fourth intercostal space and a transverse incision above the clavicle at the base of the neck. It is particularly useful in the case of subclavian artery and SVC involvement.

The improved exposure of the subclavian vessels allowed by the aforementioned approaches has contributed toward increasing the possibility of radical resection, even in cases of Pancoast tumors infiltrating vascular structures. For this reason vascular involvement itself is no longer considered to be a contraindication for surgery, as in the past. Also, the negative effect of vascular involvement on survival, observed by some investigators, has not been confirmed in those series in which high complete resection rates have been achieved.[27]

Extensive local involvement of brachial plexus is generally considered a contraindication to surgery, due to the high rate of incomplete resection and the poor prognosis.[28] However, resection of the lower part of the plexus including C8 and T1 roots has been reported by some investigators.[29,30] The neurologic consequences include diffuse weakness of the intrinsic muscles of the hand after T1 resection, and permanent paralysis of the hand muscles after C8 nerve excision.

Recent improvements in surgical techniques have also increased the possibility to achieve radical resection in the case of Pancoast tumors infiltrating the vertebrae. Some selected experiences worldwide[31-33] have reported the possibility of a multidisciplinary surgical team (thoracic surgeon, neurosurgeon, orthopedic surgeon) being able to perform laminectomy, partial vertebrectomy, and resection of whole vertebral body in association with major lung resection, obtaining significant prognostic advantages. Mazel and colleagues[33] have observed in radically resected patients a 52% 2-year survival rate, which was significantly higher than that obtained in the nonradically resected patients (13%).

Extended resections including vessels, spine, and brachial plexus are reported in the literature in fewer than 10% of all resected Pancoast tumors. It is probable that the marked tumor regression obtained with aggressive induction chemoradiotherapy regimens may have helped to reduce the rate of such extensive en bloc excisions.

RESECTION OF TUMOR INVADING THE CHEST WALL

Lung cancer has been reported to invade the chest wall in up to 5% to 8% of all resected cases in large series.[34,35] Pain represents the most common clinical presentation, with an incidence ranging between 37%[36] and 76%[37] in surgical series.

Involvement of the chest wall, which is classified as T3 disease, may include a spectrum of clinical situations ranging from isolated infiltration of the parietal pleura to invasion of soft tissue and/or bone, and even of major thoracic muscles. In other cases, a tumor with peripheral location may develop inflammatory adhesions to the parietal pleura without infiltrating it, so that a preoperative suspicion of T3 disease may be not confirmed intraoperatively or postoperatively on the surgical specimen.

The surgical treatment varies from en bloc chest wall resection associated with major lung resection to extrapleural major lung resection. The indication for en bloc resection is clearly mandated in the case of full-thickness infiltration of the chest wall. On the contrary, it is still controversial whether an extrapleural lung resection could be considered adequate for tumors apparently confined to the parietal pleura. Such operations may be advantageous in avoiding unnecessary chest wall resection when bone and soft tissue are not involved, thus reducing the risk of surgical complications, but they expose the patient to the higher risk of recurrence with nonradical resection.

It is generally difficult to define the exact limit of tumor infiltration by preoperative imaging; the intraoperative evaluation almost always determines the final decision to resect the chest wall. Standard computed tomography and magnetic resonance imaging have shown limited accuracy in the assessment of chest wall involvement when no specific signs, such as rib destruction or soft-tissue infiltration, are visible.[38] The presence of specific radiologic features of the tumor including a large contact surface with the pleura, associated pleural thickening, and obliteration of the fat pad have been reported as factors indicating an increased probability of chest wall invasion,[39] but does not provide conclusive information.

The surgical approach may vary in relation to the location of the tumor. A posterolateral thoracotomy is generally adequate in most cases, because the majority of tumors with chest wall invasion occur in the posterior and lateral district.[40,41] However, for cancer invading the chest wall anteriorly a lateral or anterolateral approach may be advisable.[34]

Careful palpation of the tumor and the chest wall intraoperatively is fundamental to achieving a radical resection with free margins. A macroscopic free margin of at least 1 cm all around the tumor is generally considered sufficient,[42,43] although there are some investigators[44,45] who recommend a 3- to 4-cm margin and one segment of noninfiltrated rib above and below the gross margin of the tumor.

In the case of tumors extending in the costovertebral sulcus, it may be preferable to disarticulate the ribs from the vertebrae. Moreover, this tumor location may be prone to increased risk of incomplete resection and of damage to the spinal cord vascularization coming from ramifications of the dorsal branches of the intercostal arteries, as emphasized by some investigators.[46]

Small posterior defects, generally less than 5 cm in diameter, and defects covered by the scapula usually do not require chest wall reconstruction. The reconstruction is usually performed for defects of 3 or more ribs, not covered by the scapula. Reconstruction is also recommended for defects located at the tip of the scapula, to avoid its entrapment on the edge of the resected chest wall. Alternatively, some investigators have performed a scapular tip resection to prevent this complication or to treat it.[45]

The need for reconstruction has been reported as from 40%[47] to 64%[48,49] of cases in different series. The chest wall reconstruction can be performed using a synthetic material prosthesis or by using autologous muscle flap with or without prosthetic repair. Most commonly used prosthetic materials include polytetrafluoroethylene (PTFE) and polypropylene. PTFE is flexible, resistant to tension, and impervious to fluids and air. Polypropylene mesh is much less expensive and is not impervious to air and fluids. In the case of large defects in which a curvature is required, this mesh can be reinforced by a methylmethacrylate matrix curved support. The use of a rigid prosthesis is generally not recommended because it can damage and penetrate the surrounding tissue with the respiratory movements.

Data from the literature present marked heterogeneity concerning the type of surgical resection performed (en bloc or extrapleural), the variable rate of N1–2 patients included, and the discrepancies in complete resection rate in different studies. Favorable results have been reported especially for N0 patients, with 5-year survival rates in this stage of more than 40% in most series.[40,45,47,48,50] The presence of positive N2 nodes represents a factor significantly worsening long-term prognosis in almost all of the published studies. On the other hand, this prognostic disadvantage has not been systematically reported for N1 patients in comparison with N0 patients (**Table 2**).[44,45,47,48,50–55]

Distant metastases are the main cause of late mortality in most surgical experiences, with local relapses generally observed in fewer than 30% of all recurrences.[44,49–51]

Results of en bloc resections are hardly comparable with those of extrapleural resections, because of the heterogeneous inclusion criteria and the different surgical indications from one study to another. Some studies published in the 1980s reported clear prognostic advantages for en bloc resection. Piehler and colleagues[52] observed a 75% 5-year survival rate after en bloc resection compared with 27.9% after extrapleural resection. McCaughan and colleagues[53] found a 5-year survival rate of 48% after en bloc resection and of 16% after extrapleural resection. More recently, Doddoli and colleagues[47] observed a better prognosis with en bloc resection. Conversely, in a study from Memorial Sloan Kettering,[56] no significant difference in survival between en bloc and extrapleural resection was reported. Akay and colleagues[49] found similar 5-year survival between patients who underwent extrapleural resection for limited parietal pleura invasion and patients who underwent en bloc resection for deeper chest wall infiltration. The lack of significant difference in survival between the two techniques has been confirmed by other investigators.[40,50,52] In other experiences the chest wall has been systematically removed also in cases of invasion limited to the parietal pleura.

Postoperative mortality after chest wall resection for lung cancer has been reported to range from 0% to 7.8%,[40,45,47,48,52] with most studies reporting a mortality rate of less than 5%. It has been estimated that the risk for death after such operations is 3 times higher than that observed after standard major lung resections.

The main cause of mortality is represented by respiratory complications (66%–75% incidence).[34,41,47] The occurrence of these complications is certainly promoted by the alterations in respiratory mechanics caused by extended chest wall resection.

Another serious complication related to surgery is local infection at the site of prosthetic reconstruction. This event usually requires the removal of the synthetic prosthesis. Paraplegia following costovertebral disarticulation caused by injury to spinal cord vascularization is a rare complication, but its remote risk has to be considered in the case of tumors invading the paravertebral sulcus.[46]

Table 2
Results of resections for lung tumors invading the chest wall

Authors, Year	No. of Patients	5-Year Overall Survival (%)	5-Year N0 Survival (%)	5-Year N1 Survival (%)	5-Year N2 Survival (%)
Chapelier et al,[44] 2000	100	18	22	9	0
Magdeleinat et al,[55] 2001	195	21	25	20	21
Facciolo et al,[45] 2001	104	61.4	67.3	100	17.9
Riquet et al,[51] 2002	125	22.5	30.5	0	11.5
Burkhart et al,[48] 2002	95	38.7	44.3	26.3	—
Matsuoka et al,[50] 2004	76	34.2	44.2	40	6.2
Doddoli et al,[47] 2005	309	30.7	40	23.8	8.4
Lin et al,[56] 2006	42	28.4	39	17.1	—

SLEEVE RESECTIONS

The indication for a sleeve resection for lung cancer is well established: a tumor arising at the origin of a lobar bronchus and/or at the origin of the lobar branches of the PA, but not infiltrating as far as to require pneumonectomy (PN). In addition, a sleeve resection may be indicated when N1 nodes infiltrate the bronchus from the outside, as is often the case in the left upper lobe tumors requiring a combined reconstruction of the bronchus and the PA. From a functional point of view, sleeve lobectomy (SL) is strictly indicated in patients who cannot withstand PN, but recent experiences have shown that the advantages of sparing lung parenchyma are evident even in patients without cardiopulmonary impairment.[57-63] The primary goal oncologically is in every case the complete resection of the tumor with free resection margins. The decision to perform PN or SL is based on both oncologic and physiologic considerations. Many investigators believe that PN, especially right PN, is a disease itself, with severe impairment of lung function and quality of life after surgery, and therefore the latter intervention should be avoided whenever possible.

The first bronchial sleeve resection was performed in 1947 for a carcinoid tumor[64] while the first SL for lung cancer was reported by Allison in 1954.[65] Since then, significant technical advances and increasing experience over time have allowed the achievement of excellent clinical and oncologic results, giving wide diffusion to this procedure.

Different techniques have been described for bronchial anastomotic reconstruction. The authors favor the use of interrupted sutures of 4-0 monofilament absorbable material.[57,66] However, the use of continuous running suture (complete or partial) has been described by others.[67,68]

The technique for the anastomotic reconstruction of the PA has been generally standardized with the use of running suture of 5-0 or 6-0 monofilament nonabsorbable material.[68-71]

Protection of the bronchial anastomosis by a viable tissue flap is recommended by most investigators.[72,73] The authors routinely use an intercostal muscle flap,[72] which has an excellent vascularization provided by the intercostal artery, favoring the preservation of the air tightness even in the case of small anastomotic dehiscence, and minimizing the risk of PA erosion especially when an associated vascular reconstruction is performed. Alternatively, the use of mediastinal fat pad,[73] or pericardial or pleural flap[68] has been reported.

For the final success of bronchial and vascular reconstructive procedures, it is essential to avoid tension on the anastomosis; this can be achieved by dividing the pulmonary ligament or, more often on the right side, by opening the pericardium around the pulmonary vein.

In unusual situations the circumferential defect after en bloc resection of the infiltrated PA may be too extensive to allow direct vascular end-to-end anastomosis. Such is usually the case of a left upper lobe tumor infiltrating the PA extensively but not the lobar bronchus, so that a bronchial sleeve is not indicated. In such cases the interposition of a conduit of biological or synthetic material can be used. The authors have described the successful deployment of an autologous pericardial or bovine pericardial conduit.[71] The use of pulmonary vein of the resected lobe has been also reported (**Fig. 3**).[74]

When analyzing survival data reported in the literature over the last 15 years, most studies show similar or better results for parenchymal sparing resections if compared with PN. Moreover, in the analysis of 5-year survival according to stage and nodal status, SL results in higher survival rates for stages I, II, and III, although the survival advantage in stage III appears to be limited (**Table 3**).[59-62,75,76]

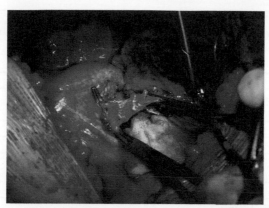

Fig. 3. Reconstruction of the pulmonary artery by pulmonary vein conduit.

In a report by Ludwig and colleagues,[62] SL results in a statistically significant favorable prognosis for long-term survival, with a survival advantage in patients with N0, N1, and N2 disease. However, this prognostic advantage for stage III N2 patients is not always confirmed. Therefore, the role of parenchymal sparing operations in patients with N2 disease still remains incompletely defined.[59,62]

Postoperative morbidity and mortality data reveal better results overall for patients undergoing SL in comparison with PN (**Table 4**).[59–62,75,76]

These results justify the increasing use of parenchymal sparing procedures for lung cancer also in patients with good cardiopulmonary function, as observed in the last years.

Table 3
Survival rates after sleeve lobectomy and pneumonectomy for lung cancer

Authors, Year	Stage I Patients	Stage II Patients	Stage III Patients	Stage I 5-Year Survival (%)	Stage II 5-Year Survival (%)	Stage III 5-Year Survival (%)
Sleeve Lobectomy						
Gaissert et al,[75] 1996	29	31	12	42	53	43
Tronc et al,[114] 2000	83	73	26	63	48	8
Fadel et al,[59] 2002	54	47	36	55	62	21
Terzi et al,[60] 2002	48	52	50	60	32	22
Deslauriers et al,[78] 2004	83	72	29	66	50	19
Kim et al,[61] 2005	14	18	15	88	52	8
Ludwig et al,[62] 2005	31	41	44	57	40	22
Takeda et al,[85] 2006	26	19	17	45[a]	45[a]	21.8
Pneumonectomy						
Gaissert et al,[75] 1996	9	25	21	—	43	—
Deslauriers et al,[78] 2004	164	361	471	50	34	22
Kim et al,[61] 2005	28	11	10	75	36	38
Ludwig et al,[62] 2005	31	52	111	45	42	13
Takeda et al,[85] 2006	24	14	70	38[a]	38[a]	52.8

[a] Stage I–II.

Table 4
Sleeve lobectomy versus pneumonectomy: postoperative morbidity and mortality

Authors, Year	Complications (%)	Postoperative Mortality (%)	Local Recurrence (%)	Distant Recurrence (%)
Sleeve Lobectomy				
Gaissert et al,[75] 1996	11	4	14	—
Tronc et al,[114] 2000	16	1.6	22	11
Fadel et al,[59] 2002	16	2.9	15	11
Terzi et al,[60] 2002	14.5	12	5	18
Deslauriers et al,[78] 2004	—	1.3	2.2	—
Kim et al,[61] 2005	74.9	6.1	22	22
Ludwig et al,[62] 2005	38	4.3	—	—
Takeda et al,[85] 2006	45.2	1.6	9.7	29
Pneumonectomy				
Gaissert et al,[75] 1996	16	9	—	—
Deslauriers et al,[78] 2004	—	5.3	35	—
Kim et al,[61] 2005	44	4.1	6	20
Ludwig et al,[62] 2005	26	4.6	—	—
Takeda et al,[85] 2006	40.9	1.8	10.9	42.7

An interesting meta-analysis[77] including 12 articles[61,62,75,76,78–85] published between 1996 and 2006 compared early and long-term outcome of SL with those of PN. A total of 2984 patients were included in this analysis, 21% undergoing SL and 79% undergoing PN. Two hundred and two patients underwent PA resection and reconstruction in association with a bronchial sleeve resection (164 patients) or not (38 patients). The evaluation of surgical morbidity including results from 8 studies[61,62,75,76,79,81,83,85] showed a pooled incidence of 31.3% in the SL group and of 31.6% in the PN group, without a statistically significant difference. Similar results were observed when limiting the analysis to studies reporting a larger experience (>50 patients) of SL (30.8% complication rate in SL group and 33.6% in PN group). The mean postoperative complication rate reported after PA reconstruction was similar (32.4%) to that reported after bronchial SL and PN. Overall postoperative mortality presented a pooled incidence of 3.5% in the SL group and 5.7% in the PN group, but this difference did not reach statistical significance. However, when considering only studies with a larger number (>50) of SL patients,[62,75,76,78,80,83–85] the mortality rate was significantly lower in the SL group than in the PN group.

Overall 5-year survival rate extracted from 10 studies[61,62,76,78–81,83–85] was 50.3% after SL and 30.6% after PN, showing a statistically significant difference. The median overall survival was 60 months for the SL group and 28 months for the PN group. This result may have been partially influenced by the higher rate of stage III patients included in the PN group in most studies. However, when considering survival according to pathologic N status (from the few studies reporting these data[62,85]), pooled 1-year and 5-year survival rates of patients with N0 or N1 disease are significantly higher after SL. In patients with pN2, a slight statistically significant advantage was observed in 1-year survival for the SL group, whereas no significant difference was shown for 5-year survival.

Data regarding locoregional recurrences have been reported in only 6[61,76,78,79,83,85] of the studies considered in this meta-analysis. The pooled locoregional recurrence rate was 16.1% in the SL group and 27.8% in the PN group, but this difference did not reach statistical significance. Alternatively, when considering only studies with a larger number of sleeve procedures,[76,78,83,85] a significantly lower incidence of local recurrence was found in the SL group in comparison with the PN group (14.5% vs 28.7%).

A previous meta-analysis published by Ferguson and Lehman[86] including 12 studies provided similar survival results, reporting a better long-term prognosis after SL, although the incidence of local recurrence appeared higher in comparison with PN.

The preservation of lung parenchyma has therefore been indicated by some investigators as the possible cause of a theoretical increased risk for locoregional recurrence after SL. However, although in some experiences[59] a higher local recurrence rate is reported for sleeve resection with advanced nodal status (N2), the few studies[59-61] analyzing risk factors for recurrence show that the tumor stage and the nodal status are the only negative predictive factors, rather than the type of operation performed.

The incidence of microscopic infiltration of the bronchial margins has strong significance when analyzing the anastomotic complication and local recurrence rate. Investigators[61] who have observed a significantly higher incidence of anastomotic leak in their SL series often report an increased rate of positive margins on frozen section.

Looking at literature data, when morbidity is evaluated according to the type of complication PN patients appear to experience a higher rate of cardiac complications, whereas SL patients show an increased incidence of pulmonary and airway complications.[59-62,75,76]

Postoperative quality of life has been advocated as one of the strongest indicators to influence the decision to perform SL rather than PN. Several studies indicate that lung parenchyma sparing improves postoperative quality of life, determining a greater cardiopulmonary reserve, less pulmonary edema, and less right ventricular dysfunction, due to a lower pulmonary vascular resistance.[60,82] In the meta-analysis by Ferguson and Lehman[86] the Quality Adjusted Years Quoted were 4.37 after SL and 2.48 after PN. Melloul and colleagues[87] analyzed postoperative forced expiratory volume in 1 second (FEV_1) in a retrospective study, reporting significantly higher values for patients undergoing SL. In a prospective study by Martin-Ucar and colleagues,[82] the reported mean FEV_1 loss after parenchymal sparing operations was 170 mL (range 0–500 mL) compared with 600 mL (range 200–1400 mL) after PN, indicating a strongly significant prognostic advantage for patients undergoing SL.

Special concern has been expressed by many thoracic surgeons when considering bronchovascular reconstructive procedures after induction therapy, because of the significantly higher risk of perioperative complications and mortality. Although only few investigators[63,88] perform sleeve resection routinely after neoadjuvant therapy, it has been proved in the authors' experience[63,89] that even complex parenchymal sparing operations can be performed safely after oncologic treatment without increased morbidity and mortality rates, observing long-term results comparable with those of the standard procedures (5-year survival: 31%; local recurrence rate:15%).

Resection and reconstruction of the main PA infiltrated by central bronchogenic carcinoma has been reported in two small series.[90,91] No patient surviving longer than 30 months has been reported in these experiences, thus indicating that tumors infiltrating the main PA have to be considered technically resectable but not biologically curable.

RESECTION FOR TUMORS INFILTRATING MAJOR THORACIC VESSELS

Major intrathoracic great vessels including the PA, SVC, and aorta may be infiltrated by primary lung tumors, or by metastatic hilar or mediastinal lymph nodes.

The feasibility of resection and reconstruction of great vessels involved by tumor has been largely proved, allowing radical surgical treatment in selected patients.

Resection and Reconstruction of Superior Vena Cava

Involvement of the SVC may be due to direct extension of a right upper lobe tumor or by lymph node metastases to stations R2, R4, and 3. The majority of these cancers are unresectable, and when feasible the resection usually includes PN or sleeve PN. Options for reconstruction include direct suture if a minimal portion of the circumference is involved, patch reconstruction (usually with bovine or autologous pericardium), and prosthetic conduit (biological or synthetic material) reconstruction.

Extended operations including resection and reconstruction of the SVC represent a major technical challenge, especially for the potential detrimental effect of clamping a patent vessel.[92] Partial caval clamping or clamping of a chronically obstructed SVC is usually well tolerated. On the other hand, during complete clamping of a patent SVC there is a marked hemodynamic imbalance. The mean venous pressure in the cephalic district increases and the mean arterial pressure decreases, thus causing a reduction of the brain arterial-venous gradient. This phenomenon may produce cerebral edema and damage, intracranial bleeding, and potentially lethal reduction of the cardiac output.

This hemodynamic derangement can be minimized by several intraoperative technical and pharmacologic solutions. From the surgical point of view, the placement of intraluminal or extraluminal shunts (between the brachiocephalic vein or the internal jugular vein and the right atrium) may reduce the effects of clamping. However, thrombosis of the shunt may occur; furthermore, these devices occupy space in the operative field, determining increased difficulties for the vascular sutures.

Intraoperative pharmacologic neuroprotection includes administration of steroids before clamping, and optimization of circulatory parameters during clamping by fluid administration and vasoconstrictive agents in order to increase the mean arterial pressure. Anticoagulation with intravenous sodium heparin (0.5 mg/kg) is administered before clamping and is continued in the postoperative period, taking into account the characteristics of the graft material used for reconstruction.

Vascular reconstruction can be performed by an SVC trunk replacement if a disease-free confluence of both of the innominate veins is present. After clamping and vascular resection, the anastomosis between the superior caval stump and the prosthetic conduit is performed first (5-0 or 6-0 polypropylene suture).

To avoid kinking of the prosthesis, the length of the conduit is adapted so that the distal anastomosis can be put under tension. In the case of neoplastic infiltration of the SVC origin at the confluence with the innominate veins, the revascularization is usually performed between the left innominate vein and the inferior SVC stump (or the right atrium) with closure of the right innominate vein, or alternatively between the right innominate vein and the inferior SVC stump (or the right atrium) with closure of the left innominate vein, according to the local invasion.

These types of reconstruction are almost always performed using synthetic materials (usually ringed PTFE grafts) or bovine pericardium. Minimal dissection, especially at the left innominate vein, is mandatory to avoid its rotation above the anastomosis. The risk of kinking is lower for revascularization of the right innominate vein because the residual venous stump is shorter and the direction of the graft is almost vertical.

Revascularization of both of the innominate veins implanted independently at the right atrium are generally not performed, because the blood flow through the graft is too low and exposes a high risk of thrombosis. Total resections of the SVC and both of the innominate veins, and reconstruction with a Y-shaped synthetic prosthesis (Dacron or PTFE) have been successfully realized and reported in the literature.[93]

Reconstructive materials

Different materials have been used for prosthetic reconstruction of the SVC, including biological (autologous or heterologous) or synthetic options.

Among the synthetic materials used for graft reconstruction of the SVC (Dacron, PTFE)), the PTFE is the preferred option. This synthetic material shows the highest long-term patency rate, and shortly after its implantation it becomes reepithelialized with autogenous epithelial cells in humans. PTFE grafts have a low risk of infection, less platelet deposition, and less thrombogenicity of the flow surface compared with Dacron grafts.[94] The risk for thrombosis with the PTFE prosthesis has been reported at around 10% in some of the largest series.[95,96] The synthetic grafts are usually reinforced with external rings.

Biological materials have achieved large acceptance in the reconstruction of low-pressure thoracic vessels because of improved biocompatibility, lower risk of infection and thrombosis, and lower costs if compared with synthetic materials.

Among the biological materials, autologous pericardium has been extensively used for either patch or conduit reconstruction. Although positive results have been obtained with both of these options, the large amount of tissue required for the replacement of a long vascular tube makes this material unsuitable for most cases of complete caval reconstruction. Conversely, autologous pericardium can be considered an ideal option for patch reconstruction of the SVC as well as of the PA. It is available on both sides of the chest; moreover, its harvesting does not require a separate procedure and offers a larger amount of tissue compared with venous patches. However, despite the high number of favorable characteristics (biocompatibility, adequate thickness and resistance, cost-free), fresh pericardium has some technical limits because it markedly shrinks and curls, making the adaptation of the patch to the vascular wall defect more difficult to achieve. To minimize this problem, the authors have described an original method of fixation of the autologous pericardium by glutaraldehyde[97] that improves the technical features of this material, providing increased rigidity to the patch.

Among the heterologous biological materials, bovine pericardium at present is certainly the most frequently used option. It displays some advantageous characteristics, such as the presence of even and stiff edges and the limited tendency to retract, facilitating its adaptation and suturing to the vascular wall. However, in the patch reconstructive procedures it has lower diffusion compared with autologous pericardium because of inferior biocompatibility and higher costs. Conversely, when total SVC replacement is required, bovine pericardium is preferred because the autologous tissue is generally not sufficient to create a long conduit. The pericardial conduit has a lower risk of infection and thrombosis, and does not necessitate long-term anticoagulation in comparison with synthetic materials.

The authors have devised and used an original technique for the construction of a pericardial conduit to be used for SVC replacement.[98] The bovine pericardial leaflet is trimmed to a rectangular shape of the resected caval segment length, wrapped around a syringe (5 mL or 10 mL) to obtain the appropriate diameter, and sutured longitudinally by a linear reloadable stapler The mechanical suture recently introduced in this technique (instead of the previously used manual suture) enables a quicker, easier, and more precise procedure, and confers a more regular shape to the vascular graft (**Fig. 4**).

In a series of 15 consecutive patients with lung or mediastinal malignancies undergoing resection and reconstruction of the SVC using this technique, the authors have observed a 100% patency rate of the prosthetic conduit at long term.[99]

Other biological options such as autologous venous grafts (saphenous, jugular, superficial femoral) have a limited diameter that is sufficient only for the reconstruction of the brachiocephalic vein, and are not suitable for SVC replacement. Saphenous vein graft of adequate diameter has been created by suturing the venous wall in a spiral fashion around a stent or a chest tube of appropriate size.[100]

There are in fact more than 10 series published in the literature, including some hundred patients who have undergone oncologic resection and reconstruction of the SVC. Prosthetic reconstructions have been performed in variable proportions, ranging between 0% and 49% in different series. Five-year survival rates have been reported in main series as between 21% and 31% with a perioperative mortality rate of 7% and 14% (**Table 5**).[91,101–108] There are no long-term survivors among patients with N2 lung cancer.

A review by the American College of Chest Physicians that considers the 4 largest studies published between 2000 and 2007, including 189 patients undergoing en bloc

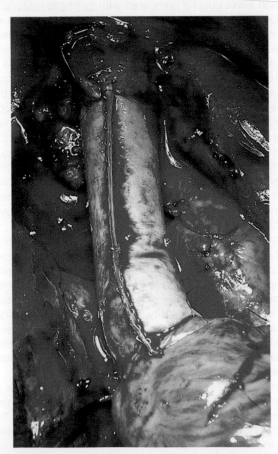

Fig. 4. Reconstruction of the superior vena cava by stapled bovine pericardial conduit.

Table 5
Resection and reconstruction of the superior vena cava for lung cancer

| | | Reconstruction | | | |
Authors, Year	Patients	Conduit (Material)	Patch (Material)	Mortality (%)	5-Year Survival (%)
Thomas et al,[101] 1994	15	4 (PTFE)	2 (PTFE)	7	24
Tsuchiya et al,[91] 1994	32	7	—	22	NR
Fukuse et al,[102] 1997	8	3 (PTFE)	—	NR	NR
Bernard et al,[103] 2001	8	2 (PTFE)	2 (PTFE)	NR	25
Spaggiari et al,[104] 2004[a]	109	28	8 (5 peric., 3 PTFE)	12	21
Shargall et al,[105] 2004	15	9 (7 PTFE, 1 jugular vein, 1 bov. peric.)	2 (peric.)	14	57 (3 y)
Suzuki et al,[106] 2004	40	11 (PTFE)	8 (aut. peric.)	10	24
Spaggiari et al,[107] 2007	52	13 (8 PTFE, 5 bov. peric., 3 n.s.)	4 (aut. peric.)	7.7	31
Yildizeli et al,[108] 2008	39	39 PTFE	—	7.7	29.4

Abbreviations: aut. peric., autologous pericardial; bov. peric., bovine pericardial; NR, not reported, n.s., not specified; peric., pericardial; PTFE, polytetrafluoroethylene.
[a] Multicenter study.

caval resection for lung cancer, reports a mean postoperative mortality of 12% and a mean 5-year survival of 25% (range: 21%–31%).[109]

A recent study[95] has shown no increased risk for overall postoperative morbidity and mortality in patients undergoing complete prosthetic replacement of SVC when compared with patients receiving direct suture repair of the vessel. However, graft reconstruction was related to a higher incidence of surgical complications in this series (17.8% vs 4.5%).

In the series published by Yildilzeli and colleagues,[110] carinal resection and squamous cell carcinoma have been found to be the most significant negative prognostic factors in patients who have undergone SVC en bloc resection for lung cancer.

Resection of Tumor Infiltrating the Aorta

Radical resections of tumors invading the aorta have been performed by intra-adventitial dissection and superficial vascular excision, by limited vascular excision requiring direct tangential suture or patch reconstruction, or by en bloc resection of portions of aorta with prosthetic replacement.

There are still few experiences reported in the literature, with a limited number of patients. The largest series[110] includes 16 patients, 10 of whom were treated by prosthetic reconstruction, 5 with patch reconstruction, and 1 by direct suture. Reported surgical mortality was 12.5% with 31% complication rate. Five-year survival rates have shown significant differences according to lymph nodal status (70% in N0 patients and 16.7% in N2–3 patients). Most patients (10) in this experience have received preoperative chemoradiotherapy and have been operated through a hemi-clamshell approach. A partial cardiopulmonary bypass (femoral vein-femoral artery) was used in 10 patients, and a passive shunt between the ascending and the descending aorta was used in 4 patients.

Table 6
Resection of the aorta for lung cancer

Authors, Year	No. of Patients	TNM	Complications (%)	Mortality	Survival (5 Years)	Survival (Median)
Mistos et al,[113] 2007	13	T4 N0–2 M0	0	0	30.7% (T4N0 100%, T4N1 37.5%, T4N2 0%)	38 ± 9 mo
De Perrot et al,[112] 2005	3	T4 N0–3 M0	66.6	0	n.s.	n.s.
Ohta et al,[111] 2005	16		37.5	12.5%	70% (N0), 16, 7% (N2–3)	n.s.
Klepetko et al,[110] 1999	7	T4 N0–2 M0	14.2	0	100% (1 y), 75% (2 y), 25% (4 y)	n.s.
Fukuse et al,[102] 1997	15		13.3	0	31.8% (3 y)	22 mo

Abbreviation: n.s., not stated.

The other published experiences of successful en bloc resections of the aorta[102,111–113] report 5-year survival rates of up to 31%, although mean follow-up times are generally limited in these studies (**Table 6**).

Different results have been reported by Tsuchiya and colleagues,[91] who published a series of 28 resected patients with aortic invasion, 21 of whom presented only adventitial involvement and 7 complete aortic wall infiltration. Intra-adventitial dissection and peeling of the lung tumor (performed in 21 patients) resulted in a high incomplete resection rate (52%). However, 3-year survival rate of patients undergoing intra-adventitial dissection was equal (14%) to that reported in the 7 patients receiving complete resection and prosthetic replacement of the aorta.

REFERENCES

1. Pancoast HK. Importance of careful Roentgen-ray investigations of apical chest tumours. JAMA 1924;83:1407–11.
2. Pancoast HK. Superior pulmonary sulcus tumor. JAMA 1932;99:1391–6.
3. Detterbeck FC. Changes in the treatment of Pancoast tumors [Review]. Ann Thorac Surg 2003;75(6):1990–7.
4. Chardack WM, MacCallum JD. Pancoast tumor; five-year survival without recurrence or metastases following radical resection and postoperative irradiation. J Thorac Surg 1956;31(5):535–42.
5. Shaw RR, Paulson DL, Kee JL. Treatment of superior sulcus tumor by irradiation followed by resection. Ann Surg 1961;154(1):29–40.
6. Shaw RR. Pancoast's tumor. Ann Thorac Surg 1984;37(4):343–5.
7. Dartevelle PG, Chapelier AR, Macchiarini P, et al. Anterior transcervical-thoracic approach for radical resection of lung tumors invading the thoracic inlet. J Thorac Cardiovasc Surg 1993;105(6):1025–34.
8. Tamura M, Hoda MA, Klepetko W. Current treatment paradigms of superior sulcus tumours [Review]. Eur J Cardiothorac Surg 2009;36(4):747–53.
9. Rusch VW, Giroux DJ, Kraut MJ, et al. Induction chemoradiation and surgical resection for superior sulcus non-small-cell lung carcinomas: long-term results

of Southwest Oncology Group Trial 9416 (Intergroup Trial 0160). J Clin Oncol 2007;25(3):313–8.

10. Kwong KF, Edelman MJ, Suntharalingam M, et al. High-dose radiotherapy in tri-modality treatment of Pancoast tumors results in high pathologic complete response rates and excellent long-term survival. J Thorac Cardiovasc Surg 2005;129(6):1250–7.

11. Marra A, Eberhardt W, Pöttgen C, et al. Induction chemotherapy, concurrent che-moradiation and surgery for Pancoast tumour. Eur Respir J 2007;29(1):117–26.

12. Pourel N, Santelmo N, Naafa N, et al. Concurrent cisplatin/etoposide plus 3D-conformal radiotherapy followed by surgery for stage IIB (superior sulcus T3N0)/III non-small cell lung cancer yields a high rate of pathological complete response. Eur J Cardiothorac Surg 2008;33(5):829–36.

13. Kunitoh H, Kato H, Tsuboi M, et al. Japan Clinical Oncology Group. Phase II trial of preoperative chemoradiotherapy followed by surgical resection in patients with superior sulcus non-small-cell lung cancers: report of Japan Clinical Oncology Group trial 9806. J Clin Oncol 2008;26(4):644–9.

14. Pitz CC, de la Rivière AB, van Swieten HA, et al. Surgical treatment of Pancoast tumours. Eur J Cardiothorac Surg 2004;26(1):202–8.

15. Ginsberg RJ, Martini N, Zaman M, et al. Influence of surgical resection and bra-chytherapy in the management of superior sulcus tumor. Ann Thorac Surg 1994; 57(6):1440–5.

16. Miyoshi S, Iuchi K, Nakamura K, et al. Induction concurrent chemoradiation therapy for invading apical non-small cell lung cancer. Jpn J Thorac Cardiovasc Surg 2004;52(3):120–6.

17. Kappers I, Belderbos JS, Burgers JA, et al. Non-small cell lung carcinoma of the superior sulcus: favourable outcomes of combined modality treatment in care-fully selected patients. Lung Cancer 2008;59(3):385–90.

18. Rusch VW, Parekh KR, Leon L, et al. Factors determining outcome after surgical resection of T3 and T4 lung cancers of the superior sulcus [Review]. J Thorac Cardiovasc Surg 2000;119(6):1147–53.

19. Alifano M, D'Aiuto M, Magdeleinat P, et al. Surgical treatment of superior sulcus tumors: results and prognostic factors. Chest 2003;124(3):996–1003.

20. Okubo K, Wada H, Fukuse T, et al. Treatment of Pancoast tumors. Combined irradiation and radical resection. Thorac Cardiovasc Surg 1995;43(5):284–6.

21. Wright CD, Moncure AC, Shepard JA, et al. Superior sulcus lung tumors. Results of combined treatment (irradiation and radical resection). J Thorac Cardiovasc Surg 1987;94(1):69–74.

22. Niwa H, Masaoka A, Yamakawa Y, et al. Surgical therapy for apical invasive lung cancer: different approaches according to tumor location. Lung Cancer 1993; 10(1–2):63–71.

23. Tatsumura T, Sato H, Mori A, et al. A new surgical approach to apical segment lung diseases, including carcinomas and inflammatory diseases. J Thorac Car-diovasc Surg 1994;107(1):32–6.

24. D'Andrilli A, Venuta F, Rendina EA. Surgical approaches for invasive tumors of the anterior mediastinum. Thorac Surg Clin 2010;20(2):265–84.

25. Grunenwald D, Spaggiari L. Transmanubrial osteomuscular sparing approach for apical chest tumors. Ann Thorac Surg 1997;63(2):563–6.

26. Masaoka A, Ito Y, Yasumitsu T. Anterior approach for tumor of the superior sulcus. J Thorac Cardiovasc Surg 1979;78(3):413–5.

27. Dartevelle PG. Herbert Sloan Lecture. Extended operations for the treatment of lung cancer. Ann Thorac Surg 1997;63(1):12–9.

28. Paulson DL. Carcinomas in the superior pulmonary sulcus. J Thorac Cardiovasc Surg 1975;70(6):1095–104.

29. Rusch VW. Management of Pancoast tumours. Lancet Oncol 2006;7(12): 997–1005.

30. Maggi G, Casadio C, Pischedda F, et al. Combined radiosurgical treatment of Pancoast tumor. Ann Thorac Surg 1994;57(1):198–202.

31. Bilsky MH, Vitaz TW, Boland PJ, et al. Surgical treatment of superior sulcus tumors with spinal and brachial plexus involvement. J Neurosurg 2002; 97(Suppl 3):301–9.

32. York JE, Walsh GL, Lang FF, et al. Combined chest wall resection with vertebrectomy and spinal reconstruction for the treatment of Pancoast tumors. J Neurosurg 1999;91(Suppl 1):74–80.

33. Mazel CH, Grunenwald D, Laudrin P, et al. Radical excision in the management of thoracic and cervicothoracic tumors involving the spine: results in a series of 36 cases. Spine 2003;28(8):782–92.

34. Stoelben E, Ludwig C. Chest wall resection for lung cancer: indications and techniques [Review]. Eur J Cardiothorac Surg 2009;35(3):450–6.

35. Mountain CF. Revisions in the international system for staging lung cancer. Chest 1997;111(6):1710–7.

36. Allen MS, Mathisen DJ, Grillo HC, et al. Bronchogenic carcinoma with chest wall invasion. Ann Thorac Surg 1999;51(6):948–51.

37. Patterson GA, Ilves R, Ginsberg RJ, et al. The role of adjuvant radiotherapy in pulmonary and chest wall resection for bronchogenic carcinoma. Ann Thorac Surg 1982;34(6):692–7.

38. Akata S, Kajiwara N, Park J, et al. Evaluation of chest wall invasion by lung cancer usingrespiratory dynamic MRI. J Med Imaging Radiat Oncol 2008; 52(1):36–9.

39. Rendina EA, Bognolo DA, Mineo TC, et al. Computed tomography for the evaluation of intrathoracic invasion by lung cancer. J Thorac Cardiovasc Surg 1987; 94(1):57–63.

40. Elia S, Griffo S, Gentile M, et al. Surgical treatment of lung cancer invading chest wall: a retrospective analysis of 110 patients. Eur J Cardiothorac Surg 2001; 20(2):356–60.

41. Martin-Ucar AE, Nicum R, Oey I, et al. En-bloc chest wall and lung resection for non-small cell lung cancer. Predictors of 60-day non-cancer related mortality. Eur J Cardiothorac Surg 2003;23(6):859–64.

42. Riquet M, Arame A, Le Pimpec-Barthes F. Non-small cell lung cancer invading the chest wall [Review]. Thorac Surg Clin 2010;20(4):519–27.

43. Allen MS. Chest wall resection and reconstruction for lung cancer [Review]. Thorac Surg Clin 2004;14(2):211–6.

44. Chapelier A, Fadel E, Macchiarini P, et al. Factors affecting long-term survival after en-bloc resection of lung cancer invading the chest wall. Eur J Cardiothorac Surg 2000;18(5):513–8.

45. Facciolo F, Cardillo G, Lopergolo M, et al. Chest wall invasion in non-small cell lung carcinoma: a rationale for en bloc resection. J Thorac Cardiovasc Surg 2001;121(4):649–56.

46. Shamji MF, Maziak DE, Shamji FM, et al. Circulation of the spinal cord: an important consideration for thoracic surgeons. Ann Thorac Surg 2003;76(1):315–21.

47. Doddoli C, D'Journo B, Le Pimpec-Barthes F, et al. Lung cancer invading the chest wall: a plea for en-bloc resection but the need for new treatment strategies. Ann Thorac Surg 2005;80(6):2032–40.

48. Burkhart HM, Allen MS, Nichols FC 3rd, et al. Results of en bloc resection for bronchogenic carcinoma with chest wall invasion. J Thorac Cardiovasc Surg 2002;123(4):670–5.
49. Akay H, Cangir AK, Kutlay H, et al. Surgical treatment of peripheral lung cancer adherent to the parietal pleura. Eur J Cardiothorac Surg 2002;22(4):615–20.
50. Matsuoka H, Nishio W, Okada M, et al. Resection of chest wall invasion in patients with non-small cell lung cancer. Eur J Cardiothorac Surg 2004;26(6):1200–4.
51. Riquet M, Lang-Lazdunski L, Le PB, et al. Characteristics and prognosis of re-sected T3 non-small cell lung cancer. Ann Thorac Surg 2002;73(1):253–8.
52. Piehler JM, Pairolero PC, Weiland LH, et al. Bronchogenic carcinoma with chest wall invasion: factors affecting survival following en bloc resection. Ann Thorac Surg 1982;34(6):684–91.
53. McCaughan BC, Martini N, Bains MS, et al. Chest wall invasion in carcinoma of the lung. Therapeutic and prognostic implications. J Thorac Cardiovasc Surg 1985;89(6):836–41.
54. Downey RJ, Martini N, Rusch VW, et al. Extent of chest wall invasion and survival in patients with lung cancer. Ann Thorac Surg 1999;68(1):188–93.
55. Magdeleinat P, Alifano M, Benbrahem C, et al. Surgical treatment of lung cancer invading the chest wall: results and prognostic factors. Ann Thorac Surg 2001; 71(4):1094–9.
56. Lin YT, Hsu PK, Hsu HS, et al. En bloc resection for lung cancer with chest wall invasion. J Chin Med Assoc 2006;69(4):157–61.
57. Rendina EA, De Giacomo T, Venuta F, et al. Lung conservation techniques: bron-chial sleeve resection and reconstruction of the pulmonary artery. Semin Surg Oncol 2000;18:165–72.
58. Van Schil PE, Brutel de la Riviere A, Knaepen PJ, et al. Long term survival after bronchial sleeve resection: univariate and multivariate analysis. Ann Thorac Surg 1996;61:1087–91.
59. Fadel E, Yldizeli B, Chapelier A, et al. Sleeve lobectomy for bronchogenic cancers: factors affecting survival. Ann Thorac Surg 2002;74:851–9.
60. Terzi A, Lonardoni A, Falezza G, et al. Sleeve lobectomy for non-small cell lung cancer and carcinoids: results in 160 cases. Eur J Cardiothorac Surg 2002;21: 888–93.
61. Kim YT, Kang CH, Sung SW, et al. Local control of disease related to lymph node involvement in non-small cell lung cancer after sleeve lobectomy compared with pneumonectomy. Ann Thorac Surg 2005;79:1153–61, 112:376–84.
62. Ludwig C, Stoelben E, Olshewski M, et al. Comparison of morbidity, 30-day mortality and long-term survival after pneumonectomy and sleeve lobectomy for non-small cell lung carcinoma. Ann Thorac Surg 2005;79:968–73.
63. Rendina EA, Venuta F, De Giacomo T, et al. Safety and efficacy of bronchovas-cular reconstruction after induction chemotherapy for lung cancer. J Thorac Cardiovasc Surg 1997;114:830–7.
64. Price-Thomas CP. Conservative resection of the bronchial tree. J R Coll Surg Edinb 1955;1(3):169–86.
65. Allison PR. Course of thoracic surgery in Groningen. Ann R Coll Surg 1954;25: 20–2.
66. Rendina EA, Venta F, Ciriaco P, et al. Bronchovascular sleeve resection. Tech-nique, perioperative management, prevention and treatment of complications. J Thorac Cardiovasc Surg 1993;106(1):73–9.
67. Gómez-Caro A, Garcia S, Reguart N, et al. Determining the appropriate sleeve lobectomy versus pneumonectomy ratio in central non-small cell lung cancer

patients: an audit of an aggressive policy of pneumonectomy avoidance. Eur J Cardiothorac Surg 2011;39(3):352–9.

68. Yildizeli B, Fadel E, Mussot S, et al. Morbidity, mortality, and long-term survival after sleeve lobectomy for non-small cell lung cancer. Eur J Cardiothorac Surg 2007;31(1):95–102.

69. Rendina EA, Venuta F, Degiacomo T, et al. Sleeve resection and prosthetic reconstruction of the pulmonary artery for lung cancer. Ann Thorac Surg 1999;68:995–1002.

70. Venuta F, Ciccone AM, Anile M, et al. Reconstruction of the pulmonary artery for lung cancer: long-term results. J Thorac Cardiovasc Surg 2009;138(5):185–91.

71. Rendina EA, Venuta F. Reconstruction of the pulmonary artery. In: Patterson GA, Deslauriers J, Lerut A, et al, editors. Pearson's thoracic and esophageal surgery. 3rd edition. Philadelphia: Churchill Livingstone; 2008. p. 909–22.

72. Rendina EA, Venuta F, Ricci P, et al. Protection and revascularization of bronchial anastomoses by the intercostal pedicle flap. J Thorac Cardiovasc Surg 1994;107(5):1251–4.

73. Tsuchiya R. Bronchoplastic techniques. In: Patterson GA, Deslauriers J, Lerut A, et al, editors. Pearson's thoracic and esophageal surgery. 2rd edition. Philadelphia: Churchill Livingstone; 2002. p. 1005.

74. Cerezo F, Cano JR, Espinosa D, et al. New technique for pulmonary artery reconstruction. Eur J Cardiothorac Surg 2009;36(2):422–3.

75. Gaissert HA, Mathisen DJ, Moncure AC, et al. Survival and function after sleeve lobectomy for lung cancer. J Thorac Cardiovasc Surg 1996;111(5):948–53.

76. Okada M, Yamagishi H, Satake S, et al. Survival related to lymph node involvement in lung cancer after sleeve lobectomy compared with pneumonectomy. J Thorac Cardiovasc Surg 2000;119(4 Pt 1):814–9.

77. Ma Z, Dong A, Fan J, et al. Does sleeve lobectomy concomitant with or without pulmonary artery reconstruction (double sleeve) have favourable results for non-small cell lung cancer compared with pneumonectomy? A meta-analysis. Eur J Cardiothorac Surg 2007;32:20–8.

78. Deslauriers J, Grégoire J, Jacques LF, et al. Sleeve lobectomy versus pneumonectomy for lung cancer: a comparative analysis of survival and sites or recurrences. Ann Thorac Surg 2004;77(4):1152–6.

79. Yoshino I, Yokoyama H, Yano T, et al. Comparison of the surgical results of lobectomy with bronchoplasty and pneumonectomy for lung cancer. J Surg Oncol 1997;64(1):32–5.

80. Suen HC, Meyers BF, Guthrie T, et al. Favorable results after sleeve lobectomy or bronchoplasty for bronchial malignancies. Ann Thorac Surg 1999;67(6):1557–62.

81. Ghiribelli C, Voltolini L, Luzzi L, et al. Survival after bronchoplastic lobectomy for non small cell lung cancer compared with pneumonectomy according to nodal status. J Cardiovasc Surg (Torino) 2002;43(1):103–8.

82. Martin-Ucar AE, Chaudhuri N, Edwards JG, et al. Can pneumonectomy for non-small cell lung cancer be avoided? An audit of parenchymal sparing lung surgery. Eur J Cardiothorac Surg 2002;21(4):601–5.

83. Bagan P, Berna P, Pereira JC, et al. Sleeve lobectomy versus pneumonectomy: tumor characteristics and comparative analysis of feasibility and results. Ann Thorac Surg 2005;80(6):2046–50.

84. Lausberg HF, Graeter TP, Tscholl D, et al. Bronchovascular versus bronchial sleeve resection for central lung tumors. Ann Thorac Surg 2005;79(4):1147–52.

85. Takeda S, Maeda H, Koma M, et al. Comparison of surgical results after pneumonectomy and sleeve lobectomy for non-small cell lung cancer: trends over

time and 20-year institutional experience. Eur J Cardiothorac Surg 2006;29(3): 276–80.

86. Ferguson MK, Lehman AG. Sleeve lobectomy or pneumonectomy: optimal management strategy using decision analysis techniques. Ann Thorac Surg 2003;76(6):1782–8.

87. Melloul E, Egger B, Krueger T, et al. Mortality, complications and loss of pulmonary function after pneumonectomy vs. sleeve lobectomy in patients younger and older than 70 years. Interact Cardiovasc Thorac Surg 2008;7(6):986–9.

88. Stamatis G, Djuric D, Eberhardt W, et al. Postoperative morbidity and mortality after induction chemoradiotherapy for locally advanced lung cancer: an analysis of 350 operated patients. Eur J Cardiothorac Surg 2002;22(2):292–7.

89. Rendina EA, Venuta F, De Giacomo T, et al. Sleeve resection after induction therapy. Thorac Surg Clin 2004;14:191–7.

90. Ricci C, Rendina EA, Venuta F, et al. Reconstruction of the pulmonary artery in patients with lung cancer. Ann Thorac Surg 1994;57(3):627–32.

91. Tsuchiya R, Asamura H, Kondo H, et al. Extended resection of the left atrium, great vessels, or both for lung cancer. Ann Thorac Surg 1994;57(4):960–5.

92. Gonzalez-Fajardo JA, Garcia-Yuste M, Florez S, et al. Hemodynamic cerebral repercussions arising from surgical interruption of the superior vena cava. Experimental model. J Thorac Cardiovasc Surg 1994;107:1044–9.

93. Chen KN, Xu SF, Gu ZD, et al. Surgical treatment of complex malignant anterior mediastinal tumors invading the superior vena cava. World J Surg 2006;30: 162–70.

94. Brewster DC. Prosthetic grafts. In: Rutherford RB, editor. Vascular surgery. Philadelphia: WB Saunders; 1995. p. 492–521.

95. Leo F, Bellini R, Conti B, et al. Superior vena cava resection in thoracic malignancies: does prosthetic replacement pose a higher risk? Eur J Cardiothorac Surg 2010;37(4):764–9.

96. Sekine Y, Suzuki H, Saitoh Y, et al. Prosthetic reconstruction of the superior vena cava for malignant disease: surgical techniques and outcomes. Ann Thorac Surg 2010;90(1):223–8.

97. D'Andrilli A, Ibrahim M, Venuta F, et al. Glutaraldehyde preserved autologous pericardium for patch reconstruction of the pulmonary artery and superior vena cava. Ann Thorac Surg 2005;80:357–8.

98. D'Andrilli A, Ciccone AM, Ibrahim M, et al. A new technique for prosthetic reconstruction of the superior vena cava. J Thorac Cardiovasc Surg 2006; 132:192–4.

99. Ciccone AM, Venuta F, D'Andrilli A, et al. Long term patency of the stapled bovine pericardial conduit for replacement of the superior vena cava. Eur J Cardiothorac Surg. [Epub ahead of print].

100. Doty DB. Bypass of superior vena cava: six years experience with spiral vein graft for obstruction of superior vena cava due to benign and malignant disease. J Thorac Cardiovasc Surg 1982;83:326.

101. Thomas P, Magnan PE, Moulin G, et al. Extended operation for lung cancer invading the superior vena cava. Eur J Cardiothorac Surg 1994;8(4):177–82.

102. Fukuse T, Wada H, Hitomi S. Extended operation for non-small cell lung cancer invading great vessels and left atrium. Eur J Cardiothorac Surg 1997;11(4): 664–9.

103. Bernard A, Bouchot O, Hagry O, et al. Risk analysis and long-term survival in patients undergoing resection of T4 lung cancer. Eur J Cardiothorac Surg 2001;20(2):344–9.

104. Spaggiari L, Magdeleinat P, Kondo H, et al. Results of superior vena cava resection for lung cancer. Analysis of prognostic factors. Lung Cancer 2004;44(3): 339–46.
105. Shargall Y, de Perrot M, Keshavjee S, et al. 15 years single center experience with surgical resection of the superior vena cava for non-small cell lung cancer. Lung Cancer 2004;45(3):357–63.
106. Suzuki K, Asamura H, Watanabe S, et al. Combined resection of superior vena cava for lung carcinoma: prognostic significance of patterns of superior vena cava invasion. Ann Thorac Surg 2004;78(4):1184–9 [discussion: 1184–9].
107. Spaggiari L, Leo F, Veronesi G, et al. Superior vena cava resection for lung and mediastinal malignancies: a single-center experience with 70 cases. Ann Thorac Surg 2007;83(1):223–9.
108. Yildizeli B, Dartevelle PG, Fadel E, et al. Results of primary surgery with T4 non-small cell lung cancer during a 25-year period in a single center: the benefit is worth the risk. Ann Thorac Surg 2008;86(4):1065–75.
109. Shen KR, Meyers BF, Larner JM, et al, American College of Chest Physicians. Special treatment issues in lung cancer: ACCP evidence-based clinical practice guidelines (2nd edition). Chest 2007;132(Suppl 3):290S–305S.
110. Klepetko W, Wisser W, Bîrsan T, et al. T4 lung tumors with infiltration of the thoracic aorta: is an operation reasonable? Ann Thorac Surg 1999;67(2):340–4.
111. Ohta M, Hirabayasi H, Shiono H, et al. Surgical resection for lung cancer with infiltration of the thoracic aorta. J Thorac Cardiovasc Surg 2005;129(4):804–8.
112. de Perrot M, Fadel E, Mussot S, et al. Resection of locally advanced (T4) non-small cell lung cancer with cardiopulmonary bypass. Ann Thorac Surg 2005; 79(5):1691–6.
113. Misthos P, Papagiannakis G, Kokotsakis J, et al. Surgical management of lung cancer invading the aorta or the superior vena cava. Lung Cancer 2007; 56(2):223–7.
114. Tronc F, Grégoire J, Rouleau J, et al. Long-term results of sleeve lobectomy for lung cancer. Eur J Cardiothorac Surg 2000;17(5):5506.

Role of Adjuvant Chemotherapy in NSCLC (Stages I to III)

Melissa H. Coleman, MD, Raphael Bueno, MD*

KEYWORDS

• Adjuvant • Chemotherapy • Early-stage • NSCLC • Treatment

Lung cancer is the leading cause of cancer mortality in the Western world with an estimated 222,520 new cases diagnosed in the United States in 2010.[1] Lung cancer is broadly subdivided into two types, small cell and non-small cell, which account for approximately 15% and 85% of cases, respectively.[1] Five-year overall survival of patients with non-small cell lung cancer (NSCLC) remains low at 17%.[1] Even in the case of patients with sufficiently early cancer to be candidates for curative surgery, long-term survival is not guaranteed. When analyzed by stage, 5-year survival rates for stage I, stage II, and stage IIIA disease are 60%, 40%, and 25%, respectively.[2] Recurrence or relapse of disease at distant sites is common and has prompted considerable research focused on chemotherapy for systematic therapy in an effort to improve long-term survival. As such, the use of adjuvant chemotherapy for early-stage NSCLC continues to evolve with the completion of numerous clinical trials and meta-analyses (Table 1), the development of novel chemotherapeutic agents, and the identification of biomarkers associated with prognosis and response to chemotherapeutic agents.

CLINICAL TRIALS EVALUATING ADJUVANT CHEMOTHERAPY

In 1995, the Non-Small Cell Lung Cancer Collaborative Group conducted a meta-analysis of 9387 patients from 52 randomized trials in an effort to address the controversial use of adjuvant chemotherapy for NSCLC.[3] For patients with early disease, 14 trials were analyzed with varying chemotherapy regimens including: cyclophosphamide, nitrosourea plus methotrexate, cisplatin, doxorubicin, and cyclophosphamide, cisplatin and vindesine, and tegafur or tegafur plus uracil (UFT). The investigators identified differences in survival benefit according to the type of chemotherapy used. Results of the analysis favored the use of more modern regimens that included cisplatin because trials using long-term alkylating agents (cyclophosphamide and

Division of Thoracic surgery, Brigham and Women's Hospital, 75 Francis Street, Boston, MA 02115, USA
* Corresponding author.
E-mail address: rbueno@partners.org

Surg Oncol Clin N Am 20 (2011) 757–767
doi:10.1016/j.soc.2011.07.011
1055-3207/11/$ – see front matter © 2011 Elsevier Inc. All rights reserved.

surgonc.theclinics.com

Table 1
Adjuvant chemotherapy trials

Trial	Number of Patients/ Accrual Dates	Stage	Chemotherapy Regimen	Radiotherapy Included	Outcome with Adjuvant Chemotherapy
ECOG (2000)	488 1991–1997	II–IIIA	Cisplatin plus etoposide	Yes	Relative likelihood of survival 0.93, 95% CI 0.74–1.18; Median survival nonsignificant ($P = .56$)
ALPI (2003)	1209 1994–1999	I–IIIA	Cisplatin, vindesine, mitomycin	Yes	Overall survival HR 0.96, 95% CI 0.81–1.13, $P = .589$ Progression-free survival HR 0.89, 95% CI 0.76–1.03, $P = .128$
IALT (2004)	1867 1995–2000	I–III	Cisplatin plus 1. Vindesine 2. Vinblastine 3. Vinorelbine 4. Etoposide	Yes	Overall survival HR 0.86, 95% CI 0.76–0.98, $P = .03$ Disease-free survival HR 0.83, 95% CI 0.74–0.94, $P<.003$
IALT Update (2010)					Median follow-up 7.5 years Overall survival HR 0.91, 95% CI 0.81–1.02, $P = .10$ Disease-free survival HR 1.33, 95% CI 0.89–2.0, $P = .16$
BLT (2004)	381 1995–2001	I–IIIB or IV	Cisplatin plus 1. Mitomycin 2. Mitomycin, vinblastine 3. Vindesine 4. Vinorelbine	Yes	Overall survival HR 1.02, 95% CI 0.77–1.35, $P = .90$ Progression-free survival HR 0.97, 95% CI 0.74–1.26, $P = .81$
JBR.10 (2005)	482 1994–2001	IB–II	Cisplatin plus vinorelbine	No	Overall survival HR 0.69, 95% CI 0.52–0.91, $P = .04$ Recurrence-free survival HR 0.60, 95% CI 0.45–0.79, $P<.001$
JBR.10 Update (2010)					9.3 year median follow-up Overall survival HR 0.78, 95% CI 0.61–0.99, $P = .04$
ANITA (2006)	840 1994–2000	IB–IIIA	Cisplatin plus vinorelbine	Yes	Adjusted risk for death with chemotherapy HR 0.80, 95%CI 0.66–0.96, $P = .017$ Overall survival at 5 years improved by 8.6%
CALGB 9633 (2008)	344 1996–2003	IB	Carboplatin plus paclitaxel	No	Overall survival HR 0.83, 90% CI 0.64–1.08, $P = .125$ Disease-free survival HR 0.80, 90% CI 0.62–1.02, $P = .65$

Abbreviations: ANITA, Adjuvant Navelbine International Trialist Association; ALPI, Adjuvant Lung Cancer Project Italy; BLT, Big Lung Trial; CALGB is Cancer and Leukemia Group B; ECOG, European Cooperative Oncology Group; IALT, International Adjuvant Lung Cancer Trial; JBR.10, The North American Intergroup Trial initiated by the National Cancer Institute of Canada Clinical Trials in 1994.

nitrosourea) were associated with an increased risk of death when compared with surgery alone. Although this analysis demonstrated a trend toward a survival benefit with the use of cisplatin-based drugs, the findings were inconclusive because the difference of 0.87 in the hazard ratio (HR) for overall survival was not significant ($P = .08$). However, this result led to subsequent trials seeking to further assess the survival benefit of cisplatin-based postoperative chemotherapy.

Based on the trends reported in the 1995 meta-analysis, in 2004 the International Adjuvant Lung Cancer Trial (IALT) Collaborative Group performed a prospective clinical trial that was designed to evaluate the effect of cisplatin-based chemotherapy on survival after complete surgical resection.[4] Patients were enrolled from 1995 to 2000, with a total of 1867 patients (stage I, II, or III; based on the 1986 American Joint Committee on Cancer classification) randomized to chemotherapy or observation in addition to surgery. Those patients randomized to the chemotherapy group received cisplatin combined with vindesine, vinblastine, vinorelbine, or etoposide; and 25% of these patients received postoperative radiotherapy (PORT). The investigators reported higher overall survival ($P<.03$) and disease-free survival rates ($P<.003$) for the group receiving chemotherapy in addition to surgery.

One year later, the North American Intergroup published the results of a randomized control trial (trial number JBR.10) that examined vinorelbine and cisplatin versus observation in stage IB and stage II NSCLC patients after complete resection.[5] In this study, 482 patients were randomized to chemotherapy versus no adjuvant treatment. The chemotherapy group had lower rates of recurrence ($P = .003$) and longer recurrence-free survival ($P<.001$) when compared with the observation group. In addition, there was an absolute survival advantage at 5 years of 15% ($P = .03$) for the surgery plus chemotherapy group. Subgroup analyses were also performed to assess survival differences based on histology, stage, and presence or absence of a *ras* mutation. Squamous cell cancer histology was found to be associated with greater recurrence-free survival ($P = .02$). When patients were analyzed by stage, those with stage II disease in the surgery plus chemotherapy group were noted to have a longer medial survival than the surgery alone group (HR 0.59, $P = .004$), whereas chemotherapy did not provide a statistically significant increase in overall survival for patients with stage IB disease ($P = .79$). However, the investigators cautioned against making conclusions based on this finding because the stage-by-treatment interaction test did not reach statistical significance ($P = .13$) and the numbers required to demonstrate a response in early-stage cancer may not have been reached. Finally, the study found that patients with wild-type (normal) *ras* seemed to benefit from adjuvant chemotherapy; however, this finding was tempered by the fact that the effect of *ras*-mutation status on treatment outcome was not statistically significant.

Two years later, the Adjuvant Navelbine International Trialist Association (ANITA) reported their results on 840 patients randomized to either observation or treatment with vinorelbine and cisplatin after surgery, with some patients in each treatment group receiving postoperative radiotherapy.[2] The results of this trial indicated a survival benefit for those patients treated with vinorelbine and cisplatin when compared with those patients in the observation group (HR 0.80, $P = .017$). The trial reported an 8.6% survival benefit at 5 years that was maintained at 8.4% at 7 years.

Following these trials, subsequent analyses building on the original 1995 meta-analysis were performed in an effort to update treatment recommendations. In 2007, Cancer Care Ontario and the American Society of Clinical Oncology published the "Adjuvant Chemotherapy and Adjuvant Radiation Therapy for Stages I-IIIA Resectable Non Small-Cell Lung Cancer Guideline."[6] In this treatment guideline, recommendations for the use of adjuvant chemotherapy were made based on eight meta-analyses and 16 randomized control trials. This guideline focused on patients who underwent an R0 resection and who were treated with a cisplatin-based chemotherapy regimen. Recommendations for treatment by stage were presented. Adjuvant cisplatin-based chemotherapy was recommended for stages IIA, IIB, and IIIA, but was not recommended for IA or IB. The use of alkylating agents as part of chemotherapy regimens was not recommended based on the conclusions of the 1995 meta-analysis. This was followed in 2008 by a pooled analysis conducted by the Lung Adjuvant Cisplatin Evaluation (LACE) Collaborative Group in which trials using adjuvant cisplatin-based chemotherapy regimens were evaluated in an effort to elucidate treatment options associated with improved survival.[7] In addition, the analysis aimed to identify subgroups of patients who derived increased benefit from the administration of adjuvant chemotherapy. This analysis focused on trials that occurred after the 1995 meta-analysis and, ultimately, five trials, with data for 4584 patients (stages IA–III) were included. Furthermore, the analysis excluded trials in which neoadjuvant chemotherapy, non–cisplatin-based regimens, or concurrent radiotherapy and chemotherapy was administered. The investigators concluded that adjuvant chemotherapy improved survival and that this effect varied with stage.

However, not all the trials conducted demonstrated a significant improvement in overall survival associated with the use of adjuvant chemotherapy. The Eastern Cooperative Oncology Group found neither significant decrease in intrathoracic recurrence ($P = .58$) nor improvement in survival ($P = .56$) with adjuvant chemotherapy plus radiotherapy versus radiotherapy alone. The trial included 488 stage II and IIIA patients with a median follow-up of 44 months and a chemotherapy regimen consisting of four cycles of cisplatin and etoposide. Of the 232 patients randomized to the chemotherapy and radiotherapy treatment arm, 69% completed all or part of the full four cycles. The investigators noted that the combination of chemotherapy and radiotherapy was associated with significant side effects that were not associated with radiotherapy alone.

In 2003 the Adjuvant Lung Project Italy/European Organization for Research and Treatment of Cancer-Lung Cancer Cooperative Group Investigators reported results of a randomized trial studying survival of stage I to IIIA NSCLC patients treated with chemotherapy versus observation.[8] Patients treated with radiotherapy were included in both the chemotherapy group (mitomycin, vindesine, and cisplatin) and the control group. Randomization was performed on 1209 patients, with a median follow-up time of 64.5 months. The investigators found no statistically significant improvement in overall survival between the adjuvant chemotherapy group and the no-treatment group ($P = .128$). Similarly, in this trial, 69% of patients in the chemotherapy group completed the planned three cycles of treatment. The following year, results of the Big Lung Trial were published and, again, no significant benefit from adjuvant chemotherapy was demonstrated ($P = .90$).[9] The 381 stage I to III patients were randomized to the treatment arms of the study at the individual treating doctor's discretion. The trial included patients who had received neoadjuvant chemotherapy or adjuvant chemotherapy, plus or minus radiotherapy, versus surgery alone. Most patients in the treatment group of the trial received adjuvant chemotherapy (97%) versus neoadjuvant chemotherapy (3%). Four options for chemotherapy regimens were used: (1) cisplatin, mitomycin, and ifosfamide; (2) cisplatin, mitomycin, and vinblastine; (3) cisplatin and vindesine; and (4) cisplatin and vinorelbine.

More recently, the Cancer and Leukemia Group B, Radiation Therapy Oncology Group, and North Central Cancer Treatment Group Study Groups (trial number CALGB 9633) reported a negative trial of adjuvant paclitaxel plus carboplatin versus observation in patients with stage IB NSCLC.[10] Three hundred and forty-four patients were randomized to adjuvant chemotherapy or observation and no radiotherapy was administered in either treatment group. There was no significant survival advantage for the patients in the chemotherapy arm after a median follow-up of 74 months (P = .12). However, the investigators did note a significant survival benefit for patients in the chemotherapy group with tumors greater than or equal to 4 cm (P = .43).

In 2010, updates of both JBR.10 and the original 1995 meta-analysis were published.[11,12] The JBR.10 update provided results after a median follow-up period of 9.3 years, compared with a median follow-up of 5.1 years in the chemotherapy group and 5.3 years in the observation group in the original report. The absolute survival benefit for the chemotherapy group continued to be observed, at 11% compared with the 15% published previously. Survival benefit was statistically significant for patients with stage II disease (P = .01); however, it failed to reach significance for stage IB patients (P = .87). In agreement with the CALGB 9633 trial, tumor size of greater than or equal to 4 cm was found to be predictive of chemotherapy effect (P = .02). The investigators found no significant interaction between ras mutation status and overall or disease-specific survival. In the 1995 meta-analysis update, the investigators analyzed updated data from previously included trials in addition to including trials that began randomization after January 1, 1965. Selection of trials for analysis was also refined to perform two meta-analyses: (1) surgery plus adjuvant chemotherapy versus surgery alone or (2) chemotherapy, surgery, and radiotherapy versus surgery plus radiotherapy. In the first meta-analysis, the investigators found a significant survival benefit for surgery plus chemotherapy compared with surgery alone (P<.0001). The second meta-analysis demonstrated a survival benefit for surgery, chemotherapy, and radiotherapy (P = .009).

ADJUVANT CHEMOTHERAPY TREATMENT BY STAGE

The recommendations for the use of adjuvant chemotherapy for early-stage NSCLC are based on evidence presented in the seminal adjuvant chemotherapy trials and meta-analyses herein reviewed. Additionally Cancer Care Ontario and the American Society of Clinical Oncology published a NSCLC guideline based on consensus drawn from the evidence published in these studies.[6]

STAGE IA

Currently, observation is recommended for patients with completely resected stage IA disease. Few adjuvant chemotherapy trials include stage IA patients. This results in limited evidence that it confers a survival benefit. In the update of the 1995 meta-analysis, the investigators reported no difference in the efficacy of platinum-based chemotherapy by stage. They reported a 3% survival advantage at 5 years with chemotherapy; however, this was not significant (P = .33).

STAGE IB

The efficacy of adjuvant chemotherapy for patients with stage IB disease varies among trials. After complete resection, adjuvant chemotherapy is not routinely recommended. However, patients who are considered to have a high risk of recurrence may benefit from the addition of chemotherapy. Although the survival advantage of adjuvant chemotherapy for stage IB disease was not statistically significant in the randomized control trials or in the meta-analyses reviewed, the CALGB 9633 and the JBR.10 update suggest a benefit for patients with tumors greater than or equal to 4 cm. Of note, a randomized trial of adjuvant chemotherapy with uracil-tegafur versus no treatment in stage IA and IB patients demonstrated a survival benefit among patients treated with the combined regimen (P = .04).[13] Further subgroup analysis showed that among patients with T2 disease, those treated with adjuvant uracil-tegafur had an 85% 5-year survival rate versus 74% in the untreated group (P = .005).

STAGE II

Following complete resection, the administration of adjuvant chemotherapy is recommended for stage II NSCLC patients. Patients with stage II disease were found to have statistically significant survival benefits when treated with adjuvant cisplatin-based chemotherapy regimens (LACE, JBR.10, ANITA).[2,5,7]

STAGE IIIA

Adjuvant cisplatin-based chemotherapy treatment is recommended for stage IIIA disease. Subgroup analysis of patients with stage IIIB disease demonstrated statistically significant survival benefits with administration of adjuvant cisplatin-based chemotherapy (LACE, IALT, ANITA).[2,4,7]

CHEMOTHERAPY REGIMENS
Alkylating Agents

Earlier trials of chemotherapy for NSCLC included the use of alkylating agents, such as cyclophosphamide and nitrosourea. Alkylating agents cause the binding of alkyl groups to DNA and lead to cross-linking events that cause cytotoxicity.[14] Currently the use of alkylating agents is not recommended because the results of the 1995 meta-analysis indicated a detrimental effect (HR = 1.15, P = .005).[3]

Platinum Compounds

Platinum compounds have been established as a mainstay of systemic therapy for various malignancies and have demonstrated efficacy in the treatment of NSCLC.[14] These compounds cause apoptosis by binding to DNA and causing cross-linking to occur.[15] Carboplatin is associated with fewer side effects than cisplatin, and numerous trials have attempted to assess the differences in efficacy of treating NSCLC.[14,16] Toxicities associated with cisplatin include anemia, neutropenia, nephrotoxicity, and neurotoxicity.[14,16] In contrast, carboplatin is less nephrotoxic and neurotoxic, as well as being associated with less nausea and vomiting when compared with cisplatin.[14] Most trials report on outcomes of adjuvant cisplatin-doublet chemotherapy.[4–7] The JBR.10 and ANITA trials studied vinorelbine and cisplatin doublet therapy and both reported overall survival benefits.[2,5,12] Cisplatin-doublet therapy has emerged as a standard of care for adjuvant chemotherapy. Based on the negative results of the CALGB 9633 trial, carboplatin is not recommended as standard treatment; however, carboplatin-doublet therapy may be considered for those patients with comorbidities that would preclude the use of cisplatin because of the toxicity profile of cisplatin.[17]

Tubulin-Binding Agents

Anti-microtubule agents target tubulins in the rapidly dividing cancer cells and disrupt the cell cycle, ultimately leading to mitotic arrest and cell death.[15] Tubulin-binding agents include the synthetic taxanes (paclitaxel and docetaxel) and the naturally occurring vinca alkaloids (vincristine and vinorelbine).[14] They are often administered in combination with a platinum compound.

Tegafur and Uracil

Combined treatment with UFT (ie, tegafur, a prodrug of 5-fluorouracil, and uracil) has been shown to be effective for early-stage NSCLC. UFT is comprised of a fixed molar ratio (1:4) of tegafur and uracil. It is administered with calcium folinate, a derivative of 5-fluorouracil, which is taken orally as a daily regimen. 5-Fluoropyrimidines exert their cytotoxic effects by inhibiting thymidylate synthase, which ultimately affects DNA synthesis and repair, as well as incorporation into RNA.[14] In a randomized trial of stage I lung adenocarcinoma, patients treated with UFT were found to have a survival benefit (P = .04).[13] Results of a subsequent meta-analysis of adjuvant UFT treatment versus surgery alone also demonstrated improved survival among patients treated with UFT (P = .001).[18,19] At present, tegafur is not approved for use in the United States.

PROGNOSTIC AND PREDICTIVE MARKERS FOR EARLY-STAGE NSCLC

Although adjuvant chemotherapy has been demonstrated to confer survival benefits for stage II to IIA NSCLC, the associated survival advantage remains modest. To date, the role of adjuvant chemotherapy for stage IB disease is less well defined. Identification of subgroups of patients at high risk for recurrence and/or identification of tumor characteristics associated with efficacy of chemotherapeutic agents has the potential to improve current treatment regimens. In addition, given the heterogeneity of histology among NSCLC tumor types, further elucidation of tumor characteristics may aid in the development of a more personalized adjuvant chemotherapy regimen.[20] Numerous studies have attempted to identify biomarkers associated with prognosis and response to specific chemotherapeutic agents.

One possible biomarker is excision repair cross-complementation group 1 (ERCC1). The International Adjuvant Lung Cancer Trial Bio Investigators study investigated ERCC1 expression in relation to cisplatin-based adjuvant chemotherapy in the patients included in the IALT.[4,21] Resistance to platinum agents is attributed, in part, to DNA repair mechanisms and ERCC1 is an enzyme involved in the repair of platinum-induced DNA damage.[15,21] Tumors of 761 of the 1867 IALT patients were analyzed for ERCC1 by immunostaining. The patients in the adjuvant chemotherapy group with ERCC1-negative tumors had significantly longer survival than did the patients in the control group (HR 0.65; 95% CI 0.50–0.86, P = .002).[21] In contrast, patients with ERCC1-positive tumors demonstrated no difference in survival when compared with the group receiving chemotherapy and the control group. A later meta-analysis evaluated the association between ERCC1 and carboplatin-based treatment.[22] The investigators reported that firm conclusions could not be drawn based on the existing trial data and that future prospective randomized trials were needed.

Similarly, BRCA1 expression has been associated with prognosis in early-stage NSCLC and with response to platinum-based therapy. An analysis of mRNA expression of BRCA1 in chemonaive NSCLC patients after complete resection found that high BRCA1 expression correlated with decreased event-free survival (P = .04).[23] The Spanish Lung Cancer Group is currently recruiting patients for a randomized trial investigating the administration of adjuvant chemotherapy based on BRCA1 mRNA levels in completely resected stage II to IIA NSCLC patients (Randomized Study of Customized Adjuvant Chemotherapy Based on BRCA1 mRNA Levels in Completely Resected Stages II-IIIA in Non-Small Cell Lung Cancer (GECP-SCAT), Spanish Lung Cancer Group, ClinicalTrials.gov identifier: NCT00478699). This is a phase III study and the chemotherapy agents will be administered as one of three regimen options: (1) docetaxel plus cisplatin, (2) docetaxel, (3) or gemcitabine plus cisplatin. Results of this trial may shed further light on the preliminary indications that patients with low BRCA1 levels may benefit from platinum-based chemotherapy agents, whereas those with high BRCA1 levels may benefit from chemotherapy using tubulin-binding agents.[23]

Expression levels of class III β-tubulin have been correlated with outcome in NSCLC.[24] Class III β-tubulin expression was measured in tumor samples from patients studied in the JBR.10 trial.[25] These patients were treated with adjuvant chemotherapy consisting of cisplatin and vinorelbine. The investigators reported that high levels of class III β-tubulin were associated with poor survival amongst patients who did not receive adjuvant chemotherapy. Among patients with high β-tubulin levels, those treated with chemotherapy had improved recurrence-free survival when compared with patients in the control arm (HR = 0.45, 95% CI 0.27–0.75, P = .002). Although the investigators concluded that high β-tubulin levels are associated with poor prognosis in early-stage disease, in advanced NSCLC disease, high β-tubulin levels are associated with improved response to chemotherapy with vinorelbine or paclitaxel. The investigators discuss the possibility that β-tubulin levels may vary in terms of prognostic implications depending on the stage of the NSCLC.

The *ras* family of genes is a subfamily of the membrane-bound guanosine triphosphate (GTP)-binding proteins (GTPases). The human *ras* genes encode 3 amino acid proteins (H-RAS, NRAS, and KRAS) that are involved in the regulation of cell differentiation, growth, and apoptosis.[26] *Ras* mutations have been found in 15% to 30% of lung cancers, with KRAS accounting for approximately 90% of *ras* mutations in lung adenocarcinoma.[27] In the JBR.10, trial, *ras* mutation status was determined in 451 of the 482 patients studied. Both in the initial trial report and in the updated analysis, chemotherapy did not have a statistically significant affect on median survival in patients with *ras* mutations. In the updated analysis, median survival for *ras* mutation-positive patients was 9.7 years with chemotherapy versus 7.8 years with observation (HR = 0.82, 95% CI 0.50–1.35, P = .44).[12] However, there was a trend toward a benefit from chemotherapy for patients with wild-type *ras* (HR = 0.72, 95% CI 0.51–1.02, P = .06). These data suggest that *ras* mutation status does not have prognostic implications in early-stage NSCLC, but that wild-type *ras* mutation status might be associated with improved response to vinorelbine plus cisplatin.[26]

CURRENT CLINICAL TRIALS

Several ongoing trials aim to further address the use of adjuvant chemotherapy for early-stage NSCLC. The CALGB-150803 trial (A Validation of the 64-Gene Signature Using Affymetrix-HG_U133A Array in Stage I NSCLC From the CALGB Lung Cancer Study (140202), Cancer and Leukemia Group B, ClinicalTrials.gov identifier: NCT00990873) aims to specifically address the question of adjuvant chemotherapy for stage I NSCLC patients. A 64-gene signature will be accessed for its ability to predict prognosis for patients with stage I NSCLC. This molecular-based test has the potential to identify the subset of stage I patients likely to benefit from adjuvant chemotherapy. Additionally, current trials are evaluating the efficacy of combination adjuvant chemotherapy. The RADIANT study (RADIANT: A Multi-center, Randomized, Double-blind, Placebo-controlled, Phase 3 Study of Single-agent Tarceva [Erlotinib] Following Complete Tumor Resection With or Without Adjuvant Chemotherapy in Patients With Stage IB-IIIA Non-small Cell Lung Carcinoma Who Have EGFR-positive Tumors, OSI Pharmaceuticals, ClinicalTrials.gov identifier: NCT00373425) is a multicentered study that includes patients with stage IB to IIIA disease and EGFR-positive tumors. In this study, patients are treated with Tarceva or placebo, with or without adjuvant chemotherapy. Similarly, ECOG-E1505 (A Phase III Randomized Trial of Adjuvant Chemotherapy With or Without Bevacizumab for Patients With Completely Resected Stage IB (>4 cm)-IIIA Non-Small Lung Cancer (NSCLC), Eastern Cooperative Oncology Group, ClinicalTrials.gov identifier: NCT00324805) is currently recruiting patients for a study of combination chemotherapy with the monoclonal antibody bevacizumab for patients with surgically resected stage IB to IIIA NSCLC. Melanoma-associated antigen A3 (MAGE-A3), found in approximately 30% of patients with stage I and 50% of patients with stage II tumors, is associated with poor prognosis and has been shown to be expressed on tumor cells but not on normal cells.[28,29] The MAGRIT trial (GSK1572932A Antigen-Specific Cancer Immunotherapeutic as Adjuvant Therapy in Patients With Resectable MAGE-A3 Positive Non-Small Cell Lung Cancer, GlaxoSmithKline, ClinicalTrials.gov identifier: NCT00480025) aims to evaluate the use of the immunotherapeutic product GSK1572932A in patients with resected stage IB to IIIA NSCLC. In this ongoing, phase III trial, disease-free survival will be measured for patients randomized to treatment with MAGE-A3 vaccine or placebo.

SUMMARY

Globally, lung cancer is the most common cancer with an estimated 1.6 million new cases worldwide in 2008.[30] Lung cancer is associated with high rates of recurrence and low long-term survival rates, which together pose a considerable challenge to the treatment of NSCLC. For early-stage NSCLC, surgical resection is the primary treatment, although the high rates of recurrence following resection call for additional systemic therapy. Although the role of adjuvant chemotherapy in NSCLC was previously a subject of some controversy, evidence from large randomized control trials and meta-analyses now demonstrate the significance of incorporating adjuvant chemotherapy as a standard of care. However, the evidence for adjuvant chemotherapy for stage IB patients remains less well defined. During the last decade, it has become clear that lung cancers represent a heterogeneous population of tumors, even within histologic subtypes, that result from the occurrence of different types of mutations. This heterogeneity depends on the racial and potentially ethnic background of the populations studied. These variables have not been controlled in the published studies described herein. The status of EGF1R is an example of this phenomenon. This may, in part, explain some of the differences in the results among the studies. As additional information becomes available regarding new targets and targeted therapies, new prognostic and predictive biomarkers have the potential to clarify the role of adjuvant chemotherapy for stage IB and, even, for stage IA patients by identifying subgroups of patients likely to respond favorably to treatment. In addition, biomarkers may play an increasing role in the selection of chemotherapy regimens in an effort to improve long-term survival for patients with early-stage NSCLC. Finally, ongoing clinical trials evaluating combination therapies and immunotherapies have the potential to further improve the efficacy of adjuvant chemotherapy.

REFERENCES

1. Jemal A, Siegel R, Xu J, et al. Cancer statistics, 2010. CA Cancer J Clin 2010; 60(5):277–300.
2. Douillard JY, Rosell R, De Lena M, et al. Adjuvant vinorelbine plus cisplatin versus observation in patients with completely resected stage IB-IIIA non-small-cell lung cancer (Adjuvant Navelbine International Trialist Association [ANITA]): a randomised controlled trial. Lancet Oncol 2006;7(9):719–27.

3. Non-small Cell Lung Cancer Collaborative Group. Chemotherapy in non-small cell lung cancer: a meta-analysis using updated data on individual patients from 52 randomised clinical trials. BMJ 1995;311(7010):899–909.

4. Arriagada R, Bergman B, Dunant A, et al. Cisplatin-based adjuvant chemotherapy in patients with completely resected non-small-cell lung cancer. N Engl J Med 2004;350(4):351–60.

5. Winton T, Livingston R, Johnson D, et al. Vinorelbine plus cisplatin vs. observation in resected non-small-cell lung cancer. N Engl J Med 2005;352(25):2589–97.

6. Pisters KM, Evans WK, Azzoli CG, et al. Cancer Care Ontario and American Society of Clinical Oncology adjuvant chemotherapy and adjuvant radiation therapy for stages I-IIIA resectable non small-cell lung cancer guideline. J Clin Oncol 2007;25(34):5506–18.

7. Pignon JP, Tribodet H, Scagliotti GV, et al. Lung adjuvant cisplatin evaluation: a pooled analysis by the LACE Collaborative Group. J Clin Oncol 2008;26(21):3552–9.

8. Scagliotti GV, Fossati R, Torri V, et al. Randomized study of adjuvant chemotherapy for completely resected stage I, II, or IIIA non-small-cell lung cancer. J Natl Cancer Inst 2003;95(19):1453–61.

9. Waller D, Peake MD, Stephens RJ, et al. Chemotherapy for patients with non-small cell lung cancer: the surgical setting of the Big Lung Trial. Eur J Cardiothorac Surg 2004;26(1):173–82.

10. Strauss GM, Herndon JE 2nd, Maddaus MA, et al. Adjuvant paclitaxel plus carboplatin compared with observation in stage IB non-small-cell lung cancer: CALGB 9633 with the Cancer and Leukemia Group B, Radiation Therapy Oncology Group, and North Central Cancer Treatment Group Study Groups. J Clin Oncol 2008;26(31):5043–51.

11. Arriagada R, Auperin A, Burdett S, et al. Adjuvant chemotherapy, with or without postoperative radiotherapy, in operable non-small-cell lung cancer: two meta-analyses of individual patient data. Lancet 2010;375(9722):1267–77.

12. Butts CA, Ding K, Seymour L, et al. Randomized phase III trial of vinorelbine plus cisplatin compared with observation in completely resected stage IB and II non-small-cell lung cancer: updated survival analysis of JBR-10. J Clin Oncol 2010; 28(1):29–34.

13. Kato H, Ichinose Y, Ohta M, et al. A randomized trial of adjuvant chemotherapy with uracil-tegafur for adenocarcinoma of the lung. N Engl J Med 2004; 350(17):1713–21.

14. Chabner B, Longo DL. Cancer chemotherapy and biotherapy: principles and practice. 4th edition. Philadelphia: Lippincott Williams & Wilkins; 2006.

15. Chang A. Chemotherapy, chemoresistance and the changing treatment landscape for NSCLC. Lung Cancer 2011;71(1):3–10.

16. Rajeswaran A, Trojan A, Burnand B, et al. Efficacy and side effects of cisplatin- and carboplatin-based doublet chemotherapeutic regimens versus non-platinum-based doublet chemotherapeutic regimens as first line treatment of metastatic non-small cell lung carcinoma: a systematic review of randomized controlled trials. Lung Cancer 2008;59(1):1–11.

17. Sangha R, Price J, Butts CA. Adjuvant therapy in non-small cell lung cancer: current and future directions. Oncologist 2010;15(8):862–72.

18. Tanaka F, Wada H, Fukushima M. UFT and S-1 for treatment of primary lung cancer. Gen Thorac Cardiovasc Surg 2010;58(1):3–13.

19. Hamada C, Tanaka F, Ohta M, et al. Meta-analysis of postoperative adjuvant chemotherapy with tegafur-uracil in non-small-cell lung cancer. J Clin Oncol 2005;23(22):4999–5006.

20. Rosell R, Taron M, Massuti B, et al. Predicting response to chemotherapy with early-stage lung cancer. Cancer J 2011;17(1):49–56.
21. Olaussen KA, Dunant A, Fouret P, et al. DNA repair by ERCC1 in non-small-cell lung cancer and cisplatin-based adjuvant chemotherapy. N Engl J Med 2006; 355(10):983–91.
22. Vilmar A, Sorensen JB. Excision repair cross-complementation group 1 (ERCC1) in platinum-based treatment of non-small cell lung cancer with special emphasis on carboplatin: a review of current literature. Lung Cancer 2009;64(2):131–9.
23. Reguart N, Cardona AF, Carrasco E, et al. BRCA1: a new genomic marker for non-small-cell lung cancer. Clin Lung Cancer 2008;9(6):331–9.
24. Seve P, Dumontet C. Is class III beta-tubulin a predictive factor in patients receiving tubulin-binding agents? Lancet Oncol 2008;9(2):168–75.
25. Seve P, Lai R, Ding K, et al. Class III beta-tubulin expression and benefit from adjuvant cisplatin/vinorelbine chemotherapy in operable non-small cell lung cancer: analysis of NCIC JBR.10. Clin Cancer Res 2007;13(3):994–9.
26. Riely GJ, Marks J, Pao W. KRAS mutations in non-small cell lung cancer. Proc Am Thorac Soc 2009;6(2):201–5.
27. Schettino C, Bareschino MA, Maione P, et al. The potential role of pharmacogenomic and genomic in the adjuvant treatment of early stage non small cell lung cancer. Curr Genomics 2008;9(4):252–62.
28. Sicnel W, Varwerk C, Linder A, et al. Melanoma associated antigen (MAGE)-A3 expression in Stages I and II non-small cell lung cancer: results of a multicenter study. Eur J Cardiothorac Surg 2004;25(1):131–4.
29. Mellstedt H, Vansteenkiste J, Thatcher N. Vaccines for the treatment of non-small cell lung cancer: investigational approaches and clinical experience. Lung Cancer 2011;73(1):11–7.
30. Ferlay J, Shin H-R, Bray F, et al. Estimates of worldwide burden of cancer in 2008: GLOBOCAN 2008. Int J Cancer 2010;127(12):2893–917.

Role of Surgery in Small Cell Lung Cancer

Seth D. Goldstein, MD[a], Stephen C. Yang, MD[b],*

KEYWORDS

• Surgery • Small cell • Lung cancer

NOMENCLATURE

Small cell lung cancer (SCLC) is estimated to account for approximately 13% of newly diagnosed lung cancers.[1] It is considered distinct from non–small cell lung cancer (NSCLC), due to different biological and clinical patterns. Specifically, SCLC is known to have a more aggressive biology with rapid growth and early spread, as well as a common association with paraneoplastic syndromes. Of all histologic types of lung cancer, SCLC is the most sensitive to chemotherapy and radiation, but prognosis remains poor, with an overall median survival following treatment of 10 months and a 5-year survival of 5%.[2]

SCLC is seen almost exclusively in smokers and is characterized by a rapid tumor doubling time, high growth fraction, and early development of metastases. The majority of patients present with extrathoracic metastases, but more sensitive imaging and screening modalities have resulted in better detection of early disease. The first staging of SCLC by severity was introduced by the Veterans' Administration Lung Study Group (VALSG) in the 1950s. In that classification, limited disease (LD) was characterized by tumor confined to the ipsilateral hemithorax that can be safely included in a single radiation port. More widespread cancer was termed extensive disease (ED). Approximately 40% of all new SCLC diagnoses are LD,[1] which historically has improved survival compared with ED, with a median survival of 16 months and a 12% 5-year survival following chemoradiotherapy.[2]

In 1989, after the introduction of TNM staging, the International Association for the Study of Lung Cancer (IASLC) described LD SCLC as consistent with TNM stages IA to IIIB, with ED describing patients with distant metastases.[3] Additionally in the IASLC nomenclature at that time, supraclavicular, hilar, and mediastinal nodes were included in LD. These modifications have been found to be somewhat more prognostic than

The authors have nothing to disclose.
[a] General Surgery, Johns Hopkins University School of Medicine, 600 North Wolfe Street, Blalock 240, Baltimore, MD 21287, USA
[b] Division of Thoracic Surgery, Johns Hopkins University School of Medicine, 600 North Wolfe Street, Blalock 240, Baltimore, MD 21287, USA
* Corresponding author. Division of Thoracic Surgery, Johns Hopkins University School of Medicine, 600 North Wolfe Street, Blalock 240, Baltimore, MD 21287.
E-mail address: syang@jhmi.edu

Surg Oncol Clin N Am 20 (2011) 769–777
doi:10.1016/j.soc.2011.08.001
1055-3207/11/$ – see front matter © 2011 Published by Elsevier Inc.
surgonc.theclinics.com

the original VALSG,[4] and continue to be used to estimate prognosis and guide treatment.

For decades, clinicians and clinical trial investigators have consistently commented that LD SCLC comprises a heterogeneous patient population, with little similarity in survival rates between patients presenting with a peripheral nodule and those with main bronchus tumors and lymphadenopathy. Recognizing this, in 1993 the Toronto Lung Oncology Group suggested relying more heavily on TNM staging rather than grossly grouping LD and ED. Patient survival in their cohort with clinical stages I and II was significantly better than those with stage III including N2 or N3 involvement.[5] The same article also proposed a "very limited disease" category defined by small tumors with a negative mediastinoscopy.

Despite these data and subsequent recognition that dichotomous LD/ED staging of SCLC may not be as predictive a framework as TNM, particularly for surgical intervention, the use of these terms has persisted in clinical practice, due to the fact that by not routinely offering resection for SCLC, it has been more difficult to validate staging accuracy. Because almost all patients with LD are candidates for chemotherapy and radiation, the two-group system has not been as problematic while investigating those modalities. Meanwhile, several reports in the surgical literature have found that TNM staging for SCLC is predictive of outcome, particularly for low-stage tumors.[6–15] For the purposes of this article, the term early stage (ES) will include clinical or pathologic stage IA through IIB.

Conventional treatment for SCLC is combination thoracic radiation and platinum-based multiagent chemotherapy (most often etoposide and cisplatin),[16] with surgery traditionally thought to have no role in disease management. However, ES SCLC may be more amenable to local control following resection, with a growing body of literature suggesting that surgery is an important component of multimodality therapy. Here the authors attempt to summarize what is currently known about ES SCLC, and outline the methods by which this controversy is actively being investigated.

HISTORY OF SURGICAL LITERATURE

Before 1970 surgical resection was often used to treat SCLC; however, surgery was supplanted by radiation following the British Medical Research Council (MRC) report that radiotherapy alone provided better survival than surgery alone as primary therapy for patients with SCLC.[17,18] Of note, despite the statistically significant difference between surgery and radiation, the mean survival was less than 1 year in both groups. Furthermore, data were analyzed by intention to treat, and included 37 patients who underwent exploratory thoracotomy only or no surgery in the analysis of the 71 patients in the surgical arm.

The Veterans Administration Surgical Oncology Group in 1982 retrospectively reviewed their experience with 132 patients with SCLC who had undergone resection, and reported as high as 60% 5-year survival for T1N0 lesions status post surgery and adjuvant chemotherapy.[19] This rate was higher than adjuvant survival rates for later-stage disease, and led the investigators to conclude that resection is definitely indicated in patients with T1N0M0 lesions and probably indicated in those with T1N1M0 or T2N0M0 lesions. This study was an early proponent of the concept of more precise staging to determine candidacy for surgery.

In 1994, the Lung Cancer Study Group published a prospective randomized trial of induction chemotherapy followed by either surgery or radiation.[20] Of the 328 patients initially treated with 5 cycles of cyclophosphamide, doxorubicin, and vincristine, 146 responders were randomized to surgery or no surgery. All patients received radiation therapy to the chest and brain. There was no difference in survival between the two arms, with a median survival time of 16 months and a 2-year survival rate of 20%. However, patients with stage I were specifically excluded from this trial. This study has been the only randomized one to date comparing surgery and chemotherapy, and is often cited as the primary rationale to not offer resection for SCLC. There have been no published randomized trials conducted using a modern chemotherapy regimen (platinum-based) in ES disease.

JUSTIFICATION FOR SURGERY

The MRC trial effectively slowed the investigation of surgery for SCLC for 2 decades following its publication. However, there have been several strong criticisms of the conclusions. Most notably, there were few ES patients in the cohort, and subgroup analysis was not performed. In the 1994 Lung Cancer Study Group randomized trial, patients with T1N0 lesions were excluded and the study was performed before the advent of platinum-based modern chemotherapy. Despite these findings historically, for many practitioners there is strong intuitive rationale for the use of surgery in ES. Accordingly it continues to be investigated, and data are emerging to support the hypothesis that when staged appropriately, there is a benefit for resection in select cases. The arguments for surgery generally revolve around efficacy of local control and uncertainties in histologic diagnosis.

LOCAL CONTROL

Local recurrence of SCLC after disease treatment can be at the primary tumor site as well as via lymphatic spread. Current chemoradiation regimens have a local failure rate approaching 50%.[21,22] However, there are data to suggest that following surgical resection, local control may approach 85% to 90%,[7,12] and when surgery has been directly compared with chemoradiation there has been a significantly lower rate of local recurrence after surgical resection.[10]

UNCERTAINTIES IN HISTOLOGIC DIAGNOSIS

Small carcinoid tumors with no nodal involvement can occasionally be misdiagnosed as ES SCLC by needle biopsy. Furthermore, as many as one-quarter of resected SCLCs are found to be histologically mixed with other types (such as NSCLC).[23] Because NSCLC tumors are less sensitive to current chemoradiotherapies, there is a risk of residual or refractory disease if treated without resection. Furthermore, after failure of chemotherapy, surgery has been shown to commonly reveal mixed histologies that are more amenable to surgery.[24] In the event of survival for 2 years or more after SCLC diagnosis, new tumors should be considered as possibly NSCLC, although resection in that context has a lower median survival than resection for primary NSCLC (25 vs 58 months, respectively).[25]

STUDIES IN THE MODERN ERA

Since the introduction of the TNM staging system, several retrospective and prospective nonrandomized reports have noted the benefits of surgical resection for patients with ES SCLC. A selection of these series is compared in **Table 1**, with patient outcomes by stage as reported. Of note, there appears to be an effect of tumor stage on 5-year survival whenever surgery is offered as a primary treatment, and the survival rates for ES patients in these studies are higher than those reported for conventional treatment with modern platinum-based chemotherapy.

Table 1
Selected studies of surgery combined with platinum-based chemotherapy for late-stage SCLC

Authors,[Ref.] Year	N	Study Design	Regimen	Overall 5-Year Survival, % by Stage (Pathologic When Available)			
				Stage I	Stage II	Stage III	Overall
Fujimori et al,[6] 1997	22	Prospective	Induction PE ± D	73 (I + II)[a]		43[a]	67[a]
Rea et al,[7] 1998	104	Prospective	CAV or PEB, adjuvant for Stage I–II, induction for Stage III	52	30	15	32
Eberhardt and Korfee,[8] 2003	46	Prospective	Induction PE		44 (IIB + IIIA)		39
Rostad et al,[9] 2004	38	Retrospective		45		6 (IIIB)	
Badzio et al,[10] 2004	67	Retrospective with case-matched control	Adjuvant PE or CAV				27
Brock et al,[11] 2005	23	Retrospective	22% induction, 55% adjuvant, 22% surgery alone or unspecified	86			68
Tsuchiya et al,[12] 2005	61	Prospective		70	38	39	57
Granetzny et al,[13] 2006	95	Retrospective		43 (I + II)			
Bischof et al,[14] 2007	39	Retrospective	Adjuvant PE	49 (I + II)			
Lim et al,[15] 2008	59	Retrospective	24% adjuvant, regimen unknown	60	50	50	52
Vallieres et al,[35] 2009	349	Retrospective (IASLC database)	Various	48	39	12	30

Abbreviations: A, adriamycin (doxorubicin); B, epirubicin; C, cyclophosphamide; D, doxorubicin (adriamycin); E, etoposide; P, cisplatin; V, vincristine.
[a] Three-year survival reported.

Badzio and colleagues[10] created a retrospective case-control series comparing 67 patients following surgery for LS SCLC with adjuvant chemotherapy with 67 pair-matched patients undergoing conventional treatment. The 2-year and 5-year survival rates were 43% and 27%, respectively, in the surgical group; and 17% and 4%, respectively, in the nonsurgical group. Local relapse occurred in 15% of those treated with surgery and in 55% of patients treated without surgery. Distant relapse rates were similar between groups. Similarly, Rostad and colleagues[9] used a lung cancer registry in Norway to compare treatment strategies and reported that specifically for stage I disease, 5-year survival was 45% in surgical and 11% in conventional treatment groups.

Brock and colleagues[11] performed a retrospective study comparing surgical outcomes in SCLC both before and after the introduction of platinum-based chemotherapy, and concluded that highly selected patients with SCLC may benefit from surgery with induction or adjuvant chemotherapy. The 82 patients with stage I lesions who underwent resection experienced a 5-year survival rate of 86%. Of note, platinum chemotherapy as the adjuvant therapy had a significant effect on survival, as did lobectomy over nonanatomic wedge resection. The patients that benefited the most in that cohort were women with completely resected T1-T2 N0 disease who went on to receive platinum chemotherapy.

The Japan Clinical Oncology Group also demonstrated a high 5-year survival for resected stage I disease (67% stage IA, 73% stage IB).[12] In their cohort of patients undergoing surgery there was a 10% local recurrence rate, which was superseded by a 15% brain failure rate, demonstrating the potential importance of prophylactic cranial irradiation.

Another retrospective study by Bischof and colleagues[14] analyzed 39 patients with ES (stage IA–IIB) SCLC, and demonstrated a 47-month median overall survival and a 47% 5-year survival for these patients who underwent resection followed by adjuvant chemotherapy. Although radiation to both the primary site and prophylactically to the brain was found to be protective, 59% of this cohort did not receive thoracic radiation and 44% no radiation at all, possibly skewing the survival rates even lower than if those measures had been applied.

In 2009, the IASLC reviewed their database of more than 100,000 lung cancer cases. Of these, 13,290 were SCLC and approximately 1% of those (n = 349) had undergone R0 resection. One-year and 5-year survival outcomes in the IASLC data were found to be inversely proportional to both T and N classification.

Recently, two studies queried the Surveillance Epidemiology and End Results (SEER) database for outcomes following resection for SCLC. Yu and colleagues[26] concluded that surgery without radiation offered reasonable survival for node-negative patients with SCLC. Outcomes were not reported by tumor stage specifically, but 5-year survival was 50% for all patients who received a lobectomy for SCLC, and there was no statistically significant advantage of adjuvant radiation compared with surgery alone. Schreiber and colleagues[27] found similar survival rates among 861 SCLC patients in the SEER database who underwent resection. Surgery was most beneficial in ES SCLC, with a 5-year survival of 53%, but conferred a benefit in all nodal status groups.

All studies have concluded that despite the lack of randomized trials comparing surgery with definitive chemoradiation for ES SCLC, resection likely plays an important role as a part of multimodality therapy as it evolves.

CLINICAL MANAGEMENT

Most patients who undergo resection for SCLC have the diagnosis made after the nodule is resected. Therefore, in those patients who have a diagnosis of SCLC based on endobronchial or transthoracic biopsy, the pathology slides should be reread. On presentation, patients should be clinically staged as accurately as possible. Computed tomography (CT) and positron-emission tomography imaging is often useful to assess for regional spread and metastatic disease. Magnetic resonance imaging of the brain should be done. In addition, in a similar fashion to NSCLC, cervical mediastinoscopy is the definitive procedure to determine nodal status of the mediastinum.[28,29] Studies using endobronchial ultrasonography to stage the nodal involvement around the tracheobronchial tree are lacking, but undoubtedly will be forthcoming in the future as data for NSCLC mature. CT imaging has a high false-negative rate in this context, making the direct surgical sampling even more important. At present, there is no role for bone marrow biopsy in patients with clinically ES disease.

The timing of surgery relative to chemotherapy and radiation has not been completely established. Although adjuvant resection was initially reported, neoadjuvant or induction therapy has been successfully reported and is thought to be at least as efficacious.[6,28,30]

Regardless of whether patients have received induction therapy or have already undergone wedge resection of a peripheral nodule, a formal lobectomy with mediastinal lymph node dissection should be performed on diagnosing SCLC. This approach has been shown to have a significant effect on survival compared with nonanatomic resections.[11]

One of the most difficult facets of SCLC treatment is its propensity for local recurrence. Although primary resection may improve local control, there is a high risk of relapse in any treatment paradigm. Salvage surgery may be an appropriate option for patients who are nonresponders or have relapsed after remission. One retrospective review offered resection, including pneumonectomy if needed, and reported a 23% 5-year survival rate.[24] Of interest, some patients in that small cohort were found to have mixed histology in their tumor pathology at salvage surgery, lending more weight to the argument for surgery based on uncertainties in histologic diagnosis as already outlined.

The American College of Chest Physicians does not currently recommend surgery as a first-line treatment for SCLC.[31] However, these guidelines state that surgery for curative intent may be performed following mediastinoscopy, while acknowledging that peripheral lesions were excluded from the single randomized trial of surgery for SCLC. The Lung Cancer Study Group trial represented state of the art in 1994, but there have been no subsequent studies of surgery with current platinum-based chemotherapy and modern radiation regimens in a randomized fashion. Furthermore, stage I tumors were specifically excluded from that cohort. In determining the role of surgery for ES disease, modern clinicians should be discouraged from using the conclusions of that trial in formulating treatment therapies.

There is a growing body of literature suggesting that for ES SCLC, surgery may indeed confer a benefit when offered along with chemotherapy and radiation. Patient selection is clearly the pivotal issue, as the historical method of staging SCLC is overly broad from a surgical perspective. This fact has been eloquently pointed out by several recent reviews.[8,32,33] The concept of LD as confined to a single hemithorax also includes regionally advanced stage III tumors that are less amenable to both local and distant control. "Early stage" or "very limited" are more practical grouping methods, comprising stages IA to IIB. Whereas the best 5-year survival rates in phase 3 trials of modern chemoradiotherapy with prophylactic cranial irradiation are less than 25%,[21,22] patients with ES SCLC treated surgically have reportedly fared far better.

If surgery is found to confer a benefit in ES SCLC, it will certainly become a cornerstone of the treatment paradigm as newer, more targeted therapies are developed. Angiogenesis inhibitors, growth factor receptor inhibitors, apoptosis promoters, and

Table 2
Randomized multimodality therapy for limited-disease SCLC

	Essen Thoracic Oncology Group	West Japan Thoracic Oncology Group	German Multicenter Randomized Trial
CT	Cisplatin, etoposide	Cisplatin, etoposide	Carboplatin, etoposide, paclitaxel
RT	Hyperfractionated 45 Gy twice daily	Hyperfractionated 45 Gy twice daily; PCI only if complete response from induction CT/RT	50 Gy, once daily; PCI
Arm A	CT × 3 + surgery + Boost CT/RT	CT × 3 + CT/RT + PCI + surgery	CT × 5 + surgery ± RT + PCI
Arm B	CT × 3/RT + surgery + Boost CT	CT × 2/RT + CT × 2 + PCI	CT × 5 + RT + PCI

Abbreviations: CT, chemotherapy; PCI, prophylactic cranial radiation; RT, radiation therapy.
Data from Eberhardt W, Korfee S. New approaches for small-cell lung cancer: local treatments. Cancer Control 2003;10:289–96.

drugs targeting immune system antibodies are all currently under investigation as novel SCLC agents.[16,34] Although a review of these molecular markers is beyond the scope of this discussion, there are proteins whose expression have been correlated with therapeutic resistance or poorer survival in SCLC, including Bcl-2, fragile histidine triad complex (FHIT), and c-kit. Other SCLC tumor signature markers that correlate with chemotherapy response similar to NSCLC include ERCC1, MYC, bcl-2, and p16.

Given that relatively few patients present with ES SCLC, a randomized trial including resection for these lesions may not be practical to perform. At present, ongoing trials in Europe and Japan (**Table 2**) will attempt to address the issue of induction chemoradiation therapy and the role of surgical resection for advanced-stage disease. Prospective intergroup trials are now being formulated to not only better define the role of surgical resection for ES disease but also to collect tissue to help in characterizing biological markers that may confer translational importance.

SUMMARY

Conventional treatment for SCLC is currently thoracic radiation and combination chemotherapy. Surgery has been traditionally stated to have little to no role in disease management. However, there is a growing body of literature suggesting that surgery is an important component of multimodality therapy for ES SCLC. Certainly in the current body of recent cohort studies, it appears that ES leads to improved 5-year survival rates following surgery with adjuvant therapy compared with chemotherapy and radiation alone. Despite negative previous data that have been much criticized, there should be a new focus of both clinical and basic science research on SCLC. As knowledge of the biology of this disease expands, it remains unclear exactly which of the clinical and biologic factors will ultimately predict long-term survival. Randomized trials comparing surgery with modern medical management are ongoing; the results will undoubtedly help to clarify the role of surgical intervention in SCLC.

REFERENCES

1. Govindan R, Page N, Morgensztern D, et al. Changing epidemiology of small-cell lung cancer in the United States over the last 30 years: analysis of the surveillance, epidemiologic, and end results database. J Clin Oncol 2006;24:4539–44.

2. Jänne PA, Freidlin B, Saxman S, et al. Twenty-five years of clinical research for patients with limited-stage small cell lung carcinoma in North America: meaningful improvements in survival. Cancer 2002;95:1528–38.
3. Stahel RA, Ginsberg R, Havemann K, et al. Staging and prognostic factors in small cell lung cancer: a consensus report. Lung Cancer 1989;5:119–26.
4. Micke P, Faldum A, Metz T, et al. Staging small cell lung cancer: Veterans Administration Lung Study Group versus International Association for the Study of Lung Cancer—what limits limited disease? Lung Cancer 2002;37:271–6.
5. Shepherd FA, Ginsberg RJ, Haddad R, et al. Importance of clinical staging in limited small-cell lung cancer: a valuable system to separate prognostic subgroups. J Clin Oncol 1993;11:1592–7.
6. Fujimori K, Yokoyama A, Kurita Y, et al. A pilot phase 2 study of surgical treatment after induction chemotherapy for resectable stage I to IIIA small cell lung cancer. Chest 1997;111:1089–93.
7. Rea F, Callegaro D, Favaretto A, et al. Long term results of surgery and chemotherapy in small cell lung cancer. Eur J Cardiothorac Surg 1998;14:398–402.
8. Eberhardt W, Korfee S. New approaches for small-cell lung cancer: local treatments. Cancer Control 2003;10:289–96.
9. Rostad H, Naalsund A, Jacobsen R, et al. Small cell lung cancer in Norway. Should more patients have been offered surgical therapy? Eur J Cardiothorac Surg 2004;26:782–6.
10. Badzio A, Kurowski K, Karnicka-Mlodkowska H, et al. A retrospective comparative study of surgery followed by chemotherapy vs. non-surgical management in limited-disease small cell lung cancer. Eur J Cardiothorac Surg 2004;26:183–8.
11. Brock MV, Hooker CM, Syphard JE, et al. Surgical resection of limited disease small cell lung cancer in the new era of platinum chemotherapy: its time has come. J Thorac Cardiovasc Surg 2005;129:64–72.
12. Tsuchiya R, Suzuki K, Ichinose Y, et al. Phase II trial of postoperative adjuvant cisplatin and etoposide in patients with completely resected stage I-IIIa small cell lung cancer: the Japan Clinical Oncology Lung Cancer Study Group Trial (JCOG9101). J Thorac Cardiovasc Surg 2005;129:977–83.
13. Granetzny A, Boseila A, Wagner W, et al. Surgery in the tri-modality treatment of small cell lung cancer. Stage-dependent survival. Eur J Cardiothorac Surg 2006; 30:212–6.
14. Bischof M, Debus J, Herfarth K, et al. Surgery and chemotherapy for small cell lung cancer in stages I-II with or without radiotherapy. Strahlenther Onkol 2007; 183:679–84.
15. Lim E, Belcher E, Yap YK, et al. The role of surgery in the treatment of limited disease small cell lung cancer: time to reevaluate. J Thorac Oncol 2008;3: 1267–71.
16. Lee CB, Morris DE, Fried DB, et al. Current and evolving treatment options for limited stage small cell lung cancer. Curr Opin Oncol 2006;18:162–72.
17. Miller AB, Fox W, Tall R. Five-year follow-up of the Medical Research Council comparative trial of surgery and radiotherapy for the primary treatment of small-celled or oat-celled carcinoma of the bronchus. Lancet 1969;2:501–5.
18. Fox W, Scadding JG. Medical Research Council comparative trial of surgery and radiotherapy for primary treatment of small celled or oat celled carcinoma of bronchus. Ten year follow up. Lancet 1973;2:63–5.
19. Shields TW, Higgins GA Jr, Matthews MJ, et al. Surgical resection in the management of small cell carcinoma of the lung. J Thorac Cardiovasc Surg 1982;84: 481–8.

20. Lad T, Piantadosi S, Thomas P, et al. A prospective randomized trial to determine the benefit of surgical resection of residual disease following response of small cell lung cancer to combination chemotherapy. Chest 1994;106:320S–3S.
21. Turrisi AT III, Kim K, Blum R, et al. Twice-daily compared with once-daily thoracic radiotherapy in limited small-cell lung cancer treated concurrently with cisplatin and etoposide. N Engl J Med 1999;340:265–71.
22. Schild SE, Bonner JA, Shanahan TG, et al. Long-term results of a phase III trial comparing once-daily radiotherapy with twice-daily radiotherapy in limited-stage small-cell lung cancer. Int J Radiat Oncol Biol Phys 2004;59:943–51.
23. Asamura H, Kameya T, Matsuno Y, et al. Neuroendocrine neoplasms of the lung: a prognostic spectrum. J Clin Oncol 2006;24:70–6.
24. Shepherd FA, Ginsberg R, Patterson GA, et al. Is there ever a role for salvage operations in limited small-cell lung cancer? J Thorac Cardiovasc Surg 1991; 101:196–200.
25. Smythe WR, Estrera AL, Swisher SG, et al. Surgical resection of non-small cell carcinoma after treatment for small cell carcinoma. Ann Thorac Surg 2001;71:962–6.
26. Yu JB, Decker RH, Detterbeck FC, et al. Surveillance epidemiology and end results evaluation of the role of surgery for stage I small cell lung cancer. J Thorac Oncol 2010;5:215–9.
27. Schreiber D, Rineer J, Weedon J, et al. Survival outcomes with the use of surgery in limited-stage small cell lung cancer: should its role be re-evaluated? Cancer 2010;116:1350–7.
28. Eberhardt W, Stamatis G, Stuschke M, et al. Prognostically orientated multimodality treatment Including surgery for selected patients of small cell lung cancer patients stages IB to IIIB: long-term results of a phase II trial. Br J Cancer 1999;81:1206–12.
29. Inoue M, Nakagawa K, Fujiwara K, et al. Results of preoperative mediastinoscopy for small cell lung cancer. Ann Thorac Surg 2000;70:1620–3.
30. Wada H, Yokomise H, Tanaka F, et al. Surgical treatment of small cell carcinoma of the lung: advantage of preoperative chemotherapy. Lung Cancer 1995;13:45–56.
31. Simon GR, Turrisi A. Management of small cell lung cancer: ACCP evidence-based clinical practice guidelines (2nd edition). Chest 2007;132:324S–39S.
32. Anraku M, Waddell TK. Surgery for small-cell lung cancer. Semin Thorac Cardiovasc Surg 2006;18:211–6.
33. Koletsis EN, Prokakis C, Karanikolas M, et al. Current role of surgery in small cell lung carcinoma. J Cardiothorac Surg 2009;4:30.
34. Blackhall FH, Shepherd FA. Small cell lung cancer and targeted therapies. Curr Opin Oncol 2007;19:103–8.
35. Vallières E, Shepherd FA, Crowley J, et al. The IASLC Lung Cancer Staging Project: proposals regarding the relevance of TNM in the pathologic staging of small cell lung cancer in the forthcoming (seventh) edition of the TNM classification for lung cancer. J Thorac Oncol 2009;4(9):1049–59.

Surgical and Endoscopic Palliation of Advanced Lung Cancer

Aaron M. Cheng, MD*, Douglas E. Wood, MD

KEYWORDS

- Lung cancer palliation • Therapeutic bronchoscopy
- Airway obstruction • Malignant pleural effusion
- Massive hemoptysis

AIRWAY OBSTRUCTION

Central airway obstruction refers to significant obstruction of the trachea and main bronchi. Patients with advanced-stage lung cancer who have this complication are likely to have significant dyspnea and hemoptysis, which can become life threatening, because the onset of stridor implies impending airway obstruction and requires immediate attention. Obstructive symptoms can be caused by intraluminal tumor obstruction, extraluminal tumor compression, or both; airway obstruction by the tumor can also produce aggravating factors due to excessive mucous production and plugging, postobstructive pneumonia, and hemoptysis. Appropriate therapeutic strategies must be anticipated to provide palliation and symptomatic relief.

Bronchoscopy remains the single most important diagnostic and therapeutic tool for managing airway obstruction. Several different bronchoscopic interventions are available to palliate airway obstruction in advanced-stage lung cancer. Choosing one bronchoscopic intervention over another is more often determined as much by physician bias as by the cause and anatomic location of the obstruction and patient comorbidities. It is very important to recognize that there are some patients with locally advanced lung cancer involving the central airways who may be amenable to a curative-intent resection involving a tracheoplastic or bronchoplastic procedure. Treatment decisions to offer only palliative endobronchial management in locally advanced lung cancer should be rigorously avoided when potential definitive tracheobronchial resection and reconstruction could be otherwise considered with complete resection. Patients with advanced non–small cell lung carcinoma (NSCLC) with

Division of Cardiothoracic Surgery, University of Washington School of Medicine, Box 356310, 1959 NE Pacific Street, AA-115, Seattle, WA 98195-6310, USA
* Corresponding author.
E-mail address: chengam@uw.edu

Surg Oncol Clin N Am 20 (2011) 779–790
doi:10.1016/j.soc.2011.07.008
1055-3207/11/$ – see front matter © 2011 Elsevier Inc. All rights reserved.

malignant central airway obstruction who undergo local treatment by therapeutic bronchoscopy do not have worse survival than those with advanced-stage lung cancer without airway obstruction.[1] Therefore, therapeutic bronchoscopy should be offered to those patients with advanced-stage NSCLC and airway obstruction as an effective palliative measure.

Patients with symptoms from central airway compromise can be offered several different bronchoscopic options. Tumors that invade into the airway can be treated by mechanical core-out, laser ablation, electrocautery, and dilatation and stent placement. Each of these approaches has the benefit of reliable and immediate improvement in appropriately selected patients. Cryotherapy, photodynamic therapy (PDT), and brachytherapy also are effective for treating endoluminal tumors but usually require several days to achieve a tumor response and so have a more limited role in the management of patients who are acutely symptomatic due to central airway obstruction. Extraluminal compression of central airways by tumor causing severe symptoms is not usually palliated well by techniques other than dilatation and stenting. When therapeutic bronchoscopy is unavailable for patients with impending death from airway compromise, endotracheal intubation passing the tube beyond the area of stenosis with the aid of flexible bronchoscopy can be temporarily lifesaving before the patient is transferred to a referral center.

Bronchoscopic debridement of intraluminal tumor obstruction can quickly and effectively palliate airway obstruction and relieve dyspnea. Rigid bronchoscopy is the preferred technique and is a safe effective method to evaluate and stabilize a patient with airway compromise from tumor invasion or compression. The rigid bronchoscope is much quicker and more effective in accomplishing this task than the flexible bronchoscope. Rigid bronchoscopes are available in different diameters; by maneuvering the bronchoscope beyond the area of obstruction, the patient can be ventilated during the intervention, and further evaluation of the nature of the obstruction can be done concomitantly. Flexible bronchoscopy can be performed through the rigid scope, which allows distal airway evaluation and treatment. In many situations, the act of performing a rigid bronchoscopy dilates the area of obstruction; however, the benefit of this method is brief in cases of obstruction from lung cancer, in which obstruction occurs predominantly from extrinsic compression of the airway. In situations in which there is an endoluminal component to airway obstruction, the rigid bronchoscope is used to core out the obstructing lesion with the beveled tip of the rigid bronchoscope applied at the base of the tumor. Retrieving the pieces with biopsy forceps piecemeal using the biopsy forceps through the rigid bronchoscope can be helpful. The benefit of such a core-out procedure is its technical simplicity and the lack of need for additional equipment beyond the standard instruments used in rigid bronchoscopy. Rigid bronchoscopy also allows access for additional therapies to palliate and alleviate the acute symptoms caused by central airway obstruction from lung cancer and has been shown to be an effective technique to permit immediate discontinuation of mechanical ventilation in patients who had required intubation for airway compromise from lung cancer.[2]

Laser resection, electrocautery, and stenting are therapeutic bronchoscopic techniques that can provide immediate relief from endoluminal airway obstruction and can be used independently or in conjunction with bronchoscopic debridement.[3] Laser resection can be performed via rigid bronchoscopy or flexible bronchoscopy and essentially has the same indications as mechanical core-out procedures for treatment of malignant airway obstruction. Laser resection is not effective in cases of dominant external compression, and a relative contraindication is hypoxemia because the risk of fire limits the inspired oxygen fraction to no greater than 40% fraction of inspired oxygen. When done using flexible bronchoscopy, laser resection using the Nd:YAG laser can be performed under topical anesthetic and is able to reach the lobar orifices more easily than mechanical debridement by rigid bronchoscopy. The main goal of laser resection is palliation of symptoms in patients with inoperable lung cancer with endobronchial manifestations, and, as such, there is little improvement in ventilation with laser resection of obstruction of the segmental bronchi. Laser resection is a substantially longer process than mechanical debridement, requires significant additional equipment and cost, and incurs the additional risks of airway fire, perforation, and fistula formation.[4,5] In general, there is little practical benefit of laser resection alone over mechanical core-out procedures in cases of malignant endoluminal obstruction, but it is often combined with other treatment modalities, especially as a means of assuring hemostasis.

Electrocautery refers to application of electrical current to produce tissue heating and coagulation as electrons are conducted to the tissue because of voltage differences between the electrocautery probe and the target tissue. Argon plasma coagulation (APC) is also a mode of electrocoagulation. In APC, the ionized argon gas jet flow conducts electrons, allowing a noncontact mode of treatment. Both methods result in coagulative necrosis of the tumor lesion. The therapeutic goal of electrocautery/APC in advanced-stage lung cancer is the same as laser resection and mechanical debridement: to achieve immediate debulking of endobronchial lesions. In contrast to laser resection, electrocautery has a more superficial effect and does not produce deep tissue necrosis, which is preferable if major vessels are in the vicinity. In addition, electrocautery/APC does not have the logistical concerns of laser, such as, special eye protection is not necessary, and it can be performed by flexible bronchoscopy. From a cost standpoint, electrocautery/APC is less expensive to perform than laser resection. The success rate of this technique is comparable to other bronchoscopic debulking techniques, and the technique is on the order of 70% to 80% effective.[6]

PDT, brachytherapy, and cryotherapy have also been used as palliative treatment in patients with advanced-stage lung cancer and obstructive central lesions.[7] However, these techniques have a delay in treatment response and therefore are not suitable in patients with acute obstructive symptoms. Cryotherapy is more limited in use than either PDT or brachytherapy in bronchoscopic palliation of primary lung cancer. All 3 modalities, like the previously discussed interventions, are applicable only to tumors that have an endoluminal component requiring treatment.

PDT is a 2-stage treatment process that produces tumor necrosis by excitation of a chemical photosensitizing agent (eg, porfimer sodium) by a specific light wavelength that matches the absorption band of the agent. The first stage is photosensitization of the bronchial tumor lesion, which is then followed by the illumination stage with exposure of the agent to the light of specific wavelength. At present, Photofrin (Axcan Pharma Inc) is licensed for use in advanced-stage lung cancer by the Food and Drug Administration and is the most commonly used photosensitizer with a long-standing safety record. The recommended dose of the drug is 2 mg/kg body weight and is administered intravenously 24 to 72 hours before the illumination stage. The light that activates the porphyrin-based photosensitizer is within the red region of the light spectrum (630 nm), and different light sources have been used, including argon dye lasers and diode lasers. Because the photosensitizer is only activated in the presence of the laser light source, specific areas for PDT can be targeted. However, indiscriminate illumination could result in collateral damage to normal tissue. The light generated by the laser is delivered to the tumor by optical fibers that are introduced via either the rigid or fiber-optic bronchoscope. The delivery fibers can be either a cylindrical diffuser, which distributes light circumferentially to be used for interstitial treatment when placed within a tumor mass or a microlens delivery fiber, which is designed for surface application. Tissue necrosis and sloughing of tissue occurs within a few days, and a follow-up rigid and flexible bronchoscopy is necessary for removal of the necrotic debris and tissue and for airway clearance, particularly infected secretions collected beyond the bronchial obstruction. Repeat treatment can also be performed after debridement but needs to be performed within the prescribed time (within 7 days of Photofrin injection) to achieve additional tumoricidal effect. Several studies have confirmed the efficacy and safety of PDT procedures for cancer, and, in those with advanced-stage cancer and endoluminal bronchial obstruction, PDT is capable of providing significant palliative improvement and may have a more durable benefit than mechanical debridement or laser resection because of its wider radial effect of tumor necrosis, which may delay tumor regrowth and obstruction.[8] In many cases of NSCLC, patients with inoperable cancer are referred for PDT following recurrence of tumor after chemotherapy/radiotherapy.[9] Although PDT may be an effective palliative therapy, its response is slow and should not be used as the primary intervention for treatment of obstructing central airway lesions with a threatened airway. Also, PDT is associated with considerably greater complexity than the other approaches, which must be considered when PDT is performed in fragile patients with limited life spans. Complications specific to light sensitivity, notably skin burn, can occur, and this skin photosensitivity can last for 4 to 6 weeks during which patients must avoid exposure to sunlight, a significant negative factor for quality-of-life considerations in patients being palliated for cancer.

Endoluminal brachytherapy remains one of the oldest techniques of interventional bronchoscopy, and, like PDT, its effect on tumor debulking is delayed; therefore this technique is not indicated in situations in which immediate tumor debulking for airway obstruction is required. However, brachytherapy can be used to treat airway obstruction caused by extraluminal cancer located immediately adjacent to the airway. The radiation source, iridium 192, is delivered through endobronchial catheters positioned under flexible bronchoscopy, and the therapy sessions can be performed on an outpatient basis with minimal short-term complications. Brachytherapy, therefore, is of benefit, particularly in patients with reduced performance status. The effects of high–dose rate brachytherapy can be initially observed after 1 week, and the peak effect is seen usually after 3 weeks. This technique has the benefit of having a longer-lasting tumoricidal effect than the other described bronchoscopic therapies and can also destroy tumor beyond the bronchial wall. However, brachytherapy only has an effective treatment range of 1 to 2 cm from the endoluminal source and so has no significant impact on bulky tumors involving the airway. Therefore, brachytherapy should not be used to replace standard external beam radiation therapy in most patients. Brachytherapy is primarily used in patients who have already received maximal doses of external beam radiation, and current evidence supports its role as a complementary therapy to palliate patients with airway obstruction rather than as primary therapy alone.[10–12] The major contraindication for this therapy is the presence or imminent danger of fistula formation between the treated bronchi and other adjacent structures. Complications associated with brachytherapy include radiation bronchitis and stenosis and can occur days or weeks after therapy. The most important adverse effect as mentioned earlier is fatal hemoptysis and bronchovascular fistula formation, which has an overall reported prevalence of 10%.[13–15]

Cryotherapy offers another modality of treating endoluminal lesions and is based on the cytotoxic effects of cold on living tissue. Cryotherapy tumor destruction relies on the formation of intracellular and extracellular ice crystals, which damage intracellular organelles and cause cellular dehydration. An additional vascular effect occurs: the cold induces an initial tissue vasoconstriction followed by a delayed vasodilation. A zone of local infarct results 6 to 12 hours later. With a 3 mm diameter cryoprobe, the area of destruction is approximately 1 cm in diameter with a depth of 3 mm. Like PDT and brachytherapy, cryotherapy has a delayed effect for tumor destruction, but it differs in that it does not induce collagen damage or risk bronchial wall perforation because collagen and cartilage are quite cryoresistant. Nonhemorrhagic necrosis of the treated lesion occurs 1 to 2 weeks after the procedure, and, generally, the necrotic tissue is expectorated or removed with follow-up bronchoscopy. Flexible cryoprobes are available and can be performed by flexible bronchoscopy; however, the cryoprobes used with rigid bronchoscopy are more powerful and less time consuming to perform. Cryotherapy has been reported to have significant palliative improvement in patients with obstructive airway symptoms from advanced-stage lung cancer, with symptomatic improvement in cough, dyspnea, chest pain, and hemoptysis as well as performance status.[16,17] Although the application of cryotherapy is less widely applied, it seems as effective as the other palliative methods that use thermal energy, such as laser and electrocautery.[18] The major disadvantage of cryotherapy is that it does require repeated applications for treatment effectiveness and therefore is not ideal for relieving acute dyspnea from airway obstruction.

None of the therapies thus far described are effective for symptomatic airway obstruction caused by extraluminal compression, which represents a high percentage of patients with advanced lung cancer. These patients often have predominant extrinsic airway compression from the disease or have endoluminal tumor obstruction with significant extrinsic compression, and, under these conditions, airway stenting is the only immediate treatment that can provide prompt symptomatic relief. The goals of tracheobronchial stenting in palliation of advanced-stage malignancy are to relieve dyspnea and improve drainage of the obstructed distal lung. Indications for airway stenting in palliation of malignant airway obstruction include the following conditions: (1) extensive tracheal or bronchial compression by the primary lung tumor or central lymph node metastasis without other treatment options, (2) airway stabilization in the acutely symptomatic or compromised patient while the tumor is treated with chemotherapy or radiation therapy, and (3) airway maintenance following tumor debulking by the various therapeutic endoluminal bronchoscopic techniques described earlier. The benefit of stenting is that it provides immediate relief of obstruction, but stenting frequently requires debulking or dilatation of the tumor lesion in order to place the largest-diameter stent possible. The primary disadvantage of airway stenting is impairment of the innate mucociliary clearance mechanisms, which can result in airway obstruction from inspissated secretions, and also obstruction from granulation tissue or tumor ingrowth can become problematic, depending on the type of stent that is deployed. Stent migration and displacement occur but are usually less problematic if an appropriate-sized stent is placed.[19]

There are a variety of commercially available tracheobronchial stents, and a full description of the various types is beyond the scope of this review. However, the selection of the optimal stent should be based on the knowledge of the advantages and disadvantages of the individual types of stent and of their method of deployment and on the anatomic location of the lesion. In general, there are 2 types of airway stents, silicone and expandable metal stents, which can be covered or uncovered. The Dumon or Hood stents are the most widely used silicone stents and come in different diameters and lengths as well as Y configuration for placement in the lower tracheal and carinal region. These stents have external silicone studs or flanges to decrease stent migration and require rigid bronchoscopy and general anesthesia for placement. Intrinsically, silicone stents have smaller inner diameter to outer diameter ratios than metal stents, but silicone stents are relatively less expensive and have minimal tissue reactivity, allowing them to be more easily removed or repositioned.

Self-expanding metal stents have gained in popularity over the years because of their ease of insertion because they can be deployed by flexible bronchoscopy with fluoroscopic guidance and under local anesthesia. Other advantages of self-expanding metal stents include their radiopaqueness, which allows radiographic visualization; the greater airway cross-sectional diameter area due to thinner walls; and the ability of these stents to conform to tortuous airways with minimal migration as the radial expansion force is distributed more uniformly across the stent. The major disadvantage of metal stents is that they are very difficult to reposition or remove and may become secondarily obstructed by tumor ingrowth or granulation tissue. Although the covered metal stents have fewer problems with tumor ingrowth or granulation, it can still occur at the bare metal ends of these stents. Third-generation stents are now available that combine much of the advantages of both expandable and solid silicone stents. These stents are expandable and easier to place yet are completely covered, allowing the option of repositioning or removal (at the cost of more dislodgement) and avoiding the complication of tumor or granulation tissue ingrowth and obstruction.

Airway stenting has been demonstrated to be beneficial in patients with severe symptomatic airway obstruction from advanced lung cancer.[20] Stenting is commonly followed by adjuvant therapy such as radiation and chemotherapy and has been associated with improved median survival.[21] However, airway stenting should also be considered as primary palliative treatment in patients with obstruction of the central airways who lack other treatment options. In one study from the Netherlands, tracheobronchial stenting as part of the palliative care of patients with terminal cancer was associated with immediate symptomatic relief and quality-of-life improvement, which was found to be worthwhile even in these patients who had very limited life expectancies.[22]

In general, a combination of all the earlier-mentioned palliative techniques can be used in a given patient. The choice and sequence of techniques used depend on availability, surgeon expertise, and longevity. Patients are often treated with one modality, receive therapy and stabilize, and then later on develop further symptoms requiring alternative techniques.

Malignant Pleural Effusion

The onset of malignant pleural effusion (MPE) in patients with NSCLC represents a dismal prognosis, with median survival after diagnosis of MPE on the order of 4 to 6 months. The International Association for the Study of Lung Cancer reclassified MPE to the M1a descriptor, recognizing its prediction for poor long-term survival with an overall 5-year survival rate of 7%.[23] Once patients are diagnosed with MPE, treatment strategies for NSCLC shift to a palliative intent, including relief of effusion-related symptoms. It becomes imperative that management strategies are aligned with the patient's informed preferences, which preferably are conducted by a multidisciplinary team that is well versed in all the different palliative modalities that can be offered to these patients.

An important consideration in managing a patient with NSCLC who develops a pleural effusion is that not all effusions are necessarily malignant. Suspected malignant effusions should be confirmed by cytologic tests or pleural biopsy unless there is other compelling evidence of unresectable stage IV disease. Patients with lung cancer and a nonmalignant effusion may still be candidates for curative-intent therapy. However, once diagnosed with an MPE, management should be guided by individualization of care that takes into account clinical factors, including the patient's functional status and estimated life expectancy, the severity of MPE-related symptoms, and the patient's preferences regarding the acceptable invasiveness of management options. Several different options are available for treatment of MPE-related symptoms and range from observation with periodic thoracocentesis to pleurodesis to various indwelling drainage catheter techniques.[24]

MPEs from NSCLC generally respond poorly to chemotherapy and radiation therapy and require intervention for management of its related symptoms. MPE from NSCLC generally are associated with shorter survival compared with MPE related to other cancer causes; however, estimated length of survival for individual patients with MPE varies.[25] Prognostic factors that are often used include pleural fluid volume, pleural imaging features, and performance level. High metabolic activity in the pleural fluid determined by fludeoxyglucose F 18 positron emission tomography has been shown to portend poor survival.[26] Performance level has also been correlated with overall survival in patients with MPE and may guide patients to undergo less invasive procedures for management of the pleural effusion. An Eastern Cooperative Oncology Group Performance Status of 2 or 3 has been shown to predict high inhospital mortality in patients who undergo surgical pleurodesis.[27]

Several options exist for management of patients with MPE-related symptoms, and familiarity with the various benefits, risks, and costs associated with different options is necessary to choose the appropriate treatment for each individual patient. Therapeutic large-volume thoracentesis is a useful initial approach for managing lung cancer patients with symptomatic MPEs. Cytologic analysis of the pleural fluid in patients with diagnosed lung cancer can confirm the M1a staging of these patients and therefore alter treatment options. The use of ultrasound guidance is preferred to guide thoracocentesis. Using ultrasound guidance, one can decrease inadvertent injury by localizing the pleural fluid, and this technique can be used to evaluate the degree of lung reexpansion with fluid removal. Therapeutic thoracocentesis is also useful in determining if a patient's respiratory complaints can be attributed to the effusion: improvement of a patient's symptoms following large-volume thoracocentesis suggests that more invasive interventions to palliate anticipated recurrence of the MPE can improve the patient's quality of life. However, if the patient's respiratory symptoms fail to improve significantly after large-volume thoracocentesis, other causes for the patient's complaints should be sought and excluded before proceeding with more invasive options to treat the MPE. Generally, we recommend repeat therapeutic thoracocentesis of patients with recurrent symptomatic MPEs to individuals with very-poor short-term survival and those in whom pleurodesis or chronic indwelling drainage catheters are not tolerated well.

The goal of pleurodesis is to obliterate the pleural space by producing adhesions between the parietal and visceral pleurae and thereby prevent pleural fluid reaccumulation. A variety of different pleurodesis protocols exist that reflect provider preferences and can range between differences in instillation of sclerosants to differences in surgical approach. No large-scale multicenter trials have compared the efficacy of different pleurodesis protocols. The most common chemical sclerosants used are talc, doxycycline, and bleomycin. Systematic reviews of primary studies indicate that talc is the most effective sclerosant in preventing nonrecurrence of effusions.[28] Concerns regarding the adverse effects from talc limit its use in patients with benign disease, but talc is not generally considered a limiting factor in patients with a malignant effusion. Reported complications include fever, chest pain, empyema, and acute lung injury leading to acute respiratory distress syndrome. Talc-related acute lung injury is thought to be caused by talc's small particle size, which can be systemically absorbed by vascular beds and thereby cause an inflammatory reaction beyond the pleural space.[29] Studies have reported lung injury from talc instillation in 3% to 8% of patients and increased oxygen requirements in up to 30% of patients.[30,31] Although the chemical sclerosant for pleurodesis can be instilled at the bedside via tube thoracostomy or by image-guided small-bore catheters, our preference is to perform pleurodesis by video-assisted thoracoscopic (VAT) talc insufflation. The VAT approach has been demonstrated to achieve higher rates of successful pleurodesis when compared with medical pleurodesis at the bedside via a chest tube and has not been associated with increased mortality. Thoracoscopy also allows the surgeon to assess whether there is a chance of reexpansion and pleural apposition. Thoracoscopic talc pleurodesis has been reported to have an overall success rate of approximately 96%.[28]

Although medical pleurodesis is quicker, simpler to perform, and less costly than VAT pleurodesis, we believe that VAT offers significant advantages by allowing more complete pleural fluid drainage, disrupts and lyses pleural adhesions, and ensures even distribution of the talc throughout the pleural surface. Most importantly, VAT allows the surgeon to thoroughly assess the completeness of lung reexpansion before proceeding with pleurodesis. The lung's ability to fully reexpand and achieve complete pleural apposition is a critical factor in predicting the effectiveness of pleurodesis.[32] In general, we reserve bedside pleurodesis in patients who are unwilling or unable to tolerate general anesthesia and single lung ventilation.

Chronic tunneled indwelling catheters offer an alternative strategy for management of symptomatic MPEs. These catheters can be inserted in the outpatient setting with or without the use of radiologic guidance or as part of the VAT procedure when the underlying lung does not reexpand completely or extensive tumor interposition in the pleural space makes pleurodesis unlikely to be successful. The patient can then intermittently drain pleural fluid in the home setting, and this management strategy offers significant improvement of symptoms. Most patients with these catheters do not require subsequent procedures. The complications associated with these catheters include catheter infection, cellulitis, empyema, catheter obstruction, and reports of tumor tracking along the catheter track. The use of chronic indwelling catheters has traditionally been used in patients with large symptomatic pleural effusions with trapped lungs, those who could not tolerate pleurodesis, or those who had failed previous pleurodesis attempts. However, spontaneous pleurodesis with the use of tunneled catheters has been reported to occur in patients with MPEs and has prompted some providers to offer chronic indwelling catheters as primary therapy for managing MPEs over pleurodesis, citing the multiple benefits of catheters with ease of placement, decreased or lack of need for hospitalization, and immediate relief of symptoms.[33] There are limited data on the cost-effectiveness of treatment of MPEs by indwelling catheters versus talc pleurodesis. One cost-effective analysis model suggested that the use of placement of a chronic indwelling catheter became more cost effective than talc pleurodesis if the life expectancy was 6 weeks or less.[34]

Again, use of throacoscopy can allow an assessment of the potential for reexpansion. If the lung reexpands adequately, then pleurodesis may be preferred. If on the other hand the lung is trapped, the port site can be used as the entry point for placement of an indwelling catheter.

Ultimately, the choice of strategy for managing symptomatic MPEs from lung cancer, pleurodesis or chronic indwelling catheter drainage, should be individualized based on the relative benefits and drawbacks of each option while taking into account patient preferences and priorities. We have found that frequently patients are amenable to either option, and, in these circumstances, we recommend a VAT approach first. Under VAT, we are able to completely drain the pleural effusion, address loculations and adhesions, and thoroughly assess the pleural space. If the lung fully expands, we proceed with talc pleurodesis; however, if there is incomplete lung expansion, we can easily place a tunneled indwelling catheter and the patient does not require additional hospitalization.

Hemoptysis

Hemoptysis occurs in about 7% to 10% of patients who have lung cancer, which most often is mild with only blood-tinged sputum resulting from erosion of small friable mucosal blood vessels; however, hemoptysis is often frightening and anxiety provoking to the patient and family members.[35–37] Hemoptysis occurs from neovascularization in and around the tumor, tumor necrosis and exfoliation with exposure of underlying blood vessels, trauma from cough or iatrogenesis, and airway-vascular fistula formation. In those patients with advanced stages of bronchogenic carcinoma, severe hemoptysis can be life threatening because of malignant invasion of central pulmonary and bronchial vessels and is associated with a very high mortality.[38] Radiation therapy is effective in treating hemoptysis due to friable tumor and small vessel erosion but obviously is ineffective for major fistula or emergency control of life-threatening hemoptysis. Other treatment options exist for management of nonmassive hemoptysis, including the various therapeutic bronchoscopic techniques previously described, namely, laser coagulation and APC/electrocautery.[6] However, these bronchoscopic interventions are not feasible in the setting of life-threatening hemoptysis.

The management of massive life-threatening hemoptysis takes on greater urgency because the major acute threat to the patient's life lies in asphyxiation from blood flooding the tracheobronchial tree. The patient needs to be admitted to the critical care unit, and immediate management mandates securing the airway, isolating the bleeding lung, reversing any coagulopathy, and providing fluid resuscitation. Most often in patients with already-known advanced lung cancer, the side of bleeding is presumed, and the patient should be placed with the (tumor) bleeding side down. If the site of bleeding is uncertain, flexible bronchoscopy can be performed urgently to localize the bleeding source once the patient is intubated, preferably with a large-diameter endotracheal tube. A single-lumen cuffed endotracheal tube is generally more beneficial than a double-lumen tube, which is more difficult to place in the proper position and has lumens that are too small in diameter in general to allow adequate toilet bronchoscopy. Flexible bronchoscopy can be undertaken immediately bedside, but it is preferable to perform further bronchoscopic evaluation in the operating room for obvious reasons. One should be prepared to perform both flexible and rigid bronchoscopy. In cases of ongoing massive hemoptysis, performing a rigid bronchoscopy can facilitate suctioning and irrigation of large blood clots. The rigid scope can also be advanced into the nonbleeding side and allow ventilation and oxygenation of the patient as pulmonary toilet of the nonbleeding side is conducted.

Once the airway is secure, temporary hemorrhage control is attempted. A variety of different methods are available, which include iced-cold saline lavage in 50 mL aliquots alternating with dilute epinephrine (1 mL of 1:1000 epinephrine diluted in 10 mL of normal saline) instilled to the bleeding lung side. Topical hemostatic agents have also been applied by bronchoscopic guidance to arrest severe hemoptysis. In one study, 56 of 57 patients who continued to have persistent endobronchial bleeding despite bronchoscopic wedging with iced-cold saline lavage and instillation of vasoconstrictive agents were successfully treated by topical hemostatic tamponade using oxidized regenerated cellulose mesh.[39] If the bronchial site of bleeding can be located, placement of an endobronchial blocker through an endotracheal tube using flexible bronchoscopy can be useful to isolate the bleeding site from further soiling the nonbleeding lung, and this blocker can be left in place in the intubated patient to allow for tamponade of the bleeding.[40] There also has been a successful case report of endoscopic stenting to tamponade bleeding in a patient with central lung cancer presenting with massive hemoptysis.[41]

If temporary control of the bleeding cannot be achieved, the patient can be considered for percutaneous embolization of the bleeding vessel to try to temporize bleeding. Massive hemoptysis into the tracheobronchial tree can arise from 2 vascular systems, the systemic bronchial arteries or the pulmonary artery vasculature, and, therefore if the bronchial arteriography is normal, a pulmonary arteriogram should also be performed. Embolization of the bleeding vessels can be performed using absorbable gelatin sponge and can effectively control bleeding; however, most reports of embolization in massive hemoptysis from lung cancer are limited.[42,43] Rarely, a central pulmonary artery bleeding source can be controlled by intravascular pulmonary artery stenting. Surgical resection is generally not an option in these patients with advanced stages of lung cancer who present with massive hemoptysis because there is no long-term benefit.

REFERENCES

1. Chhajed PN, Baty F, Pless M, et al. Outcome of treated advanced non-small cell lung cancer with and without central airway obstruction. Chest 2006;130(6): 1803–7.
2. Colt HG, Harrell JH. Therapeutic rigid bronchoscopy allows level of care changes in patients with acute respiratory failure from central airways obstruction. Chest 1997;112(1):202–6.
3. Bolliger CT, Sutedja TG, Strausz J, et al. Therapeutic bronchoscopy with immediate effect: laser, electrocautery, argon plasma coagulation and stents. Eur Respir J 2006;27(6):1258–71.
4. Cavaliere S, Foccoli P, Farina PL. Nd:YAG laser bronchoscopy. A five-year experience with 1,396 applications in 1,000 patients. Chest 1988;94(1):15–21.
5. Cavaliere S, Venuta F, Foccoli P, et al. Endoscopic treatment of malignant airway obstructions in 2,008 patients. Chest 1996;110(6):1536–42.
6. Morice RC, Ece T, Ece F, et al. Endobronchial argon plasma coagulation for treatment of hemoptysis and neoplastic airway obstruction. Chest 2001;119(3):781–7.
7. Vergnon JM, Huber RM, Moghissi K. Place of cryotherapy, brachytherapy and photodynamic therapy in therapeutic bronchoscopy of lung cancers. Eur Respir J 2006;28(1):200–18.
8. Jones BU, Helmy M, Brenner M, et al. Photodynamic therapy for patients with advanced non-small-cell carcinoma of the lung. Clin Lung Cancer 2001;3(1): 37–41 [discussion: 42].
9. Moghissi K, Dixon K, Stringer M, et al. The place of bronchoscopic photodynamic therapy in advanced unresectable lung cancer: experience of 100 cases. Eur J Cardiothorac Surg 1999;15(1):1–6.
10. Anacak Y, Mogulkoc N, Ozkok S, et al. High dose rate endobronchial brachytherapy in combination with external beam radiotherapy for stage III non-small cell lung cancer. Lung Cancer 2001;34(2):253–9.
11. Huber RM, Fischer R, Hautmann H, et al. Palliative endobronchial brachytherapy for central lung tumors. A prospective, randomized comparison of two fractionation schedules. Chest 1995;107(2):463–70.
12. Nori D, Allison R, Kaplan B, et al. High dose-rate intraluminal irradiation in bronchogenic carcinoma. Technique and results. Chest 1993;104(4):1006–11.

13. Langendijk H, de Jong J, Tjwa M, et al. External irradiation versus external irradiation plus endobronchial brachytherapy in inoperable non-small cell lung cancer: a prospective randomized study. Radiother Oncol 2001;58(3):257–68.

14. Yao MS, Koh WJ. Endobronchial brachytherapy. Chest Surg Clin N Am 2001; 11(4):813–27.

15. Kelly JF, Delclos ME, Morice RC, et al. High-dose-rate endobronchial brachytherapy effectively palliates symptoms due to airway tumors: the 10-year M. D. Anderson Cancer Center experience. Int J Radiat Oncol Biol Phys 2000;48(3): 697–702.

16. Maiwand MO. The role of cryosurgery in palliation of tracheo-bronchial carcinoma. Eur J Cardiothorac Surg 1999;15(6):764–8.

17. Maiwand MO, Evans JM, Beeson JE. The application of cryosurgery in the treatment of lung cancer. Cryobiology 2004;48(1):55–61.

18. Walsh DA, Maiwand MO, Nath AR, et al. Bronchoscopic cryotherapy for advanced bronchial carcinoma. Thorax 1990;45(7):509–13.

19. Wood DE. Management of malignant tracheobronchial obstruction. Surg Clin North Am 2002;82(3):621–42.

20. Wood DE, Liu YH, Vallieres E, et al. Airway stenting for malignant and benign tracheobronchial stenosis. Ann Thorac Surg 2003;76(1):167–72 [discussion: 173–4].

21. Furukawa K, Ishida J, Yamaguchi G, et al. The role of airway stent placement in the management of tracheobronchial stenosis caused by inoperable advanced lung cancer. Surg Today 2010;40(4):315 20.

22. Vonk-Noordegraaf A, Postmus PE, Sutedja TG. Tracheobronchial stenting in the terminal care of cancer patients with central airways obstruction. Chest 2001; 120(6):1811–4.

23. Detterbeck FC, Boffa DJ, Tanoue LT. The new lung cancer staging system. Chest 2009;136(1):260–71.

24. Heffner JE. Management of the patient with a malignant pleural effusion. Seminars in respiratory and critical care medicine. Semin Respir Crit Care Med 2010;31(6):723–33.

25. Dresler CM, Olak J, Herndon JE, et al. Phase III intergroup study of talc poudrage vs talc slurry sclerosis for malignant pleural effusion. Chest 2005;127(3):909–15.

26. Duysinx B, Corhay JL, Larock MP, et al. Prognostic value of metabolic imaging in non-small cell lung cancers with neoplasic pleural effusion. Nucl Med Commun 2008;29(11):982–6.

27. Bernard A, de Dompsure RB, Hagry O, et al. Early and late mortality after pleurodesis for malignant pleural effusion. Ann Thorac Surg 2002;74(1):213–7.

28. Shaw P, Agarwal R. Pleurodesis for malignant pleural effusions. Cochrane Database Syst Rev 2004;1:CD002916.

29. Rossi VF, Vargas FS, Marchi E, et al. Acute inflammatory response secondary to intrapleural administration of two types of talc. Eur Respir J 2010;35(2):396–401.

30. Kuzniar TJ, Blum MG, Kasibowska-Kuzniar K, et al. Predictors of acute lung injury and severe hypoxemia in patients undergoing operative talc pleurodesis. Ann Thorac Surg 2006;82(6):1976–81.

31. Gonzalez AV, Bezwada V, Beamis JF, et al. Lung injury following thoracoscopic talc insufflation: experience of a single North American center. Chest 2010; 137(6):1375–81.

32. Steger V, Mika U, Toomes H, et al. Who gains most? A 10-year experience with 611 thoracoscopic talc pleurodeses. Ann Thorac Surg 2007;83(6):1940–5.

33. Warren WH, Kalimi R, Khodadadian LM, et al. Management of malignant pleural effusions using the Pleur(x) catheter. Ann Thorac Surg 2008;85(3):1049–55.

34. Olden AM, Holloway R. Treatment of malignant pleural effusion: PleuRx catheter or talc pleurodesis? A cost-effectiveness analysis. J Palliat Med 2010;13(1):59–65.
35. Hyde L, Hyde CI. Clinical manifestations of lung cancer. Chest 1974;65(3):299–306.
36. Chute CG, Greenberg ER, Baron J, et al. Presenting conditions of 1539 population-based lung cancer patients by cell type and stage in New Hampshire and Vermont. Cancer 1985;56(8):2107–11.
37. Corner J, Hopkinson J, Fitzsimmons D, et al. Is late diagnosis of lung cancer inevitable? Interview study of patients' recollections of symptoms before diagnosis. Thorax 2005;60(4):314–9.
38. Corey R, Hla KM. Major and massive hemoptysis: reassessment of conservative management. Am J Med Sci 1987;294(5):301–9.
39. Valipour A, Kreuzer A, Koller H, et al. Bronchoscopy-guided topical hemostatic tamponade therapy for the management of life-threatening hemoptysis. Chest 2005;127(6):2113–8.
40. Saw EC, Gottlieb LS, Yokoyama T, et al. Flexible fiberoptic bronchoscopy and endobronchial tamponade in the management of massive hemoptysis. Chest 1976;70(5):589–91.
41. Chung IH, Park MH, Kim DH, et al. Endobronchial stent insertion to manage hemoptysis caused by lung cancer. J Korean Med Sci 2010;25(8):1253–5.
42. Knott-Craig CJ, Oostuizen JG, Rossouw G, et al. Management and prognosis of massive hemoptysis. Recent experience with 120 patients. J Thorac Cardiovasc Surg 1993;105(3):394–7.
43. Mal H, Rullon I, Mellot F, et al. Immediate and long-term results of bronchial artery embolization for life-threatening hemoptysis. Chest 1999;115(4):996–1001.

Index

Note: Page numbers of article titles are in **boldface** type.

doi:10.1016/S1055-3207(11)00058-5
1055-3207/11/$ – see front matter © 2011 Elsevier Inc. All rights reserved.
surgonc.theclinics.com

United States Postal Service

Statement of Ownership, Management, and Circulation
(All Periodicals Publications Except Requester Publications)

1. Publication Title	2. Publication Number	3. Filing Date
Surgical Oncology Clinics of North America	0 1 2 - 5 6 5	9/16/11

4. Issue Frequency	5. Number of Issues Published Annually	6. Annual Subscription Price
Jan, Apr, Jul, Oct	4	$241.00

7. Complete Mailing Address of Known Office of Publication (Not printer) (Street, city, county, state, and ZIP+4®)

Elsevier Inc.
360 Park Avenue South
New York, NY 10010-1710

Contact Person
Stephen Bushing

Telephone (Include area code)
215-239-3688

8. Complete Mailing Address of Headquarters or General Business Office of Publisher (Not printer)

Elsevier Inc., 360 Park Avenue South, New York, NY 10010-1710

9. Full Names and Complete Mailing Addresses of Publisher, Editor, and Managing Editor (Do not leave blank)

Publisher (Name and complete mailing address)

Kim Murphy, Elsevier, Inc., 1600 John F. Kennedy Blvd. Suite 1800, Philadelphia, PA 19103-2899

Editor (Name and complete mailing address)

Jessica McCool, Elsevier, Inc., 1600 John F. Kennedy Blvd. Suite 1800, Philadelphia, PA 19103-2899

Managing Editor (Name and complete mailing address)

Barbara Cohen-Kligerman, Elsevier, Inc., 1600 John F. Kennedy Blvd. Suite 1800, Philadelphia, PA 19103-2899

10. Owner (Do not leave blank. If the publication is owned by a corporation, give the name and address of the corporation immediately followed by the names and addresses of all stockholders owning or holding 1 percent or more of the total amount of stock. If not owned by a corporation, give the names and addresses of the individual owners. If owned by a partnership or other unincorporated firm, give its name and address as well as those of each individual owner. If the publication is published by a nonprofit organization, give its name and address.)

Full Name	Complete Mailing Address
Wholly owned subsidiary of	4520 East-West Highway
Reed/Elsevier, US holdings	Bethesda, MD 20814

11. Known Bondholders, Mortgagees, and Other Security Holders Owning or Holding 1 Percent or More of Total Amount of Bonds, Mortgages, or Other Securities. If none, check box ☑ None

Full Name	Complete Mailing Address
N/A	

12. Tax Status (For completion by nonprofit organizations authorized to mail at nonprofit rates) (Check one)
The purpose, function, and nonprofit status of this organization and the exempt status for federal income tax purposes:
☐ Has Not Changed During Preceding 12 Months
☐ Has Changed During Preceding 12 Months (Publisher must submit explanation of change with this statement)

PS Form 3526, September 2007 (Page 1 of 3 (Instructions Page 3)) PSN 7530-01-000-9931 PRIVACY NOTICE: See our Privacy policy in www.usps.com

13. Publication Title		14. Issue Date for Circulation Data Below
Surgical Oncology Clinics of North America		July 2011

15. Extent and Nature of Circulation		Average No. Copies Each Issue During Preceding 12 Months	No. Copies of Single Issue Published Nearest to Filing Date
a. Total Number of Copies (Net press run)		813	750
b. Paid Circulation (By Mail and Outside the Mail)	(1) Mailed Outside-County Paid Subscriptions Stated on PS Form 3541. (Include paid distribution above nominal rate, advertiser's proof copies, and exchange copies)	281	263
	(2) Mailed In-County Paid Subscriptions Stated on PS Form 3541 (Include paid distribution above nominal rate, advertiser's proof copies, and exchange copies)		
	(3) Paid Distribution Outside the Mails Including Sales Through Dealers and Carriers, Street Vendors, Counter Sales, and Other Paid Distribution Outside USPS®	97	102
	(4) Paid Distribution by Other Classes Mailed Through the USPS (e.g. First-Class Mail®)		
c. Total Paid Distribution (Sum of 15b (1), (2), (3), and (4))	▲	378	365
d. Free or Nominal Rate Distribution (By Mail and Outside the Mail)	(1) Free or Nominal Rate Outside-County Copies Included on PS Form 3541	55	55
	(2) Free or Nominal Rate In-County Copies Included on PS Form 3541		
	(3) Free or Nominal Rate Copies Mailed at Other Classes Through the USPS (e.g. First-Class Mail)		
	(4) Free or Nominal Rate Distribution Outside the Mail (Carriers or other means)		
e. Total Free or Nominal Rate Distribution (Sum of 15d (1), (2), (3) and (4))	▲	55	55
f. Total Distribution (Sum of 15c and 15e)	▲	433	420
g. Copies not Distributed (See instructions to publishers #4 (page #3))	▲	380	330
h. Total (Sum of 15f and g)	▲	813	750
i. Percent Paid (15c divided by 15f times 100)		87.30%	86.90%

16. Publication of Statement of Ownership
☐ If the publication is a general publication, publication of this statement is required. Will be printed in the October 2011 issue of this publication. ☐ Publication not required

17. Signature and Title of Editor, Publisher, Business Manager, or Owner

Stephen R. Bushing — Inventory/Distribution Coordinator

Stephen R. Bushing –Inventory/Distribution Coordinator

Date
September 16, 2011

I certify that all information furnished on this form is true and complete. I understand that anyone who furnishes false or misleading information on this form or who omits material or information requested on the form may be subject to criminal sanctions (including fines and imprisonment) and/or civil sanctions (including civil penalties).

PS Form 3526, September 2007 (Page 2 of 3)

Moving?

Make sure your subscription moves with you!

To notify us of your new address, find your **Clinics Account Number** (located on your mailing label above your name), and contact customer service at:

Email: journalscustomerservice-usa@elsevier.com

800-654-2452 (subscribers in the U.S. & Canada)
314-447-8871 (subscribers outside of the U.S. & Canada)

Fax number: 314-447-8029

Elsevier Health Sciences Division
Subscription Customer Service
3251 Riverport Lane
Maryland Heights, MO 63043

*To ensure uninterrupted delivery of your subscription, please notify us at least 4 weeks in advance of move.

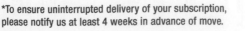
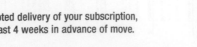

Printed and bound by CPI Group (UK) Ltd, Croydon, CR0 4YY

03/10/2024

01040461-0019